THE COMPLETE
BOOK OF
BODY
MAINTENANCE

THE COMPLETE
BOOK OF BODY MAINTENANCE

EDITED BY OLIVER GILLIE AND DERRIK MERCER

W · W · NORTON & COMPANY
New York · London

Library of Congress Cataloging in Publication Data
Main entry under title:

The Complete book of body maintenance.

   Previous edition published in 1978 under title: The
Sunday times book of body maintenance.
   Bibliography: p.
   Includes index.
   1. Health.   2. Medicine, Popular.   I. Gillie,
Oliver.   II. Mercer, Derrik.   III. The Sunday times
book of body maintenance.
RA776.S926   1979   613   79–13165
ISBN 0–393–01267–0
ISBN 0–393–00941–6 pbk.

1 2 3 4 5 6 7 8 9 0

To the memory of John H. Knowles, M. D., whose counsel in the preparation of this book was, in keeping with all his work, invaluable.

Foreword

Most of us were born with bodies in reasonably good working order. They are the only ones we will ever have. Even with the growing ability of medical science to perform successful organ transplants, there is no likelihood that we will ever be able to trade in at the end of thirty-five years or 100,000 miles for a newer, better model. Yet most people know far less about the way their own bodies operate than they do about what goes on under the hood of their car, and far less about how to keep them in good running condition.

It has always been assumed that each of us should know the rudiments of health care: how to bandage a cut hand, soothe an upset stomach, treat the symptoms of the flu—what to do until you can get to the doctor and how to follow his or her instructions afterward. We should know much more: how to use the Heimlich maneuver or cardiovascular resuscitation; how to apply a tourniquet, brace a broken bone, preserve a severed limb; how to spot the symptoms of diseases like diabetes or cancer; what immunization shots our children need, and when; how often to see the doctor, dentist, or ophthalmologist; how to use our complex system of medical care.

Beyond that, the evidence is very clear that, on us, as individuals, rests much of the responsibility for the practice of preventive medicine. By becoming informed about risks and the importance of day-to-day habits and lifestyles, we can make a major contribution to our own and our family's continued physical well-being.

Over the last century, in the industrialized nations many of the infectious diseases, particularly the diseases of childhood, that once assumed epidemic proportions have been almost totally eradicated. Leprosy, influenza, tuberculosis, diphtheria, typhoid, streptococcal infections, whooping cough, measles—all have ceased to be major causes of death. Although we think of this as entirely due to the discoveries of science, in fact their incidence began to decline before the development of rational, scientifically based medical treatments. Improvements in general dietary, environmental, and health conditions were even more important than medication.

Similarly, rickets, pellagra, goiter, xerophthalmia (the disease of Vitamin A deficiency that destroys vision), and beriberi have essentially disappeared from the developed world. We know today that these diseases are caused by nutritional deficiencies, not by infection, as was once supposed and that they can be prevented by dietary changes and by government-mandated enrichment and fortification programs.

Most children now live to grow up. The United States' infant mortality rate, although still not low enough, is at its lowest in our history; 13.6 per thousand live births. In addition, a boy or girl born today can expect to live about twenty-five years longer than if he or she had been born at the beginning of the century. As we grow older, and our population as a whole grows older—the median age is now twenty-nine: it will be thirty-six by the year 2000—we are faced with the new epidemic of the chronic degenerative diseases of middle life that have replaced the conquered infectious and deficiency diseases as major causes of death. Coronary heart disease, cancer, and stroke rank first, second, and third of our ten leading killers. Adult-onset diabetes, cirrhosis of the liver, and arteriosclerosis (hardening of the arteries) rank sixth, seventh, and eighth, right after accidents and influenza and pneumonia. By the time they reach middle age, more than 10 million Americans have some degree of physical limitations due to injury or to the effects of chronic disease.

As yet, the cause (or more likely, multiple causes) of these diseases is not known. In general, they begin at an earlier age, developing slowly and insidiously. They are hard to treat, difficult if not impossible to cure. Prevention is both better and easier, and while no one can guarantee success, a number of the risk factors associated with their development, like diet, smoking, overweight, lack of exercise, drinking to excess are certainly within our individual control. In the recently released *First Surgeon General's Report on Health Promotion and Disease Prevention*, Surgeon General of the United States Dr. Julius Richmond, the distinguished pediatrician, recommends to the American people

- a leaner diet, one lower in alcohol, salt, sugar, and total fat, particularly saturated fat,
- vigorous exercise at least three times a week,
- cutting out—or at least way down on—cigarette smoking,
- getting to a doctor or health center for regular checkups,
- obeying speed laws, using seat belts and motorcycle helmets, staying away from a car after using alcohol or a mood-altering drug.

If most people followed this and other advice contained in the *Report*, says Dr. Richmond, by 1990 the United States could cut death rates in various age groups from 20 to 35 percent, and reduce illness in older persons by 20 percent. That is worth striving for, particularly when a healthy life is so much more worth living!

In addition, there are things we should do as a community. First, no one can be counted as educated if he or she is ignorant of the basic facts of health. We can make health education a part of the standard curriculum in our secondary schools and universities and see that health information is readily available to every citizen. We need to provide more facilities—and instructors—for exercise in our schools and in the community: swimming pools; tennis and squash courts; special paths for walking, jogging, and hiking; special provision for the safety of cyclists. And, I hope we will keep in mind, as we develop alternative sources of energy and rules for their use, that as individuals and as a nation we pay a heavy social and economic price for environmental pollution.

With sufficient understanding of the science of health, a person can often prevent diseases and can certainly make full use of our system of health care. This book is a fine step in that direction: a body owners' manual for the care and maintenance of the only one you'll ever have, and a chance to influence the health of others by your example. Read it—and use it—in good health.

JEAN MAYER
PRESIDENT
TUFTS UNIVERSITY

Contents

Introduction

At the turn of the century one in four non-white Americans failed to reach his or her first birthday. White babies were slightly luckier: just one in seven died in their first year of life. If they did survive those hazardous months, they would live on average until about 55 if they were white or 43 for non-whites – to use official government terminology. Today the expectation of life *from birth* is among whites 77.3 for women, 69.7 for men; among non-whites it is 72.6 for women, 64.1 for men. The birth rate has fallen but the population has quadrupled since 1900. Some of this increase has stemmed from continuing immigration into the United States, but this is not the only factor. From the maternity ward to the geriatric wing, new skills and equipment are enabling lives to be saved that once would have been irretrievably lost. New drugs are warding off illness and sometimes death. Better housing and sanitary standards are removing the conditions in which disease festered. Vaccination programs have made generations of children largely immune from illnesses which once claimed thousands of victims every year.

The top ten killers in the United States
The table below lists the ten most common causes of death in the United States. The figures show the rate of death per 100,000 people – first the average figure for the country as a whole and then for different groups within the US expressed as the variation per 100,000 people above or below this national average. The degree of variation, as well as the nature of some of these causes of death, illustrates the scope for improvement.

Cause of death	National average	White male	White female	Other male	Other female
Heart diseases	337.2	+62.2	−31.7	−60.7	−121.3
Cancer	175.8	+23.4	−13.8	+ 3.4	− 58.0
Stroke	87.9	−11.1	+12.6	− 8.6	− 5.6
Accidents – motor	21.9	+10.6	−10.8	+11.0	− 11.9
other	25.0	+ 8.0	− 9.2	+20.8	− 8.7
Influenza and pneumonia	28.8	+ 2.2	− 1.0	+ 3.4	− 9.5
Diabetes	16.1	− 3.0	+ 1.6	− 0.6	+ 8.4
Cirrhosis of liver	14.7	+ 4.2	− 5.4	+10.7	− 1.6
Arteriosclerosis	13.7	− 1.7	+ 3.5	− 6.9	− 5.9
Suicide	12.5	+ 7.3	− 5.3	− 1.5	− 9.2
Certain diseases of early infancy	11.6	− 0.6	− 4.0	+19.5	+ 10.9

Today there are new problems. Sometimes they are consequences of past successes; the conquest of disease has greatly increased the numbers of people who now survive not merely into their fifties but into their seventies and beyond. Other problems stem from scientific or chemical processes which were unknown at the turn of the century, such as radiation. Most common of all, though, are illnesses which were comparatively rare fifty years ago, notably heart disease and cancer. There are, inevitably, many variations as people grow older, but add all the deaths together and you find that two in three are caused by heart disease, cancer and strokes. To some extent these, too, are a consequence of ageing populations: the incidence of each increases with age. Increasingly, however, they are claiming younger and younger victims. Heart disease is now a middle-aged obsession, while cancer is a major killer even in childhood. Age alone cannot therefore be their cause; it can only increase their likelihood. If this gives hope that these modern killers may be prevented or averted, it is not the sole ground for optimism. Why should death rates vary so dramatically from country to country? What can explain the difference within countries between regions and income groups? The existence of these differences shows clearly that illness and death are caused by factors other than some intrinsic failing in the human body.

Genetic or climatic factors might contribute to international differences but not to those within nations. Nor would climatic factors alone explain the differences between the health of, say, Japanese people living in Japan and Japanese immigrants in the United States. Economic differences go some way towards explaining variations in health between income groups but cannot be the major cause of health differences between broadly comparable countries. Environmental factors, such as differing occupational hazards, have a direct relationship to health differences between income groups. Health services also vary in their quality and availability. Sweden's low infant mortality rate, for instance, is largely attributed to the excellence of their hospital care. No nation is so advanced in medical knowledge, however, for this to be the dominant factor. Nor could it explain variations within a country. This leaves one other potential variable: lifestyles.

Lifestyles have received increasing attention from doctors and medical scientists in recent years. To some extent this is a response to the elusive search for cures to non-infectious diseases such as heart disease, cancer and strokes. If they cannot be cured, how can they be prevented? What is their cause? Why are they rampant today yet more rare eighty years ago? Why are they more common in some countries than others? The detective work involved in this medical quest is known as epidemiology. Its disciples are increasingly singling out the lifestyle of the Western world, notably our diet and lack of exercise, as the most likely root cause of our problems.

The evidence is advanced in detail elsewhere in this book but it does mean that we have it in our power to influence our own health and that of our family. But this book is neither a substitute for your family doctor nor an encyclopedia of medical knowledge; whole volumes have been written about individual sections of this book, and we have not covered mental health or drug addiction at all. There will also inevitably be some generalizations that do not apply to some individuals. If in doubt, see a physician.

This book promises no miracle cures, but its message is

Bronchitis. emphysema and asthma figure among the ten most common killers of white males; homicide in the top ten among non-white men and women; nephritis and nephrosis in the top ten among non-white women. (Source: National Center for Health Statistics, HEW.)

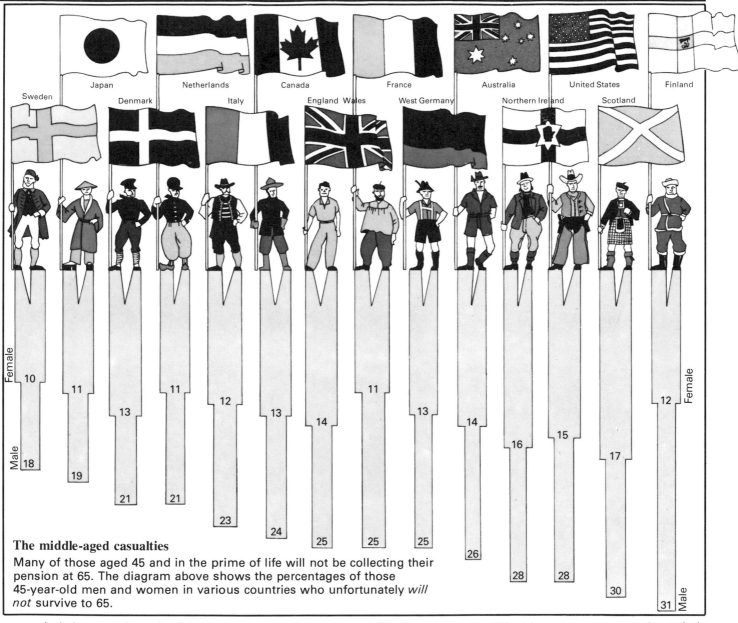

The middle-aged casualties

Many of those aged 45 and in the prime of life will not be collecting their pension at 65. The diagram above shows the percentages of those 45-year-old men and women in various countries who unfortunately *will not* survive to 65.

an optimistic one: there is abundant evidence that our health can be improved as much in the future as it has over the past hundred years. Its inspiration is the increasing belief of medical scientists that our hopes of living longer and living better depend more upon ourselves than any technical or pharmaceutical wonders now being developed in laboratories. Only charlatans guarantee good health, and we do not propose to join their number, but we can outline a lifestyle which according to the best available information should keep you fit and improve your health. Americans can draw particular encouragement from the 30 per cent decline in heart disease mortality over the last decade. In other Western countries, where there have been fewer changes in personal habits such as nutrition, smoking and exercise, the death rate is still increasing.

That prevention is better than cure, nobody would dispute. But it is not easy to put into practise. So much recent research into preventive health seems not only very confusing but also opposed to previously accepted wisdom. Foods such as milk and eggs, which we have been brought up to believe were "good", are in some cases now labeled "bad" if eaten in more than moderate quantities. Office jobs to which many people so often aspire are blamed for contributing to unfitness. Indeed, many fundamental aspects

of modern life – cars, television, elevators – now have their detractors. Scarcely a year goes by without some new theory, some new fad, which claims to undermine the "American way of life". Yet it is clearly impractical nonsense to pine for a rural heaven where somehow disease would be unknown. It is also unnecessary; it is how human beings cope with modern life that matters, not the fabric of modern life itself. This book is dedicated to no single theory and offers few medical "truths". We have attempted to present a simple and undogmatic assessment of current medical thinking about all the prime problems of physical health. It is a layman's guide not to what doctors can do for our health but to what we can do to help ourselves.

However, concentrating on illness and what *not* to do would be a depressing way to live. Life is to be enjoyed rather than just grimly survived. We have therefore tried to present a positive attitude to food, exercise, stress and general health. By learning how to maintain the body in good running order, life in any case becomes more enjoyable, as well as lasting longer. Death comes to all of us in time but today we can do more than ever before to postpone its arrival. This consoling, even cheering, thought marks a fundamental change from the world of medicine fifty or a hundred years ago.

CHILDHOOD:

Pregnancy
Protecting the Unborn Child

Birth is a time of great hope but also a time of danger. A good birth is the best omen there is for a healthy, happy life ahead. A distressing birth may take months or even years for mother and baby to overcome. Each new baby is a miracle. The newborn baby has already survived the most difficult period of life: something like a third of babies are lost in the first two months following conception, many so early that a woman scarcely notices.

The most critical stage in the development of a baby – the formation of the spinal cord and brain – is complete by the time a woman notices that her menstrual period is two weeks overdue and she is just six weeks pregnant. But the following six to eight weeks of pregnancy are equally crucial. During this time, eyes, ears and limbs are being formed. By the end of the twelfth week of pregnancy the baby is about one inch long and its shape and sex have been decided.

A baby inherits from parents the genes which decide eye and hair color, blood group and body chemistry. But the hereditary process sometimes makes mistakes and then the growing baby is usually miscarried. The majority of miscarried babies prove to have abnormal numbers of chromosomes – the minute strings of DNA which carry the inherited genes.

It is usually impossible to determine why a baby is born malformed after a normal pregnancy – the cause of eight out of ten birth malformations is still unknown. The cause is sometimes hereditary, but more often some factor in the environment as yet unidentified. Infectious diseases, drugs or perhaps some deficiency in the diet of the mother are recognized causes of birth malformation. In the majority of cases there is nothing she could have done to prevent it. However, there are many things that a woman should know and do if she is to have the best chance of giving birth to a healthy baby.

The most important single thing a woman can do to ensure the best outcome of her pregnancy is to register with a doctor at an early stage so that she can receive the full benefits of ante-natal care. Doctors are able to keep a look out for the telltale signs that a pregnancy is running into trouble. They may then act swiftly to restore the balance and prevent disaster. However, there are also some important measures a woman can take herself to give the best chance of a healthy baby.

You may well find it impossible to follow all the guidelines which we suggest here in order to give your baby the best chance. Or you may have "broken" one or more of the guidelines before you knew you were pregnant. *Do not panic.* It is always worth remembering that many pregnancies turn out well even when a woman has ignored all the best advice. If you have not done some of the things we recommend here, you should not worry too much about it. The chance of anything going wrong in an individual case as a result of one individual act – taking aspirins or tranquilizers, for example – are too small to be calculated. Indeed, these drugs may be harmless in normal circumstances – no one is certain. Nevertheless the consensus of medical opinion is that drugs should always be avoided in pregnancy where possible. These and other precautions are therefore worth taking even though the effect of any one of them is probably quite small. We are simply presenting current medical thinking so that women can decide for themselves what, if anything, they should or should not do.

If you really want a baby and things seem to have gone wrong, there are only a few circumstances when an abortion might be the best recourse. Termination of pregnancy may be seriously considered when a mother has German measles in the first three months of pregnancy, or when a doctor diagnoses some defect such as Mongolism (Down's syndrome) or spina bifida (see below), but the decision can only be taken by the parents themselves. There are few other circumstances when an abortion might reasonably be considered to be the best course of action on medical grounds alone.

TOBACCO
The greatest precaution a woman can take by herself to ensure the best outcome of her pregnancy is to give up smoking for the whole nine-month period. Husbands should also stop smoking because a woman who is sitting in a smoke-filled room absorbs smoke in the air which is in turn passed to the baby. Smoking increases the likelihood of miscarriage, abortion, poor health of the baby causing "fetal distress," premature birth, and stunting of the baby's growth. These conclusions have been reached by Professor Stanley M. Garn at the University of Michigan after an analysis of 18,000 births for the National Institute of Neurological and Communicative Disorders and Stroke. He found that low birthweight is four times as common when a mother smokes.

Ideally, a mother should also not smoke during the first year of the baby's life. Babies whose mothers smoke are

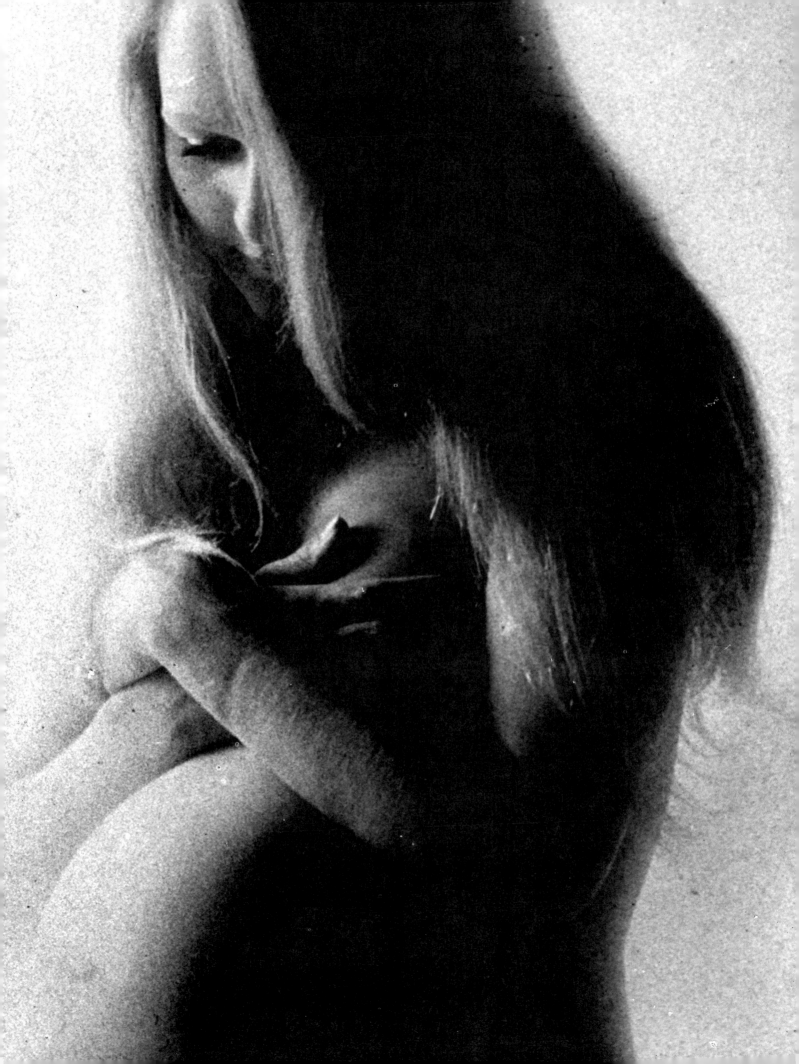

EXERCISE IN PREGNANCY

It is important to continue with normal exercise in pregnancy provided you feel well and your doctor does not advise rest. Sometimes certain types of exercise such as horse-riding are advised against in pregnancy, but there is no reason why an experienced horsewoman should not continue to ride during pregnancy so long as she does not take risks. Special exercises during pregnancy can help to overcome bad posture which will make the last months of pregnancy, when the baby becomes heavy, difficult and tiring.

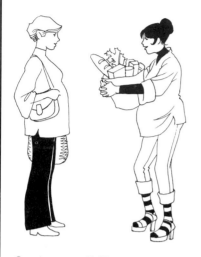

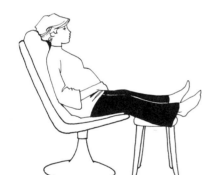

Good posture (*left*) is very important. Don't sag (*right*). Keep weight evenly between the heels and the balls of the feet, use abdomen and buttock muscles, and walk tall.

Sitting: support the back to avoid strain. Whenever possible, rest with legs raised and fully supported.

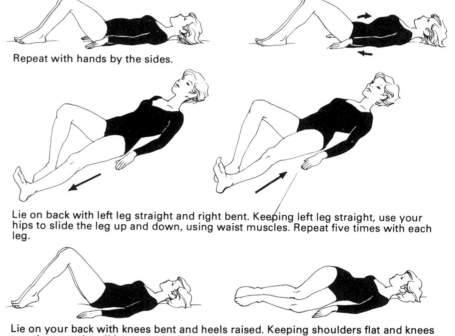

Lie on back as above. Press back against floor and pull knees up with hands. Tighten buttock muscles, then relax. Repeat five times.

With hands above head (*left*) arch the back, then press back against floor and pull up on pelvis at the same time. Feel rotation of the pelvis. Relax. Repeat five times.

Repeat with hands by the sides.

Lie on back with left leg straight and right bent. Keeping left leg straight, use your hips to slide the leg up and down, using waist muscles. Repeat five times with each leg.

Lie on your back with knees bent and heels raised. Keeping shoulders flat and knees together, gently roll knees to the left as far as is comfortably possible. This will raise your right hip, and you will feel a turning movement at your waist. Return to original position and repeat five times for each side.

more frequently admitted to the hospital with chest infections in the first year of life than those with mothers who do not smoke, according to research by doctors at the Hadassah University in Israel. It is still not clear whether the cause of the baby's chest infections is the cigarette smoke or the germs coughed by the mother, who is more prone to chest infection as a result of smoking.

ALCOHOL

There is no harm in normal social drinking, but avoid excess. A link has recently been established between excessive drinking in alcoholic women and certain birth malformations which include poor growth, small head and mental retardation. This type of malformation may be much commoner than is realized. *The Lancet* – a weekly journal for doctors – has advised in an editorial that alcoholism may be considered as a reason for abortion.

These malformations are almost certainly caused by alcohol itself rather than any particular kind of alcoholic drink. But try to drink the lighter beers and wines, and avoid spirits. Particularly avoid heavy spirits such as brandy and whisky, which contain congeners – the chemicals which are responsible for making a hangover that much worse. If you are at a party where everyone is drinking cocktails, ask for a screwdriver – a small vodka and lots of fresh orange juice – and make it last a long time. Some doctors recommend avoiding tonic waters and bitter lemon drinks in pregnancy because these drinks contain small quantities of quinine, but an occasional one will do no harm.

SEX

Women used to be advised to avoid sexual intercourse for six weeks before and six weeks after birth. Today it is accepted that a pregnant woman may have intercourse throughout pregnancy as long as it is comfortable and enjoyable and there is no pain in the vagina or abdomen. Sex should be avoided if there has been any bleeding from the vagina, as there is then a danger of infection of the womb. Once the waters have broken, birth is imminent and sex is not advisable because of the risk of infection.

Intercourse in the conventional "missionary position" with the man on top becomes awkward once the womb begins to enlarge, and the man must avoid putting his whole weight on it. Other positions are generally preferable. For example, the woman may be on top or the couple may lie on their sides with the man behind. Making love with what Sheila Kitzinger (author of *The Experience of Childbirth*) calls "careful tenderness" may help a couple's relationship to develop and increase their awareness of the baby. However, some women are naturally frightened about intercourse during pregnancy. There is no danger that intercourse will cause a miscarriage under normal circumstances, but a woman who has previously had a miscarriage should consult her doctor about sex in pregnancy.

When planning a pregnancy, it is best to change from the contraceptive pill to a mechanical method of contraception such as the diaphragm, cap or condom for two or three months before attempting to conceive. This allows regular cycles to establish themselves and time for body chemistry to readjust after taking the pill. Regular cycles help to allow the pregnancy to be dated precisely, which helps the doctor to monitor pregnancy. If a woman becomes pregnant with an intra-uterine device (IUD) in position, then it is wise to consult a doctor with a view to its removal.

PREMATURE BIRTH

Premature birth is a major cause of death in the first month of life. Advances in medicine allow most of those premature babies who survive to develop perfectly normally, but prematurity is still a major cause of cerebral palsy and is also associated with an increased risk of epilepsy, blindness, deafness and mental handicap. However, the causes of prematurity are not well understood – except for a strong link with smoking. One in fourteen newborns in the US weighs under 5½lb, and partly because of this the US has a higher infant death rate than sixteen other countries.

Attempting to reduce weight during pregnancy may cause premature birth, and so may poor nutrition, but no one seems to know just how important a factor poor diet is in the United States. As many as a quarter of pregnant mothers might be at risk from **inadequate diet** judging by the experience in Canada where nutritional counseling of women by the Montreal Diet Dispensary reduced the number of premature births by a third. Check the recommended diet (see p. 19) to see if you are eating properly.

Some doctors believe that **stress** may also cause miscarriages and premature births, although it is difficult to measure stress accurately, or even be certain that different people mean the same thing when they use the word. However, it makes sense to slow down during pregnancy and to learn to relax – particularly if you feel tense and worried. Relaxation classes and preparation for childbirth are often run by hospitals and charities (see Appendix 2). Avoid unnecessary stress, such as moving house or strenuous work during pregnancy, if you possibly can.

INFECTION

If a pregnant woman catches a virus infection which enters the blood stream, there is a chance that the virus will cross the placenta and infect the baby. The baby's body is much less able to resist this attack than an adult because the immune defenses are not yet developed, and the virus may interfere with the delicate sequence of development.

Rubella (German measles) causes defects in up to 50 per cent of babies if the mother catches the infection for the first time during the first three months of pregnancy. There is a slight risk in the fourth or fifth month. Affected babies may be born with damage to the heart, cataract and other eye abnormalities, deafness in varying degree, mental retardation, brain damage or delayed growth; and this depressing list is not complete. In the United States thousands of babies each year die or are born with malformations caused by rubella. Vaccination against the disease is now available but still one in seven US women of childbearing age is susceptible to the disease.

If a mother gets a mild infection of German measles during pregnancy it is unlikely to spread to the baby if she has already been vaccinated or previously had the disease. Doctors therefore recommend that teenage girls are vaccinated. Vaccination against German measles or use of other

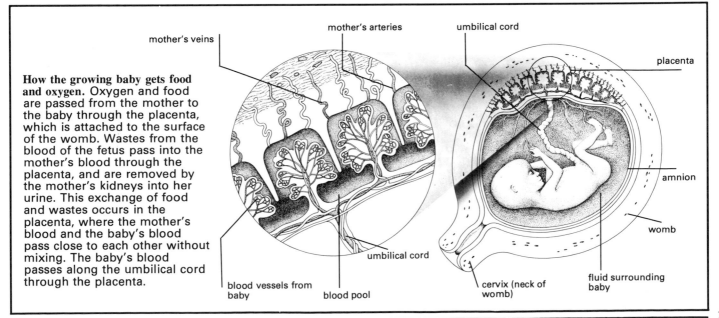

How the growing baby gets food and oxygen. Oxygen and food are passed from the mother to the baby through the placenta, which is attached to the surface of the womb. Wastes from the blood of the fetus pass into the mother's blood through the placenta, and are removed by the mother's kidneys into her urine. This exchange of food and wastes occurs in the placenta, where the mother's blood and the baby's blood pass close to each other without mixing. The baby's blood passes along the umbilical cord through the placenta.

mother's veins

mother's arteries

umbilical cord

placenta

amnion

womb

blood vessels from baby

blood pool

umbilical cord

cervix (neck of womb)

fluid surrounding baby

live vaccines should be avoided during pregnancy, because the live viruses in these vaccines can infect and damage the growing baby.

Cytomegalovirus is another common virus infection which causes hundreds of malformations a year. However, it causes scarcely any recognizable symptoms in adults and a pregnant woman is therefore unlikely to notice anything unusual. Cytomegalovirus may cause low birthweight, prematurity, deafness or mental retardation similar to the results of German measles infection. Nevertheless, probably only one in ten babies infected in the womb suffers any permanent damage.

Cytomegalovirus is spread from one adult to another by close personal contact, including kissing and sexual intercourse. Babies and children spread it in their urine. The virus is so common that it has been isolated from the neck of the womb in up to a quarter of women during pregnancy. It is, however, only when a woman gets her first infection of cytomegalovirus during pregnancy that the baby is likely to be affected.

Particular attention to hygiene – handwashing, for example – should help to avoid infection. Both husband and wife should also avoid intercourse with other partners during pregnancy. Other factors in a woman's general health may also make her vulnerable to virus infections, so avoid stress if you can. At present, no vaccine is available against cytomegalovirus.

Herpes virus infection of the vagina or cervix (see page 169) may be transmitted to the baby during delivery, and if the baby is infected the virus will damage or kill it. Women with herpes are also more likely to suffer miscarriage. Herpes is difficult to treat. If you have had an attack in the past inform your obstetrician. If tests show it is still active, then it will be advisable to deliver the baby by Cesarian.

Influenza infection during pregnancy can, in rare cases, also cause malformations. Since the influenza virus does not usually enter the blood and does not normally reach the baby, it may be that damage results from the high temperature which often occurs in influenza. Aspirin which is, of course, often taken for flu and colds is also suspected as a possible cause of malformation when women take it during pregnancy. However, no one is sure whether aspirin itself may occasionally cause malformations or if the illness which people take it for is the cause. So should a pregnant woman take aspirin when she has flu? Doctors disagree. But the sensible solution is to take aspirin for genuine flu which threatens to cause a rise in temperature, but not for minor colds and headaches.

Other virus infections such as **mumps** and **chickenpox** are also suspected of causing occasional birth defects, and **syphilis** remains an important cause of malformations, responsible for hundreds of cases a year in the US.

A parasite called **Toxoplasma** found in raw meat and animal droppings is also responsible for causing certain rare malformations. These include eye defects, brain damage and mental retardation. Women may avoid the disease by not eating raw or rare meat and avoiding animals, particularly cats, during pregnancy. A woman who has always kept animals is likely to have been exposed to the disease and be resistant. The main point to watch is that this is not the time to start keeping a cat for the first time. There is no vaccine against Toxoplasma, and it is therefore a good idea to encourage young girls to play with cats so that they can develop immunity before there is any chance of pregnancy.

It is also possible to pick up Toxoplasma from cat-droppings. Pregnant women should therefore take care to wash fastidiously after gardening. As with other attacks on the fetus, damage is most likely to be sustained within the first three months of pregnancy and so some people think it best to farm out cats with friends during that period.

Women in certain jobs are exposed to chemicals at work which may cause birth abnormalities. For example, ethylene thiourea, used until recently in the rubber industry, has been found to cause birth abnormalities as well as cancer in rats. In many industries, women may be unknowingly at risk from chemicals which they breathe in or absorb through their skin or from chemicals on food eaten on the factory floor. A pregnant woman who has a job which exposes her to chemicals and who has had a miscarriage might consider changing her work. Also avoid dyeing your hair in pregnancy (see page 108).

PRESCRIPTION DRUGS

Many women take prescribed drugs during pregnancy which are not really necessary. The safest advice is to avoid drugs altogether unless you are really ill, and then rely on the doctor's advice. Sumner J. Yaffe, Professor of Pediatrics at the State University of New York at Buffalo, says that conclusive evidence of safety is unavailable for between 75 and 85 per cent of all drugs, yet figures from a recent survey in Texas show that over eight out of ten women take at least one prescribed drug during pregnancy.

Although all new drugs must be tested on pregnant animals before they are passed by the Federal Drug Administration, this can never guarantee that they are completely safe in human pregnancy. It is well established that a drug which does not cause malformations in animals can still cause human malformations. In any case, there are thousands of drugs on the market which have never been tested for effects in pregnancy because they were first sold before these potential dangers were realized.

There is a long list of drugs known to be associated with abnormalities although it is often unclear whether the drugs actually cause the abnormality or are just indirectly involved. *Tetracycline*, for instance, is an antibiotic drug widely used to treat infections ranging from pneumonia to cystitis. It is sold under at least a dozen different trade-names and should be avoided during pregnancy because it may interfere with the growth of the baby's bones and discolor the baby's primary teeth. The drug is absorbed into bone and it is not yet known what happens in later life to babies exposed to tetracycline in the womb. There may occasionally be good reason to take tetracycline during pregnancy but it is best avoided.

Barbiturate drugs and *phenytoin* – a drug given to epileptic women to prevent convulsions – have also been suspected of causing birth defects such as cleft lip or palate or mental retardation. However, following two studies, one in the USA and one in Finland, it was discovered that the birth of abnormal babies to epileptic mothers was unrelated to drugs. It seems that a mother who suffers from epilepsy is twice as likely to have an abnormal baby whether or not she takes drugs. It would therefore be quite wrong for epileptic women not to take the drugs which help to control their illness. In any case, epileptic mothers still have excellent prospects of having a normal baby.

Illegal drugs such as *LSD*, *marijuana* and *heroin* should all be avoided in pregnancy if for no other reason than that

Different parts of the growing fetus are vulnerable to damage at different stages. The heart, eyes and limbs are already formed by the time that most women begin to realize that they are pregnant. The genital organs in both sexes continue to be vulnerable for much longer. The nervous system and brain continue to develop throughout pregnancy and afterwards, but are most vulnerable during formation.

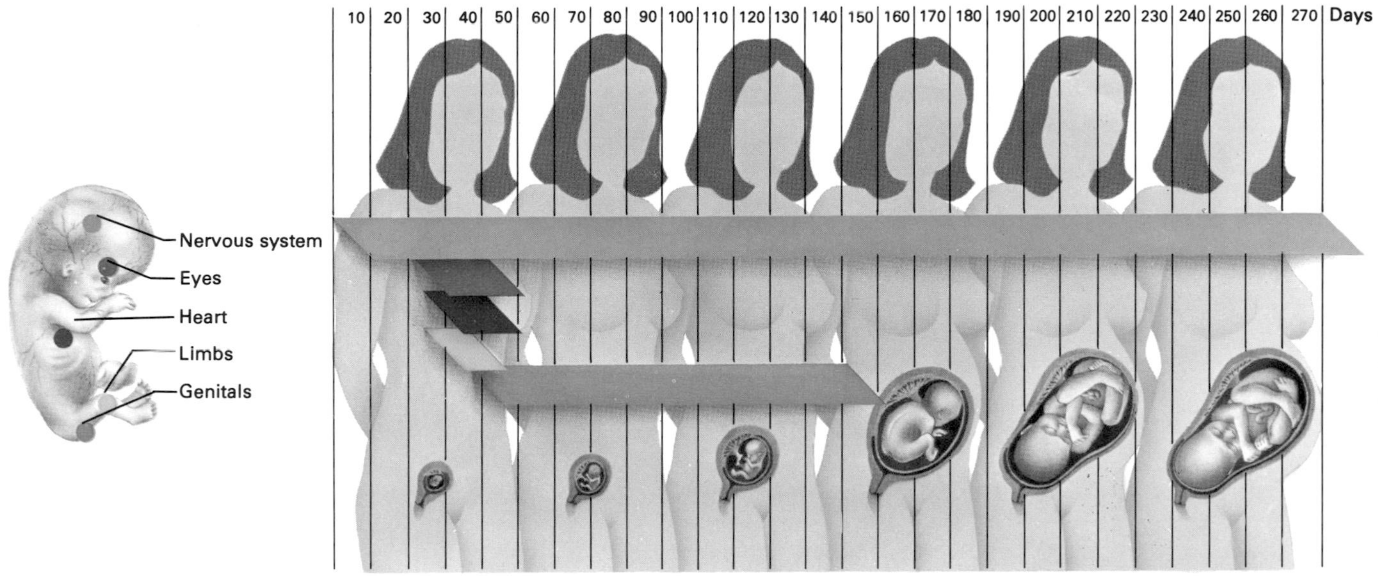

| 10 | 20 | 30 | 40 | 50 | 60 | 70 | 80 | 90 | 100 | 110 | 120 | 130 | 140 | 150 | 160 | 170 | 180 | 190 | 200 | 210 | 220 | 230 | 240 | 250 | 260 | 270 | Days |

— Nervous system
— Eyes
— Heart
— Limbs
— Genitals

they may have harmful effects on the baby.

The following additional effects of drugs in pregnancy are known or suspected: certain *sex hormones* may cause masculinization of the fetus and an increase in bone age. Certain *anti-thyroid* drugs may cause the infant to develop goitre – a swelling of the thyroid gland in the neck. Certain drugs given against cancer, leukemia and severe psoriasis may cause abnormal development of the skull and abortion. *Blood anti-coagulants* may cause bleeding of the baby in the womb with subsequent abnormalities or death. *Sulfonamide antibiotics*, used to treat many common infections, may cause pigment to be deposited in the nervous system which may possibly cause mental retardation. Some drugs used to treat blood pressure are believed to cause bowel spasm or pneumonia in babies after birth. Even *anti-histamine*, used to treat motion sickness and allergies, has been implicated as a cause of malformations; but there is no proof. *Tranquilizers* such as Librium and Valium have been suspected of causing birth defects but there is no hard evidence against them.

If you want to start a family and are on regular drug treatment, therefore, check with your doctor whether it might be better to wait; if you become unexpectedly pregnant while undergoing drug treatment, also consult your doctor.

NON-PRESCRIPTION DRUGS

Aspirin in large doses may cause a baby to bleed in the womb, which may in turn cause local abnormalities such as irregular development of limbs or fingers. Regular consumption of large quantities of aspirin during pregnancy has been found in Australia to be associated with stillbirths, low birthweight and bleeding after birth, but not with abnormalities. The tendency to bleed of babies whose mothers take a lot of aspirin is a direct result of aspirin interfering with the normal clotting process. Many patent headache tablets contain aspirin, which is usually listed in the contents under the scientific name acetylsalicylic acid. An occasional aspirin need be no cause of worry, but do not dose yourself with them regularly: see your doctor.

Antacids taken for indigestion are also associated in a number of surveys with increased abnormalities. There is as yet no evidence that the antacids actually cause the abnormalities. Nevertheless, some experts suggest that antacids are best avoided in pregnancy. Some dentists recommend that pregnant women take fluoride tablets to give a baby good teeth. However, later research suggests that fluoride does not cross the placenta and get into the baby – so the exercise is pointless.

Herbal home remedies should not be taken during pregnancy, as plants often contain powerful drugs whose effects are even less well understood than those of chemical drugs.

Vitamin tablets should not be taken unless specifically suggested by your doctor. Vitamin A, for example, is known to cause malformations when given in excessive amounts to pregnant animals.

OPERATIONS AND X-RAYS

Unnecessary medical operations and X-ray examinations of the abdomen should be avoided if there is a possibility of pregnancy. Dentistry involving general anesthetics should also be avoided if at all possible during pregnancy.

All the commonly used *anesthetics* can cause spontaneous abortion or abnormal development in animals, and are a recognized hazard for women who work in operating rooms where they may be exposed to small doses of escaped gases. *X-rays* of pregnant women may increase the risk of the baby getting leukemia in later life and can also induce mutations in the sex cells (ovary or testis) of both mother and baby.

Routine tests of pregnancy are seldom available until two weeks after the last menstrual period is due. So it can be difficult for the doctor to definitely exclude pregnancy before the decision is taken to operate, and in any case a woman may easily become pregnant while waiting for a scheduled operation. It makes sense to take stringent precautions against pregnancy while waiting for an operation and to avoid any non-urgent surgery while pregnant. Some obstetricians are trigger happy when it comes to X-raying babies in the womb. Tell your doctor that you would rather not have an abdominal X-ray during pregnancy unless he is sure that it is really necessary. Remember that the risk is minute, almost infinitesimal, but if it is avoidable why take it?

The American College of Obstetricians and Gynecologists has issued the following guidelines:
1. The use of X-ray examinations should be considered on an individual basis. Concern over harmful effects should not prevent the proper use of radiation exposure when significant diagnostic information can be obtained. Pre-examination consultation with a radiologist may be useful in obtaining optimal information from X-ray exposure.
2. There is no measurable advantage to scheduling diagnostic X-ray examinations at any particular time during a normal menstrual cycle.
3. The degree of risk involved in an X-ray examination if the person is pregnant, or should become pregnant, ought to be explained to the patient and documented in her record.

SPINA BIFIDA AND MONGOLISM

Two of the commonest birth malformations are *spina bifida* and *anencephaly*. They are both defects of the formation of the nervous system, and affect up to one in 200 babies depending on race. It is commonest in the Irish, least common in Negroes and Jews. The spinal cord and brain are formed in the growing embryo by a folding of a sheet of tissue to form a tube – the neural tube – which closes up at the top end to form the brain and closes at the bottom to form the end of the spinal cord. When the bottom end fails to close properly the baby may develop with an open spine – spina bifida – which interferes with nervous control of the lower limbs and the nervous reflexes controlling the bladder. When the top end of the neural tube fails to form a complete brain – anencephaly – the baby usually dies shortly after birth.

Babies with spina bifida vary greatly in the degree of their affliction. Some develop hydrocephalus – swelling of the head as a result of accumulation of fluid – but this can often be controlled by inserting a plastic tube (shunt) which allows the excess fluid to drain back into the body. Others are born with a deformed spine which together with partial paralysis of the legs makes walking difficult, or sometimes impossible.

Although a small proportion of spina bifida babies – perhaps one or two in ten – may have a normal life, the majority are confined to wheelchairs and spend most of their lives in institutions. As a result, some pediatricians do not think that it is right to take extraordinary surgical measures to keep them alive, and only operate on those spina bifida babies who are mildly affected.

A woman who has had one spina bifida or anencephalic baby has a one in twenty chance of having another; a woman who has had two spina bifida or anencephalic babies has a one in ten chance of having another. However, the condition is not inherited in any simple way. A susceptibility to having babies with defects of the spinal cord or brain may be inherited but it is only a susceptibility, and

doctors are searching for a factor in the environment which may cause the condition. Suspicion focused a few years ago on the eating of green potatoes or potatoes affected by blight fungus. However, women who avoid potatoes scrupulously throughout pregnancy can still have spina bifida babies, and most experts now think that the potato theory is mistaken.

According to one theory spina bifida may be caused by some parts of the conception remaining in the womb after the miscarriage, and interfering with the normal growth of the following pregnancy. This suggests some good practical advice. Any woman who has a miscarriage should consult her doctor with a view to having a D and C (dilatation and curettage) – that is, a scraping of the womb to remove any remaining products of conception – before attempting to become pregnant again. It is advisable to consult a doctor in any case after a miscarriage. A woman who has already had one spina bifida or anencephalic baby should watch carefully for a miscarriage, which can easily be overlooked in the early stages of pregnancy, and consult her doctor if she suspects she has had one.

A new way of detecting some spina bifida or anencephalic babies in the first few months of pregnancy is now available in most large hospitals. It is called *amniocentesis* and involves taking a sample of the liquid from the womb through a long needle pushed through the skin below the navel. The fluid is then analyzed for the presence of a substance called alpha-fetoprotein, which is made by the baby and in the case of babies with defective formation of the nervous system leaks out into the liquid in the womb.

Amniocentesis is not usually done before the sixteenth week of pregnancy, which means that if the baby is found to be suffering from spina bifida it may be aborted by about the twentieth week. There has been some success in several hospitals in developing a test which will work on the mother's blood and may make earlier abortion of a defective baby possible. This test is not yet generally available.

Amniocentesis can also be used to diagnose *Down's syndrome (Mongolism)*, the commonest cause of severe mental retardation in the US. About one in 500 babies is born with Down's syndrome, but a mother aged 45 is about a hundred times more likely to have a Down's baby than a mother aged 16. Most obstetricians recommend that all women over 40, or sometimes over 35, who are pregnant should have amniocentesis so that a Down's baby may be avoided.

Cells from the baby are present in the fluid which is withdrawn from the womb by amniocentesis. These cells can be grown in the laboratory and used to identify a baby with Down's syndrome. Down's syndrome is caused by the chance inheritance of an extra small chromosome – the tiny strand of DNA which carries the genes determining heredity. This extra small chromosome can be seen in dividing cells under a microscope.

As a result of some mistake, the extra small chromosome is not eliminated from the egg when it divides before fertilization and the presence of the chromosome in every cell of the body interferes with normal development. It is not known why the extra chromosome is not eliminated from the egg, and at present there are no special measures a woman can take – other than amniocentesis – to avoid a Down's baby. Down's syndrome is not usually inherited, but occasionally it can be. Special tests can identify parents who carry the factor for the rare hereditary form when this is suspected.

Amniocentesis itself may cause a baby to miscarry, and may even cause damage to the baby if the needle is not correctly placed, so it is not a procedure to be undertaken lightly. Cells obtained by amniocentesis can be used to tell the sex of the baby, which may sometimes be important, for example, to avoid inherited defects which are sex-linked – that is, show up only in boys. But it would involve an unjustified risk to use amniocentesis simply in order to have advance knowledge of a baby's sex. About twenty-five different rare inherited conditions can be identified by amniocentesis, and affected babies may in that case be aborted.

THE PREGNANT DIET

It is common sense to eat well in pregnancy, but there is little scientific evidence to show that women on poor diets are any more likely to have malformed babies than women on normal diets. Women suffering from malnutrition in Third World countries do have babies which are underweight and which may as a result suffer a permanent reduction in intelligence. However, this is thought to be rare in Western countries. The growing baby – like a parasite – will if necessary get its food at the expense of the mother.

Doctors believe that balanced nutrition during pregnancy is important, but there is a lack of precise scientific information. One survey suggests that a shortage of folic acid – one of the B vitamins – may play a part in causing spina bifida and anencephaly. Further support for the theory comes from the observation that drugs which interfere with the normal action of folic acid in the body may cause human malformations. According to another theory, chemicals called nitrites and nitrosamincs, present in preserved meats such as ham, corned beef and hot dogs, may have an association with spina bifida and anencephaly, so some people would say it is safer to avoid these preserved meats during pregnancy.

For you and your baby
1. Always choose fresh foods in preference to processed or canned foods; bread to cookies or crackers. Never eat mouldy food.
2. Limit weight-gain to about 20–28lb (9–13kg) at most. If weight-gain is too much, cut down first on cookies, crackers, sugar, jam, candy and sweetened drinks. Do not cut down on bread and potatoes, unless advised by your doctor, because these are valuable sources of nutrients and protein as well as energy.
3. Only take vitamin pills under doctor's instructions. Extra vitamins should not be necessary for a normal woman observing the following diet.

A recommended daily diet
1. A pint of milk – or half a pint of milk and 2oz cheese (50g) – for protein and calcium. Milk and a cracker half an hour before bed helps to prevent heartburn (a common complaint in pregnancy) and promotes sleep.
2. A portion of meat, fish or an egg to provide protein, iron and B vitamins.
3. A helping of root or raw green vegetables to provide vitamin C and folic acid.
4. Fruit, frozen orange juice or potatoes to provide further vitamin C.
5. Bread to provide energy and vitamins – preferably wholewheat bread, which will prevent constipation. Alternatively, eat a bran or wholegrain breakfast cereal to avoid constipation.
6. Plenty of water – about a pint – in addition to coffee and tea in normal amounts.
7. Eat liver or an oily fish (e.g., herrings, mackerel, sardines) once a week for vitamins A and D; white fish once a week for iodine.

If you don't feel hungry
Women who suffer sickness and vomiting during pregnancy are most at risk nutritionally because they may find that tea and crackers are all that they can keep down. If instead they are able to substitute milk and bread or dry toast, their intake of essential nutrients will be much improved. Another trick is to eat cold foods. Not all women feel nauseous on rising; some find that the early evening, when everyone else is having a large meal, is their worst time to eat. For these women, a good breakfast is the best answer.

SLEEP, RELAXATION AND STRESS

Try to get all the sleep you feel you need. This will be about eight hours every night and you will probably need an additional period of rest during the day, especially in the later months. Remember your body is working harder than usual feeding the baby, and you have extra weight to carry around. Relaxation is helpful so that you have time to think about the future. Try to avoid any unnecessary new projects at this time. (For more information on relaxation and sleep, see pages 92–5).

If your pregnancy is proceeding normally and you do not have any special problems (check with your doctor), then there is no reason why you should not carry on doing most of the things you usually do, including traveling and many sports, provided you feel comfortable and confident while doing them. You may find that you become uncomfortable on long journeys and it is a good idea to stop and move around after an hour or two. Avoid having your legs crossed for long periods, because this slows the circulation of the blood.

If children are conceived and born in close succession it puts a much greater stress on the mother, both during pregnancy and afterwards. A two-year gap between births usually gives a mother the chance to recover fully and give the next baby the best chance, but a longer gap may be advantageous in some cases. A longer gap also has the advantage of avoiding the more extreme rivalry and competition between children that can develop in brothers and sisters born close together.

WARNING SIGNALS
Notify your doctor at once if any of the following signs appear:
Bleeding from the vagina.
Severe or continuous nausea and vomiting.
Continuing or severe headache.
Swelling or puffiness of the face or hands, or marked swelling of the feet or ankles.
Blurring of vision or spots before the eyes.
A marked decrease in the amount of urine passed.
Pain or burning on passing urine.
Chills and fever.
Sharp or continuous abdominal pain.
Sudden gush of water from the vagina before the baby is due.

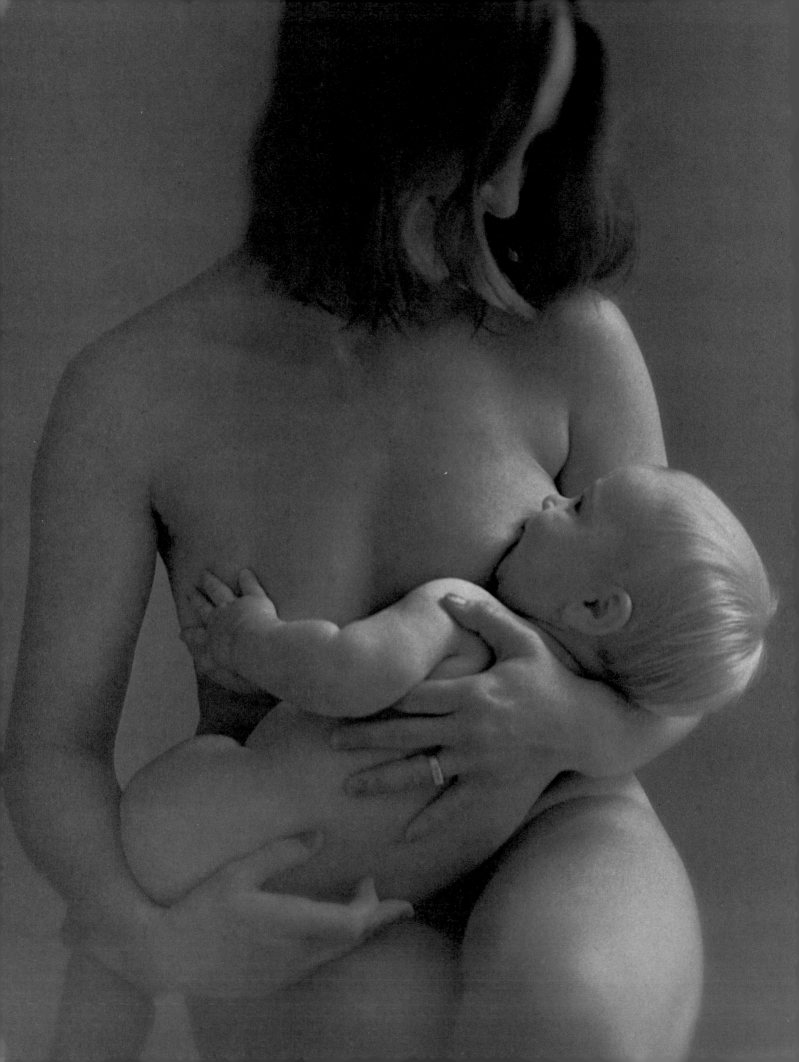

Childbirth

A mother usually knows instinctively the importance (and difficulty) of the birth she is expecting. But for the world around her it is commonplace – just another baby. Parents often have to argue to have their special needs and interests understood. Expert though doctors and maternity services are in saving life, their understanding of emotional needs has too often been dismal. So what can a prospective mother and father do for themselves?

CHOOSING THE DOCTOR
When a woman's last menstrual period is two or more weeks overdue she can ask her doctor to arrange for a pregnancy test. If this proves positive, she can then begin to consider who she wants to look after her during the pregnancy. It is a good idea to choose a doctor who takes a special interest in maternity. Good ante-natal care is most important to ensure the best outcome of the pregnancy.

ANTICIPATING PROBLEMS
The safest place to have your baby is in a hospital which is large enough to employ at least three fully qualified obstetricians, so that if you have problems in the middle of the night, at the weekend, or when one of them is on holiday, there is still an expert ready to help. However, it is often convenient for a mother to have her baby in a small hospital near her home. The atmosphere of a small hospital may be informal, and it is often easier for friends and children to visit. If there is any suggestion that the birth may be complicated, make sure that you go to one of the larger hospitals. If you score two or less on the risk chart, you are in a low-risk category and can afford to let your personal preference influence your decision. However, any change in your health later in the pregnancy might make it advisable to change plans.

RISK CHART
Score for each category which includes you. If the total is two or less, you are among 70 per cent of women who have a low risk of complications.

Unmarried (single, divorced or stable union)	1
More than 30 years old	1
Non-European descent	1
Previous baby died before or after birth	2
Three or more abortions	2
Previous Cesarean delivery	1
Previous malformed child	1
First baby	1
Fourth or later baby	1
Kidney or heart disease	4
High blood pressure	2
Diabetes	4
Anemia	1
Rhesus blood complication possible	3
Height less than 62 inches	1

Childbirth classes
Some classes in hospitals simply provide information while others involve active preparation for the birth. Active preparation has been found to help women use fewer drugs during delivery and give a better chance of a spontaneous birth without the use of forceps. Although it is difficult to prove, this probably benefits the baby; certainly many women find it more satisfying. (See Appendix 2 for organizations which arrange classes.)

The father's presence
If you want your husband or a friend to be with you during the birth, arrange this with your doctor and the hospital authorities well in advance. Most hospitals now expect and encourage fathers to be present during labor, but a few may ask husband and wife to sign a statement that they will agree to observe hospital authority. Fathers may be asked to leave while examinations are made and decisions taken about what will happen next. If a wife does not mind, there is no reason why the father should not be there during examinations. He may be able to calm his wife if the doctor has to report poor progress, or be able to arbitrate if a decision has to be made about induction. Quite often fathers are soothed into believing that nothing much is happening and find that the baby is born while they are sent home for a nap or out for a meal. It is best to wait and take snacks in the hospital.

INDUCTION
There has been a major debate within the medical profession on the ethics and safety of induced childbirth over the last few years. Induction is not necessary simply because a woman has reached the date at which the baby is expected or gone a week or two beyond it. It is difficult for a doctor to know precisely when a baby is due and a mother's dates are often not reliable, especially if she has been on the pill. If a baby is induced there is a risk that it may be premature. If the baby has to be induced – and sometimes it is necessary – then it is reasonable to expect the doctor to discuss the reasons and to consider waiting to see if circumstances change. The FDA have ruled that birth should only be induced with drugs for genuinely medical reasons.

ANESTHETICS
Some doctors will give epidural anesthetics – a local anesthetic applied to the spinal cord – to any woman who wants one, but an epidural is only really necessary when a birth is expected to be difficult. An epidural is more likely to prevent a woman from fully participating, because full sensation is lost from the waist down. It can also rarely have side effects such as causing severe headache or constipation for some days afterwards; but it does provide complete relief of pain in the majority of cases. Many women complain that they are given unwanted anesthetics – injections or gas – which make them dopey. It is often difficult to refuse an injection, but the staff have no right to give them against your will. If they do, then technically they are assaulting you.

POSITION
Women in labor usually find it uncomfortable to lie on their back for any length of time, and it can be bad for the baby because it may interfere with the supply of blood to the womb. However, women in the hospital are still told to lie

on their backs because this is most convenient for medical staff. You should not normally be asked to lie on your back for more than five to ten minutes. Most women lie on their sides but there is no reason why a woman should not sit supported by pillows with her legs bent – or even squat on the floor.

CUTTING THE VAGINA

It has become common to make a cut in the skin at the entrance to the vagina – episiotomy – to get the baby out quickly. Sometimes this is necessary when the baby is in distress, or to prevent an awkward tear. Sometimes it is done simply out of routine. Episiotomy cuts must be sewn up and the repair is not always satisfactory. It is worth telling your obstetrician that you would prefer not to have an episiotomy if it can be avoided.

LEBOYER DELIVERY

The French doctor, Frederick Leboyer (see Appendix 2) suggests that the emotional well-being of the baby is over-looked in the modern atmosphere of the delivery room with its bright lights and noise. He says lights should be low, the baby should be put on the mother's stomach after it is born and the cord cut only after it has stopped pulsating. Some obstetricians are prepared to use some of Leboyer's methods on request.

FEEDING THE BABY

If delivery is normal, there is no reason why the baby should not be put immediately to the breast – before it is cleaned and wrapped – if the mother wishes. The sooner the baby is put to the breast the better, because this stimulates the flow of milk and assists the delivery of the after-birth. Many doctors or nurses appreciate this now and are willing to do so if the mother asks. However, you must ask because it is not yet normal procedure. The baby will not get cold – the mother's skin is hot after the exertions of the delivery – and this is the natural place for the baby. Research shows that the vital bond between mother and child is formed most easily in the first few hours after birth, and that delay in giving a mother her baby can affect their relationship for years. Some mothers manage to overcome the most appalling difficulties with premature babies who cannot breast-feed, but it is so much better if these difficulties can be avoided.

Development

Few activities are as natural as bringing up children, yet few responsibilities can sometimes appear so daunting. New-born infants have always been frail and vulnerable. A century ago parents had many children but did not expect them all to live to adulthood; parents today, in the western world especially, have fewer children but greater expectations. And their optimism is largely justified. Childbirth is safer, while improvements in housing, sanitary standards and immunization have virtually eradicated diseases which once claimed tens of thousands of young lives.

The advance of medical knowledge has thus saved countless lives and eased the pain of countless more. But it has also produced a welter of research and conflicting theories

about child-care which can bemuse as much as enlighten. The trend towards smaller families has intensified parental unease. Today's new parents are likely to have been children in small families with little experience of babies or children. Unfamiliarity breeds uncertainty, so no wonder they join the millions of readers of Dr Spock and other child-care specialists.

Nor are books the only source of expertise available to parents today. Special child-care clinics help to monitor children's health and development on an almost weekly basis through the early years. The best and most experienced of parents will need such medical advice from time to time, advice based on the knowledge of hundreds of babies. However, parents should not be overawed by their new responsibilities. People have been bringing up children for thousands of years in far less propitious circumstances than today. And it is significant that the experts themselves urge parents to trust more to their instincts.

For instance, your instinct will tell you to cuddle your child and your instinct will be right. The sensation of touch is the only message from the outside world which is comprehensible to a baby: he* understands being held close and the touch of another skin. He needs human contact as spontaneously and freely and nakedly as the temperature permits. Physically and emotionally, baby needs cuddling and crooning and cooing and talking. It gives him a feeling of love and security that will be etched into his personality. And a secure child has an increased chance of becoming a healthy adult.

It is little wonder therefore that Dr Spock regarded his advice as "common sense" or that a child-care specialist of a younger generation, Penelope Leach in *Baby and Child*, should be similarly reassuring. "You are all on the same side," writes Dr Leach of parents and their children. "The side that wants to be happy, to have fun." Do things by the baby, she says, not by the book.

This book's concern for child development is restricted to matters of physical health, with the emphasis, as throughout the book, on what can be done to prevent illness and promote good health. More general guides to child development are listed in Appendix 2. We have divided this section into three age groups – the first six months; from six months until five; and the early school years – but in many cases the detailed advice on topics and diet and teeth overlap from one section to another. One piece of common sense that all parents surely know is that children cannot be divided into neat little categories. Children are individuals and they develop differently.

THE FIRST SIX MONTHS
Feeding

Babies have been "designed" to live on human milk. Cows' milk was likewise intended for calves, not young humans. Breast-feeding is therefore the ideal form of feeding young babies. The mixture is right, which is not guaranteed when a harassed mother makes up a bottle; the quantity is usually right, since milk is normally produced on a demand-and-supply basis which only a few women fail to achieve if they wish to breast-feed; and by every test, breast-feeding protects a child from disease, since the human milk carries antibodies against infection at a time when the child has not yet developed his own. Breast-feeding is particularly advisable for mothers traveling to, or living in, warm countries. This is because the water supply is more likely to be

*No male chauvinism is intended: "him" the baby helps us to differentiate the baby from "her" the mother.

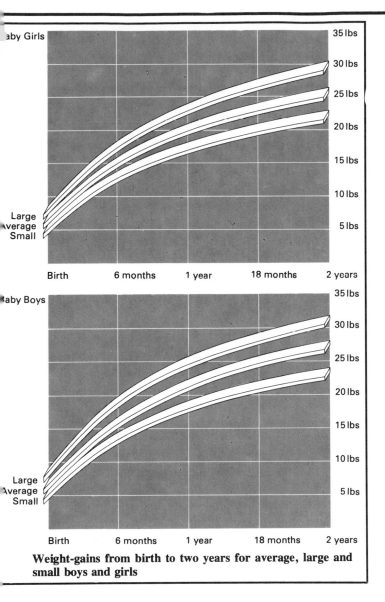

Baby Girls

35 lbs
30 lbs
25 lbs
20 lbs
15 lbs
10 lbs
5 lbs

Large
Average
Small

Birth　　6 months　　1 year　　18 months　　2 years

Baby Boys

35 lbs
30 lbs
25 lbs
20 lbs
15 lbs
10 lbs
5 lbs

Large
Average
Small

Birth　　6 months　　1 year　　18 months　　2 years

Weight-gains from birth to two years for average, large and small boys and girls

months. They should not worry about its adequacy. Modern formulae are available which are much closer to human milk than they used to be; baby will receive all the nutrition he needs for healthy development. The bottle must be clean and sterilized, of course, and the mixture made *precisely* in accordance with the instructions on the package or can. Making it stronger is making it worse rather than better. It not only leads to overfeeding and overweight but may overload the baby's body with sodium, which can have serious consequences. Never add salt, since this can harm a baby's kidneys, and never add sugar: you will only start the process of tooth decay.

But whether breast-feeding or bottle-feeding, do consult your doctor or baby clinic about whether or not to add any extra vitamins. Breast milk contains insufficient vitamin D, fresh cows' milk insufficient vitamins C and D. Powdered formulae usually contain all the necessary vitamins.

One routine part of a baby's visit to a health clinic is to be weighed. The only feeding problem which makes children ill and may cause them to die is a shortage of good food. It is a common, desperate problem in many parts of the world. In the more affluent western countries, feeding problems have a different character. Doctors here are increasingly more worried about babies being overweight than underweight. The two graphs on these pages show average weight-gains for the first year of life. As you can see, this can vary considerably depending on the size of the child, and no baby has yet been born whose weight will increase at such constant average rates. In real life, babies' weights go up at varying rates, sometimes spurting, sometimes slowing. Weight *is* important if your child appears to be exceptionally heavy or light but parents should not be too obsessive about it. Whether it concerns sleeping, feeding, teething or anything else, babies are individuals and as such will vary from one another.

You can help avoid overfeeding by sticking to milk only for the first few months. Opinions vary about the best time to introduce mixed feeding (with solids as well as milk) but it is probably best to make the change gradually between the fourth and sixth month. Babies have survived and thrived on any number of different diets (and theories) so do not be dogmatic about right and wrong times. Be flexible and introduce mixed feeding gradually. It is not a competition with targets to be achieved by this or that date. But do not start too early: milk supplies all a baby's nutritional needs in the first few months in the most easily digestible form. Adding solids or cereals too soon will lead to overweight; adding cereals may also lead to digestion difficulties in later life, so vegetables, meat, fish and cheese should form the most important elements of a baby's mixed diet. This should certainly be introduced by about six months, because baby will then need the extra iron in egg yolks, vegetables and meat that milk alone cannot supply.

Feeding-time is also important because it satisfies baby's need for comfort as well as food. It is impossible not to hold a baby close while breast-feeding, of course, but if bottle-feeding try to make sure you also cuddle baby closely. Feeding is a deeply emotional activity to a child. When he feels hungry, he feels distress: he is quite unable to reason, "It's all right, I'll get enough food in due course." All he can do is to express his distress by shrieking. If mother comes quickly to feed him, he feels secure and happy. He associates mother as food provider with mother as source of love. It is part of learning to love.

unhygienic in such countries and even if feeds can be prepared hygienically, gastroenteritis is so common that infection of the baby from other sources is much more likely. Breast-feeding gives positive protection against gastroenteritis, which can be extremely serious in young infants.

Breast-feeding has other advantages, too. These range from a lower incidence of diaper rash to fewer crib deaths (where children are found inexplicably and suddenly dead), although nobody really knows why this should be so. Even when children cease to be children it has been suggested that some illnesses are less common among those who were breast-fed than those who were bottle-fed. Such future protection could also stem from the fact that breast-fed babies are much less likely to be overfed and overweight. Mother's milk is thus the best by far, and the longer you can continue breast-feeding the better. Even a short period – the first two weeks or a month – is invaluable for a baby. Women commonly stop when baby's first teeth appear around six months, although breast-feeding can usually be continued without pain from the baby's teeth, supplemented by solid food, until the child is a year old or even older.

Although breast-feeding is the ideal, some mothers will produce insufficient milk and have no option but to bottle-feed from the earliest days. For a variety of reasons many mothers will switch to bottle-feeding during baby's first

Mother, too, can associate food with love and this can lead to a dangerous trap. A child who is not hungry at one mealtime will not want to eat much. The statement seems banal but as feeding her own baby is an emotional experience for the mother, she may feel rejected if her child declines food for which he has no appetite. She may then attempt to persuade him to make more food which will probably make him cross and possibly make him sick. It is never right to quarrel with a child about his food. Healthy normal children do not starve themselves, so try not to worry. Accept that baby will sometimes be more or less hungry than usual and that some children, like some grown-ups, have smaller appetites than others. But consult your doctor if loss of appetite persists for several days and you are at all uneasy. Never worry if a child misses one meal: he will usually make up for it at the next.

Crying

Crying is part – a large part – of a baby's language. It is used neither to annoy nor to exercise his lungs; it is used to say something. It is the baby's form of vocal communication. It can reflect a yearning for physical contact or play as well as hunger or distress. A mother's natural reaction is to pick baby up and cuddle him. This is the proper reaction. Her only problem is to work out whether baby is thirsty, hungry, too hot, too cold, frightened, lonely or bored. But she soon learns to distinguish between the different cries, which means baby has successfully communicated his feelings.

There is a school of thought which argues that mothers who rush to their babies as soon as they cry will spoil them. But psychological research shows the contrary: babies who are left to cry for a long time become more difficult and tearful children. So again the mother's instinct is right. The cry should not be ignored and mothers should not worry about whether they are doing the "right" thing by comforting their crying child.

A worried mother – worried for any reason – can transmit her worry to the child and trigger another problem. Her emotional state, whether it be worry, tension or unhappiness, may even be enough to set the child crying again. A tense, unhappy mother will also find it difficult to comfort the baby and this will only make her more tense. It is all too easy for a potentially disastrous cycle to begin this way and it is all too common for new mothers to be tense and worried. They have so much to do and so little time. If mothers do feel run down, then for their sake and their baby's they should seek help from their doctor, or try and find someone who can help to give them an occasional break.

Playing

Playing is a vital aspect of learning and growing up. Parents often think that children can only play when they are six months or older. By this they tend to mean play with toys or romp around a room. But play begins – or should begin – in the very earliest days. A baby who strokes his mother's breast during feeding is playing and learning to use his hands; a baby lying on the floor and kicking his legs is playing and learning how to exercise his body; a baby watching and later touching a mobile strung across his cot is similarly playing and learning. As baby grows older his play becomes more ambitious, so much so that you have to think constantly about safety. He does then begin to play with toys but often will gain as much fun through an improvised

toy as one bought expensively in the shops. Play helps to develop control of the body, including sight and hearing as well as muscular co-ordination and other physical skills. It is therefore an integral part of a child's physical development. It is also an opportunity for parents to talk to their children as they play with them. Baby will not understand the words but he needs to hear the noise of the human voice. The more a baby hears words, the more readily he will learn to use them himself. So do not be shy or self-conscious: talk and sing to your baby often. It should be as natural and spontaneous as smiling.

Daily routine

Mothers should not make themselves anxious by fretting unduly about a daily routine. Babies do not work like clockwork. How much they eat and how much they sleep will vary enormously from one baby to another, right from the earliest days. Feeding has already been discussed. Sleeping should be even less of a problem, at least for the baby. Babies will sleep for as long or as little as they need. Parents of wakeful children should try consoling themselves with the knowledge that there is some evidence that babies who need the least sleep are on average brighter children. The only other essential part of any baby's day is playing. A daily bath is useful but not essential; high standards of general hygiene *are* essential.

Eyesight

The first six months of life are crucial in the development of eyesight. Vision is not fully developed before three months, which means that eyes are very vulnerable throughout this period. Any sign of damage or infection should be reported to the doctor immediately. It is only as a baby's eyes develop that he begins to align the eyes together and see properly. During the first six months he begins to develop binocular vision, which means using both eyes together to see objects in depth. Until he manages this, he may look a little cross-eyed or have a "wandering eye". But if a baby over three months old still squints and looks cross-eyed, the cause is usually some fault in learning how to interpret depth. He should be seen promptly by a doctor or a specialist. At this stage, steps an be taken to rectify squints so it is important not to delay. If you are worrying unnecessarily, the doctor will not mind; if there is some cause to worry, he will welcome the opportunity of dealing with the squint at the best time. Early detection is vital.

STAGES OF GROWTH

Babies develop at such different rates that it is impossible to suggest states or stages of development which should be reached at specific ages. A very wide range is normal. But it is natural for parents to worry if a child seems slow in certain skills. Parents should always be alert to any problem which may need medical help but generally they should regard "stages of development" as no more than useful or interesting guidelines. Not only do babies vary so greatly but the child who is first to reach one given stage may not necessarily be the first to reach another. There is certainly no guarantee that he will grow up into the most intelligent or most agile or most successful of any group of babies. Many an early developer has been overtaken by a late starter.

Ultimately it does not really matter that much if he smiles at six or eight weeks, crawls at seven or nine months and so on. But if you think your child's development is way outside the norm, consult your doctor. These are some approximate milestones in the first months of life:

1. Most babies *smile* at around six weeks, rarely more than a week earlier or more than four weeks later.
2. Most babies *sit up* by around six months but they will not be able to hold themselves in this position for very long or be particularly maneuverable – this comes one to three months later.
3. Most babies will be *rolling over* from stomach to back by six months. Rolling the other way comes one to four weeks later.
4. Most babies cut their first *teeth* – the lower central incisor – at six months. By the time he is a year old he will have six incisors; they may come regularly or in sudden bursts. (See below for further information on young teeth.)
5. Most babies will *crawl* at around nine months and *walk* on their own at some time between twelve and eighteen months. A few babies omit the crawling stage altogether. Babies begin to pull themselves to their feet to *stand up* at around seven months. But variations are huge in all three skills.
6. Most babies will *speak* two or three words when they are one year old and be able to construct simple sentences one year later. But they will be "vocalizing" much earlier. Between six and nine months they will make sounds like "ma" or "pa" or "da", which thrills their parents but does not mean they have understood these common abbreviations for mother and father. (See below for further information on speech and hearing.)
7. Most babies will be able to use their hands to grasp, pull and push when *playing* by the time they are one year old. Skills such as using building blocks develop in the following year.

FROM SIX MONTHS ONWARDS
Diet
By six months "feeds" become "meals" which are taken more or less at adult times – breakfast, lunch and supper. By a year the times remain the same but the meals are taken with the rest of the family – an important part of any child's social development. The child will also then start eating normal – meaning adult – food. The habits established then are likely to remain for the rest of his life.

Children learn marvelously quickly about food from their parents, but this can also mean they learn the wrong habits and values. Children are more impressed by what their parents do than what they say. If parents start the day on a cup of coffee and a piece of buttered toast, there is no point in their extolling to their six- or seven-year-old the virtues of starting the day with a "proper" breakfast. Childhood can be a fine opportunity for the parents to develop good dietary habits for their own benefit as well as their children's. Just what this involves in terms both of what we eat and how we cook it is spelled out in the next chapter; it is never too late – or too early – to start.

Generally, what is good for adults is good for children. So fresh foods are better than convenience foods, although tired and harassed mothers are bound to use some convenience meals. This will do no harm but they should not become the corner-stone of anyone's diet. One particular way in which parents can help their children is to keep them away from sugar and candies; both are attractive to children but reduce their appetite for nutritious food and have the distinct disadvantage of rotting the teeth.

Teeth
Good teeth start in infancy and an alarming number of not-so-good ones finish there. In the US, 80 per cent of pre-school children have some decayed milk-teeth (as the first teeth are known). The rot then continues because the bacteria which are consuming the milk-teeth can attack the adult teeth already developing in the jaw. Two terrible statistics result. Between eighteen and twenty-four years of age the average American has lost 4.7 teeth and has 2.1 teeth decayed but unfilled, and some twenty million adults have no teeth of their own left.

If you want your child to avoid this painful fate, restrict sugar and candies as mentioned above and explained further in the section on teeth later in this book. Eating only at mealtimes has a double value. It is better nutritionally and better for the teeth. Anything eaten between meals tends to be sugary, and sugar is the breeding ground for the bacteria which form the acids that rot teeth. If sweets are to be eaten, have them at the end of meals.

You can also help your child's teeth by trying to brush as soon as the first milk-tooth appears. It does not matter particularly at this stage whether you brush up and down or side to side or, as dentists eventually recommend, in small circular movements. From the age of three or four, children can start brushing their own teeth but you should still supervise this. By nine or ten you will not need to supervise, but make sure they do not start skipping it. Whatever the age, teeth should be cleaned at least twice a day.

Three in five Americans drink fluoridated water, but dentists recommend fluoride toothpastes for everyone, particularly children, since fluoride can be incorporated into teeth as they grow during the first ten years of life. This is one reason why toothbrushing must become part of the daily routine from the earliest possible days. But your dentist can increase the protection by using a fluoride toothpaste, while fluoride tablets, available from drug stores, help further. With luck, the tooth-preserving habits of a lifetime will be established in childhood.

Eyesight and hearing
Whereas teeth usually start life in good condition and are then destroyed by their owners, eyes and ears, or rather sight and hearing, may be poor from the start. If your child holds toys unusually close or far away when playing, get expert advice. And if a child does not seem to notice what you say when he cannot see you, also consult a doctor.

Either or both of these defects may show up clearly when a child starts going to school. A child who wants to sit at the front of the class may be short-sighted, and teachers who report that "he doesn't listen to anything" may really be describing a child whose hearing is bad, possibly because there is wax in his ears. However, it may be more serious. Poor hearing should be detected as soon as possible because it will affect the development of a child's ability to talk. An experienced doctor can sometimes detect the problem from the more limited vocalizing and babbling of a six-month-old baby with hearing difficulties. A baby can use a hearing aid from the age of about six months and this will help him develop better speech than he otherwise would. But this is something on which parents will need specialist guidance.

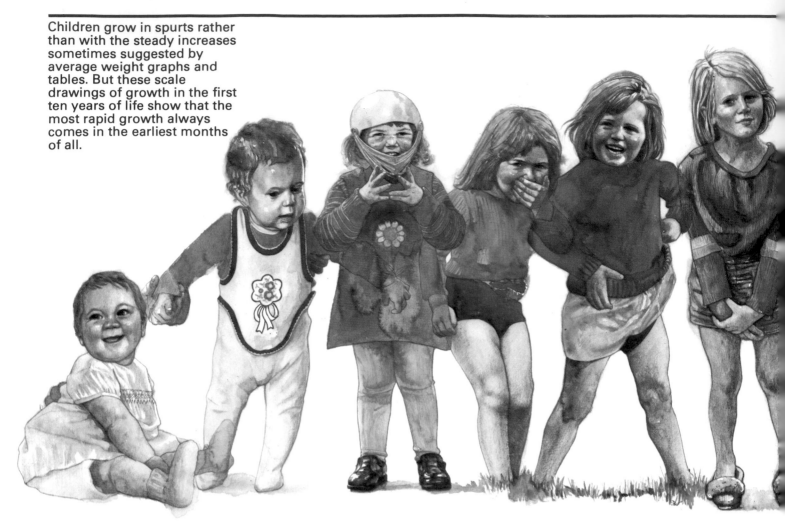

Children grow in spurts rather than with the steady increases sometimes suggested by average weight graphs and tables. But these scale drawings of growth in the first ten years of life show that the most rapid growth always comes in the earliest months of all.

If a child squints – one eye going repeatedly into a corner – then he should be seen by a specialist. If parents or close relatives have squints, the child should have a routine eye test between 2½ and 3 years; if any irregularity is observed, tests may be repeated at six-month intervals. Ideally, every child should have their eyes tested between three and five before going to school. If nothing is wrong, another examination is not necessary for perhaps two years and at two-year intervals afterwards.

Speech

Speech – the deliberate use of words in original sentences – is a unique human achievement. Other animals can learn a very limited version of the human language in signs and symbols, but none can match human skill and sensitivity. Yet simply because speech is our best means of communication, we sometimes forget just what an achievement it is and expect too much of our children.

Children develop the ability to talk, like they develop every other ability, at their own rates, and a very wide range is normal. A child will *on average* be able to use a few words, singly but with meaning, between twelve and eighteen months. Some time between the second and third year he will manage to put sentences together and hold simple conversations. By about five he will have a mastery of the technique of the spoken language.

You can help your child to speak if you remember how he learns. Speaking can be learned only by imitation, so the parent should take every opportunity of talking to a child. But a child has limitations. He can deal with short, simple sentences only. The advantage of this kind of sentence is

that every word is part of the simple message. "Don't take that" is simple. "You know you shouldn't touch my knitting" is so complicated that the child will gain virtually nothing from the words, although the *tone* will convey the message of exasperation.

For the same reason, you should speak slowly to a child. As he has no language of his own at this stage, what he is really doing is learning a foreign language. And we all know how difficult it is to pick out individual words from the rapid flow of a foreign language, even though we may actually know many of the words that are being used.

Children do not say much that is of riveting interest at first. We are fascinated by their first words but tend afterwards to let them chatter on without paying much attention. But if we want to help them learn the skills of speech and communication, we must help them by listening, by answering them in sentences they can follow, and eventually by correcting their grammar and pronunciation. The art of correction is delicate. If you are too ready to correct, conversation grinds to a halt. It is difficult, even for an adult, to continue conversations that are interspersed with sentences like "You mean sausage, dear. Now what were you saying?" On the other hand, a child can easily develop bad speech habits that can take root. This is obviously a risk if you continue to allow very bad pronunciation. But it also happens if you continue to allow them to use a pronunciation or phrase which you find amusing; children are very willing to entertain you with what eventually becomes fossilized baby-talk. Simply because a child is not fluent we are sometimes tempted to finish his sentences for him. But to do his talking for him handicaps his learning. This problem can also arise if there is an elder brother or sister who is over-ready to show off their expertise.

The importance of speech makes it inevitable that parents worry over apparent delays and difficulties in mastering this essential art of communication. Usually a late start is not serious; children, as we have said before, vary as greatly in mastering the ability to speak as they do in all other abilities. Some problems such as stuttering or lisping are often temporary. If not, speech therapy can "cure" many children and improve all of them. However, sometimes speech difficulties are symptoms of deafness or the result of a genuine disorder. So if in any doubt, consult your doctor and seek specialist advice.

Fitness

Baby will be crawling or even walking by around his first birthday. Movement is obviously another crucial skill. It is important for a child's psychological as well as physical development, so try not to worry, induce fear or interfere. This is the way a child finds out about the world, and children are much more sensible and safe than parents often credit. They explore cautiously, extending their range bit by bit. But they are as rattled by cries of "Look out!" and "Be careful!" as you would be when driving a car. They will also learn from the occasional bump and bruise, but innate caution and relatively tough skins cannot preclude every hazard. Childhood accidents are a major source of injury and even death. Children need protection from some hazards both inside and outside the home (see the next section in this chapter).

Later in this book we devote much of a chapter to the message that the health of the adult greatly depends on getting enough exercise. This habit is almost certainly born young and, unfortunately, in some children it dies young too. Parents should do what they can to get a child to be active. Babies will vary as to when they start crawling or walking, but consult the doctor if your baby seems particularly late starting. It may well be nothing, but it does no harm to ask. As children grow older they should be encouraged to use their own feet for getting about. Do not take them by car to palces they can reach under their own toddler power. A four-year-old can walk a couple of miles on a shopping expedition; a nine-year-old can cycle ten miles (but should for safety reasons be accompanied by a parent and avoid main roads); an eleven-year-old can go on lengthy camping expeditions. Schools are another obvious source of fitness and will help to keep them active with organized sports.

Feet

If a child is to enjoy moving on his own two feet, these must be kept sound and undeformed. A growing foot needs as much freedom as possible. Let your child go barefoot as much as possible and remember that tight socks (or tight stretch-suits) can be as harmful as tight shoes. When he does have to wear shoes, make sure they are comfortable and fit well. Shoes are outgrown so quickly at this age that fit matters far more than quality. *Never* buy children's shoes from a shop that asks you the size: children's feet should be remeasured every time, so look for shops which specialize in supplying – and fitting – children's shoes. (For further information on foot care, see page 106.)

VACCINATION

Vaccination or immunization has played an essential part in the decline in infectious diseases over the last fifty years. Some have declined to such an extent that immunization is no longer carried out on all children – smallpox, for example. However, in Europe the risks of whooping cough vaccination have been assessed by some doctors as not much less than the risks of the disease itself, and in Germany medical authorities no longer recommend whooping cough as a routine vaccination. It is generally accepted that whooping cough vaccination can cause serious brain damage, but there is no agreement among experts on how often this happens. The US Department of Health, Education and Welfare puts the risk of "encephalitis (inflammation of the brain) or brain damage" from vaccine containing pertussis at one in every 100,000 *doses*. Children who have any history of damage to the brain, such as epilepsy, and children who have had a particularly difficult birth which might have caused some minor brain injury should not have this vaccination, because they are believed to be vulnerable to side effects. Whooping cough vaccination (pertussis) may give valuable protection for people living in crowded conditions, particularly in countries outside Europe, North America and Australasia where the disease is much more common and much more serious.

The US Department of Health, Education and Welfare recommends the following vaccination schedules, depending on starting age. The schedules for different vaccinations are only approximate and are sometimes varied by individual doctors. For further information on infectious diseases generally – their prevention and treatment – see page 152.

If your child is 2 months old, HEW recommends beginning DPT (diphtheria, pertussis and tetanus) and polio vaccination. Booster shots of DPT and polio should be given at four and six months. Measles, rubella (German measles) and mumps vaccines can be given together as a single injection at 15 months of age (measles may not be effective if given earlier). Booster shots of DPT and polio should be given again at 18 months and 4–6 years.

If your child is 1 to 5 years of age, HEW recommends DPT and polio followed one month later by measles, rubella and mumps; then at 2, 4 and 10–16 months after first visit by DPT and polio.

If your child is older and has missed vaccinations, he or she can still have them – consult your doctor or clinic.

After 10 years: All children should have booster tetanus-diphtheria shots at age 14 to 16 years which should be repeated every 10 years. Tuberculosis vaccination (BCG) is valuable for all children who show no natural immunity after testing. Girls who have not had rubella vaccination should have it now before the reproductive years begin.

OFF TO SCHOOL

The change in a child's life when he starts school is enormous. Unless he has been going to playgroup or a nursery, this may be the first time he has spent a day, regularly, away from home and parents. Playgroup or nursery is obviously a good way of acclimatizing himself to the change as well as a good way of learning sociability and other early educational skills. But if a child has not had this opportunity, his parents should help him to prepare for his first days at school.

Whatever the parents think of their own schooldays, they should emphasize the pleasures of school when they tell him about it. Stress the adventure. Tell him what a big grown-up boy he has become. Do not say things like "At last, I'm free to get on with something". It may be a relief to have the child away from home all day but the child need not know this. It certainly will not help him adjust to his new life.

This life will be much more energetic than he is used to, so he will need plenty of sleep; the household day may need to be slightly rearranged to fit in with the school hours. Sleep is important not merely because you do not want your child to be sleepy at school but because of fundamental health reasons. A child who is short of sleep may grow slower than he should and is more likely to be underweight. There are no firm rules for bedtimes, however. If a child is bright and willing to get up in the morning, he is getting enough sleep; if he is still tired in the morning, then he is not getting enough sleep. But as a rough guide, a child between five and seven should be in bed by 7 o'clock during school semesters and the child between eight and eleven in bed by 8 o'clock.

The new demands of school also make proper diet and feeding especially important. Children, even more than the rest of us, need a good meal to start the day. Breakfast should include wholemeal cereal and some fruit. One egg, broiled bacon or some fish can be valuable, but not even small children should eat too many eggs or too much meat (see Chapter 2). Baked beans on toast or broiled tomatoes are a quick alternative. If they want some toast and marmalade or jelly too, so much the better. They should not be encouraged to hurry their food, which means that they (and their cook) must get on the move at a suitably early hour in the morning.

Most children eat their mid-day meal at school during the school year and there is a tradition of not liking school food. It obviously will not be as good as home cooking but they should be encouraged to eat something, especially as it has to sustain a child throughout the afternoon. If possible, try and call at the school to see what they are eating. A lot of schools allow automatic food machines on the premises, which serve the children candy bars, potato chips and other sweet and salty snacks that are basically unsatisfying and bad for health in the long run (see next chapter). If school food is unsatisfactory, give your child sandwiches and fruit instead.

Children usually want something to eat when they get home from school. If they do have anything, it should be light enough not to spoil their appetite for the main evening meal an hour or so later. Everybody should have three proper meals a day for their health's sake; they are more likely to do so if the habit starts young.

Hygienic behavior, to use a euphemistic phrase, is also a habit which should be started young. Children should wash their hands after using the toilet and before eating food. If they are told the reason and supervised carefully the habit will take root.

Young children generally do not need to be told to take exercise, as any parent will testify. But as they reach adolescence young people, girls probably more frequently than boys, sometimes decide that sport and exercise in general is not for them. It is not glamorous enough, they say, or they may say it will spoil their glamor by making them too muscular. It is difficult for adults to influence adolescents very effectively, but any success in getting them to realize that exercise, on the contrary, makes them more attractive (as well as generally fitter) will pay dividends in later life. It helps to imbue healthy habits if the parents appear to be speaking from experience and practicing what they preach.

WHAT PARENTS SHOULD NOT DO

A child learns a lot from his parents – for good or ill. Smoking is the most obvious bad example. It may be that a baby does not learn to smoke from watching his parents but it is not safe to rely on even that. From the age of a few months the child will accept the idea that smoking is something that adults normally do – like walking and talking – and therefore admirable and to be imitated. If you do not smoke, your child is much less likely to take up smoking himself, and you will also be protecting him in the early months by not polluting the atmosphere in which he must breathe.

A parent can also introduce a child to heavy drinking if this again seems to be normal adult behavior. The children of alcoholics are more likely to become alcoholics themselves. This is not an inherited trait but an imitated one. The most constant examples to a child are its parents, however caring or careless they may prove to be. Children should be introduced to alcohol gradually. Learning to cope with alcohol is a long way from learning to roll over from stomach to back, but it is all part of the development from baby to adulthood.

Accidents

Accidents are the most common cause of death in children and cause twice as many deaths in under-sixteens than the next two most common causes of death combined – birth abnormalities and cancers. About two in every five children suffer injury through an accident each year, and of those approximately 85 per cent need medical attention. Boys are more accident-prone than girls: 461 boys in every 1,000 are injured, for instance, compared to 320 girls. Many are left with severe disabilities, many die.

Much more could be done by government, local legislatures and parents to prevent many of these accidents from happening. Many people do not realize that there is greater danger to a child of dying in the home or garden than there is of dying on the roads. The first step in prevention is to recognize the source of danger.

Falls are by far the most common cause of injury among US children. No fewer than 6½ million children under sixteen are hurt each year in falls sufficiently seriously to involve medical attention or to cause at least temporary restricted activity. Children under six are particularly prone to falls. But these do not cause the most deaths. In 1976, traffic accidents killed a total of 1,291 children aged one to five in the US, fires or burns 680 and drownings 650, compared to the 136 who died from falls. These are also the principal causes of death from accidents among children aged five to sixteen. And although the chances of a fatal accident may appear slim statistically, far higher numbers are injured with sometimes crippling results.

Children under one year old are especially liable to choke or suffocate on food, toys or small objects such as buttons, beads or coins. These should be kept out of the children's reach, and infants' food should not contain lumps until they are old enough to chew properly. Babies suck until about six months of age, when they gradually learn to chew. Ideally, infants should be given only liquid food or smooth spoon-foods until six months of age. They can then be introduced slowly to soft solid foods until they have all their chewing teeth and are able to manage most things, although it is still wise not to give infants anything which is at all tough.

Around the age of one year old, when children become mobile, they begin to find all sorts of things on the floor and on tables which they could not reach before which could choke, poison or suffocate them – beware particularly of plastic bags. And at this age they begin to be able to reach hot pans on stoves or coffee pots on tables. Burns and scalds are one of the commonest causes of moderate to severe injury in children. Also the child, still uncertain and inexpert in movement, is likely to pull over his high chair, or fall from furniture. Fractures and concussion are another common cause of moderate to severe injury, and each year infants tragically drown while left unattended in a bath.

By the age of three or four, the child is exploring more on his own and begins to discover where the bleach, turpentine, paraffin – and the nail-polish remover – have been hidden unless they are out of reach. The fact that these substances do not taste nice seems to make no difference. The child discovers things hidden in the garage or may fall in the pool; or has learnt to switch on an electric socket and may start a fire by poking paper into the heater, or by fiddling with the pilot light on the stove.

By the time the child gets to school age, road accidents become an increasing danger. A child has a one in fifty chance of being involved in a road accident before the age of sixteen.

It is no good trying to insulate children totally from danger. They must be exposed to dangers before they can learn to avoid them. But exposure to danger must be made in a carefully calculated way at an age when a child is fully able to understand it.

HOW TO AVOID ACCIDENTS

1. **In the home**

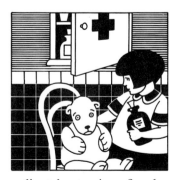

Heating. Radiant electric fires can give an inquisitive child who grasps the element a terrible burn, or may ignite inflammable clothing or furniture when placed too close. In small rooms, radiant fires should be at a high level attached to a wall. Alternatively, use a convector heater or place the radiant heater in a fireplace surrounded by a childproof guard attached to the wall. Do not use gas or oil heaters in small unventilated rooms. Get any old gas appliances inspected by your local gas company.

Kitchen. Pilot lights on a stove are a potential danger. Choose a stove without pilot lights, and use an electric lighter for the gas. Keep the lighter on a high shelf. Use a guard around the stove to prevent pans being pulled off. Always turn handles in, use the burners at the back whenever possible and if you are buying new pans, try to get short-handled ones. Keep a small fire extinguisher near the stove to deal with burning fat. Always put coffee pots and hot pans well out of reach of children. Keep matches out of reach, and instruct children in the dangers of fire with outdoor camp-fires. Only buy electric gadgets, including fires, which say they conform to safety standards approved by a recognized testing organization such as Underwriters Laboratories of New York. Never keep cleaning materials, soap powders, bleach, paints or paraffin under the sink or at floor level.

Living room and bedroom. Falls from furniture are a real danger. Never leave a small baby propped up unattended or out of reach on a chair. The baby may wriggle and fall off the chair or get into some awkward position where he may be smothered. Arrange furniture as far as possible so that it does not enable young children to climb high. Bunk-beds require special care since every year children are killed or injured through falling out while asleep. Make sure that the guards are used to make it as difficult as possible to fall out, and remove any furniture the child might collide with on the way down. Make sure that the floor beside the bunks is covered with a soft rug. Do not give pillows to babies under twelve months, since they may cause suffocation. Beware of projections on cribs which may catch children's clothing so that they may hang. Never tie anything such as a pacifier on a cord around a child's neck.

Windows. Make sure that children cannot open windows more than 100mm (about four inches). Fittings designed to make windows burglar-proof are often suitable for preventing windows from being opened too far by children inside the house, and the window can still be opened wide on a hot day when adults are in the room.

Bathrooms. Locks which can be opened from the outside with a screwdriver or in some other way are a great advantage in case of emergency. Medicines should always be locked in a cupboard or childproof medicine cabinet. Do not take tablets in front of the children because this encourages them to imitate you. Never encourage children to think of drugs as candy in order to get them to take them. If your children need medicine, ask the doctor not to provide it in the form of a sweet flavored syrup. Children sometimes drink the whole bottle because they like it and believe that a whole bottle may do them more good. It may of course be necessary to use a syrup to get your child to take essential medicine, but try an ordinary formulation first. Flush old drugs down the toilet.

2. In the garden

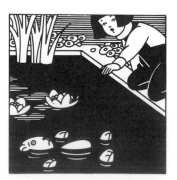

The garage or shed is a fascinating place full of mysteries for children. Chemicals used in the garden, however, are much more dangerous than most of those in your bathroom cupboard. Garden chemicals should therefore be kept under lock and key. Never transfer garden chemicals to old lemonade or whisky bottles, as this has proved a death trap not only for children. The pond or pool

How to make your home childproof: 23 ways of cutting the risk

Radiators: very hot radiators present an obvious hazard to adventuring young hands. Consult central heating specialists to see if your system can be adapted to lower temperatures.

Windows: safety catch to stop children opening them sufficiently to be able to fall out. Essential of course, for upstairs windows but desirable downstairs, too.

Stairs: should be well-lit with a light switch at top and bottom. The banisters should be firm, the stairs unobstructed. Nothing flammable should be stored underneath the stairs in case of fire.

Shelving: must be securely fixed to walls, preferably with rounded edges and ends to avoid sharp, dangerous corners. From the safety point of view this is the prime consideration but to protect adult property, such as books and records, it's often better to keep all shelving high and out of a child's reach.

Safety gate: keeps crawling youngsters safely downstairs (or upstairs). Ideally have one at both top and bottom of the stairs.

Flooring: fitted carpets are ideal because they lessen the chance of children slipping. If carpets or rugs are not fitted, make sure they are laid – and preferably fixed – on non-polished floors.

Toys: give big toys to small children so that they cannot swallow small items like beads or marbles.

Electric appliances: keep cord short without connections and where possible out of children's reach. Don't allow it to run under carpets and if possible run only one appliance per outlet. No bare wire must show.

Dining table: keep hot drinks from the edge. If you can manage without a tablecloth this will lessen the chance of a child tugging the cloth – and all that rests on it – off the table on to the floor.

Fire: fit a fixed guard to all gas and electric fires. Open solid fuel fires should also have a guard secured to the fireplace surround.

Matches: should always be kept out of children's reach in a high cupboard or on a high shelf.

Stove: turn handles of saucepans to the side if stove has a worktop on each side; if not, prevent children from pulling over pots and pans by fitting a safety guard.

Deep fat fryer: never leave pan unattended. In the event of fire never use water, always smother with a damp cloth.

Kettle: cord for all electric equipment should be kept short, but especially for electric kettles. Hook it up if necessary to make it less likely that a child can pull a kettle off a kitchen worktop and pour boiling water all over him or herself.

Storage under sink: keep bleach and other poisonous cleaning agents away from children by putting these items in a high cupboard. Turpentine, paint and other decorating materials should, where possible, be kept in a lockable outside shed.

First-aid cabinet: useful to keep in the kitchen since this is where many accidents happen and where children are more likely to be under surveillance. Must be lockable. Don't also use it to store foodstuffs.

Flooring: non-slip flooring such as vinyl or cork is particularly important in a kitchen where people carry hot food and liquids. Use non-slip polishes, too, but keep floor clean; wipe up spilt liquids at once.

Chairs: children should always be secured by a safety harness when in a high chair.

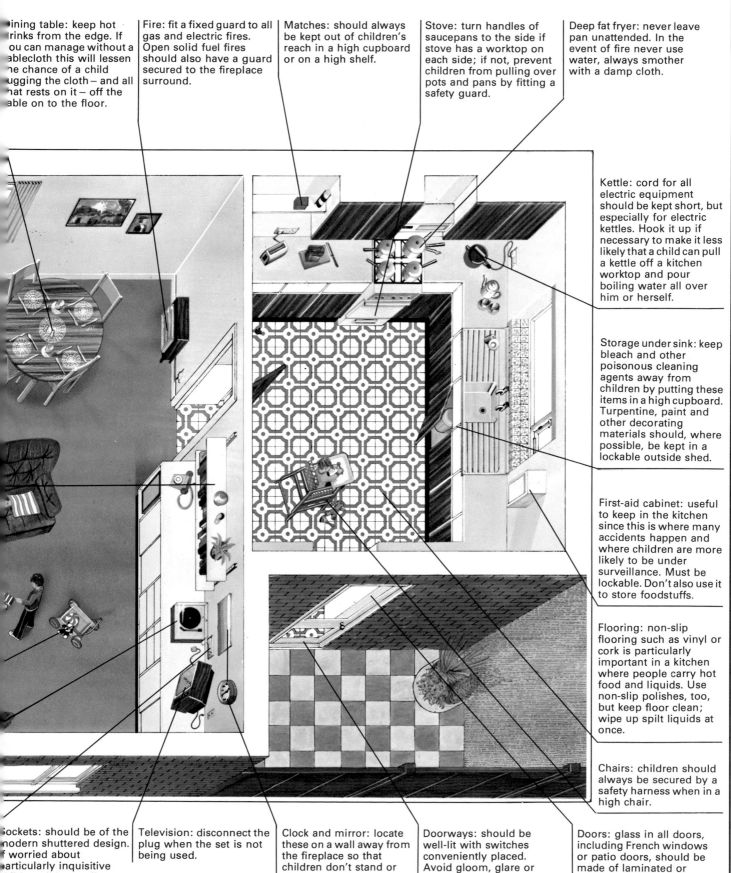

Sockets: should be of the modern shuttered design. If worried about particularly inquisitive children, "dummy" or blind plugs can be bought to fill the tempting holes.

Television: disconnect the plug when the set is not being used.

Clock and mirror: locate these on a wall away from the fireplace so that children don't stand or climb near a fire to see them.

Doorways: should be well-lit with switches conveniently placed. Avoid gloom, glare or shadows. "Sink" the doormat wherever possible.

Doors: glass in all doors, including French windows or patio doors, should be made of laminated or tempered glass.

Hazards in the country

The plants that grow in the country and by the roadside can look mouth-wateringly attractive — especially to children at play. But many are also extremely dangerous and, if eaten, can cause serious illness or even death. The variety of poisons is startling and by no means confined to the countryside: every year children are poisoned by plants which grow in their own gardens. Often the most serious hazard is the least likely. The foxglove, for instance, has such a nasty taste that if children

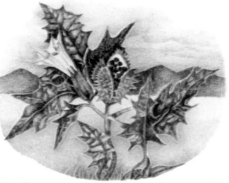

1. *Jimsonweed*, also known as thorn apple, thrives in the hot dry locations of the South and West, releasing poisonous black seeds when ripe. Symptoms include dry skin, dilated pupils.

eat a little they spit it out quickly. Poisoning is much more likely to result from less toxic but more "attractive" and edible plants such as the five common American hazards shown here. Many other plants can cause serious poisoning. The other two plants illustrated here — poison sumac and poison ivy — can cause skin irritations. Wild fungi looking like mushrooms can also be poisonous, so beware. If in doubt, leave alone; if poisonous plants have been eaten, consult a physician.

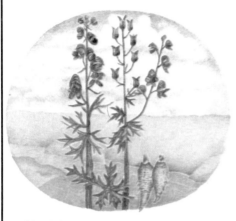

2. *Monkshood*, or aconite, is a garden species. Western monkshood is a native US plant found in mountains from Arizona to Canada. Roots not to be mistaken for horse radish.

3. *Poison ivy*. Common throughout US and Canada except West Coast, superficially the same as poison oak which is found in the West. Both can cause serious skin problems.

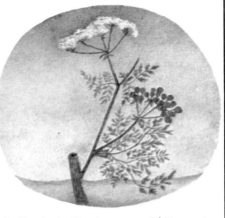

4. *Hemlock.* Also known as fool's parsley because its leaves have been mistaken for parsley. A dangerous masquerader — its roots look like parsnips, its seeds like the herb anise.

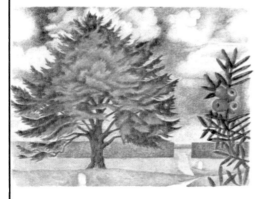

5. *Yew.* Found in America as both a tree and a shrub (ground hemlock). Its brilliant red berries can cause serious heart problems, sometimes even death.

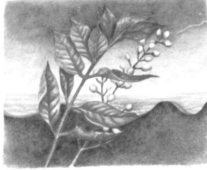

6. *Poison sumac.* It can cause extreme skin irritation on contact. Native in swampy areas, it is distinguishable from non-poisonous sumacs by its white berries.

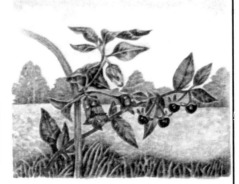

7. *Deadly nightshade.* The fruits are purple or black when ripe. Two or three can kill a child. Other nightshade species are broadly similar in appearance and danger.

is another potential source of danger, and should be fenced off if young children are allowed to play unsupervised in the garden — 300 children under five died from drowning in 1976 *in or around their homes*. Special care needs to be taken with lawn mowers: do not let children play around you while you are mowing.

Even suburban gardens can contain poisonous plants, and so children must be taught never to eat anything from the garden without being told that it is all right. Their attention should be brought to brightly colored berries, and they should be told that these are not good to eat. The

message can be reinforced by fairy tales such as Snow White, which includes descriptions of poisoning. Snow White went into a coma after eating a poisoned apple and only awoke after receiving the attentions of the prince; nowadays a doctor has to suffice. Plants pose four different hazards: allergies spread by wind-blown pollen; dermatitis or skin irritations from direct or even indirect contact with certain plants (see also Allergies, page 142); cuts or injuries from prickly plants; and poisoning from eating plants. The latter is the most serious, as it is the only hazard which can have fatal results. Children are especially vulnerable because of their natural curiosity and because smaller amounts of a poison are needed to cause harm. No fewer than twenty-nine plants which grow in US gardens or yards have caused fatalities, including the common species azalea, oleander, and rhododendron.

Parents should attempt to teach their children to recognize the plants or fungi which grow in their area, but the only safe rule is never to eat anything unless *positive* of its identification. Although poisonous plants are clearly the most serious hazard, skin irritation is more common. Poison sumac, poison ivy and poison oak alone injure an estimated two million people a year. Symptoms are a reddening of the skin with blisters that itch intensely and are easily spread.

3. In the playground

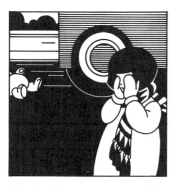

Although playgrounds have dangers, they are much safer for children than playing on the street, and provide children with invaluable training in the judgement of moving objects. However, around 100,000 US children a year receive medical treatment after playground accidents. Two-thirds of these are caused by falls, with up to three-quarters of the total occurring among children under six.

So children of this age should play under the supervision of an adult. Swings, roundabouts, slides and climbing-frames all need careful watching. Some playgrounds have supervisors in attendance. These are likely to be safer, probably because the supervisor controls dangerous use of equipment. Risks could be cut by improvements in equipment – particularly by providing impact-absorbing swings, placing climbing-frames on sand, rubber or wood chips which will help to break a fall, and improved design generally.

4. In the car

To safeguard children while driving, provide them with their own special seat and harness. A special seat will also help prevent travel sickness, because the child can see out of the window more easily. Provide over-fives with normal seat belts. Never allow children to ride next to the driver, which is the most dangerous seat in the car.

5. On the road

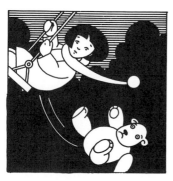

Parents often greatly underestimate the difficulties children have in learning to cross the road safely. Children under seven years old, and many older children, cannot be expected to be able to deal with all the circumstances which may arise when crossing a road. Children under five may not be able to fasten their coat buttons and talk at the same time – they need all their concentration to do one task. Older children often have the same problem when faced with crossing the road. Dr Stina Sandels, director of the Institute for Child Development Research in Stockholm, and a leading authority on children and traffic, says: "We have seen six to seven year olds who are unable to cross the road and watch out at the same time but who instead try to look first and then walk". Young children are not able to divide their attention.

The flow of traffic is variable and may change suddenly so that it becomes extremely difficult for children to follow what is happening and deduce when it is safe to cross. Adults generally find it safest to cross the road at junctions. However, Dr Sandels's research has found that children often find it more confusing at junctions, and prefer to cross on straight stretches. The situation at road junctions is too complicated for children's understanding of traffic, and they seem to realize it. Children only see the traffic from their own egocentric point of view, and do not usually learn to understand what a driver may do next until they are teenagers.

The basic problem children have, according to Dr Sandels, is developing insight into what is happening on the road. They do not see the quick glance to right and left which adults make, so they cannot imitate it. They are too small to look over the tops of cars and grasp the traffic situation. Most children are naturally cautious of dangers they are able to appreciate, but they must be taught to appreciate the special dangers of traffic.

Children must be taught much more than just how to cross the highway. They should be taught from an early age never to play in traffic areas such as parking lots, garage exits, sidewalks of busy roads or streets. They must be taught not to play beside cars and never to hang on to moving vehicles.

Point out to children the features of traffic which are important. Get them to look at cars which are near and distant, approaching and receding, and at the same time to listen to the noise they make. Point out traffic-lights and explain what they do.

Always walk beside your children when crossing the road. Never call to a child to cross the road, but cross over to the child. If you drop a child off from a car, put the child down on the side where the child is going. Teach your children to walk on the inside of the sidewalk, so that they do not stumble into the road with the chance of hitting a passing car.

Teach your children the following safety curb drill for crossing the road:

A. First find a safe place to cross.
B. Stand on the pavement near the curb.
C. Look all round for traffic and listen.
D. If traffic is coming, let it pass. Look all round again.
E. When there is no traffic near, walk straight across the road.
F. Keep looking and listening for traffic while you cross.

Also teach them to choose a place where drivers can see them. Or in crowded parking conditions to check first that there is no one at the wheel of the cars they must pass between, and then to walk out until they can see if anything is coming.

If your children must come home from school in the dark, provide them with reflective material on their coats, and advise them to pull down their hoods (if they wear them) when crossing the road, so that they can see properly. Tell them that policemen will always help them to cross the road. Never threaten them with the police, which will destroy their confidence in seeking help in traffic.

NUTRITION

Using the right fuel

One in every three deaths among people over thirty-five could be postponed if dietary theories now widely accepted by the medical profession were put into practise. This might mean another ten years of life for those people who are at present picked off before their time by heart disease or cancer.

Man, it seems, is not adapted to eating the large quantities of fat and meat he now consumes. It has been known for some time that the accumulation of fats in the blood vessels makes us prone to heart attacks and strokes. But it now appears that poor adaptation to large quantities of fat in the diet also makes us vulnerable to certain cancers.

A "Prudent (low-fat) Diet" was first publicized in 1957 by a New York doctor when he launched the Anti-Coronary Club. It was also endorsed by the American Heart Association, and more recently in Britain by the Royal College of Physicians. Expert committees in some fourteen countries have now endorsed the low-fat diet for prevention of heart disease. And now the low-fat diet has won further approval from cancer experts as well.

In addition to eating too much fat, we also eat too much sugar and too little roughage – the indigestible fibre in vegetables and grains. Too much sugar rots the teeth (see page 116) and may also have an adverse effect on the heart. Too little roughage causes slow bowel movements and constipation, which may eventually cause piles and diverticular disease, a common disease of the bowel in Western countries which is almost unknown in people living on unprocessed foods. Lack of roughage in the diet leads to these and other consequences, which Dr Denis Burkitt, British Medical Research Council scientist, has called diseases of civilization.

According to all these ideas, the majority of people in Western countries are eating an unhealthy diet which can only be put right by a diet revolution..This revolution has already begun: wholewheat bread and margarine made with polyunsaturated vegetable oils are now available in most food shops. But most people need more information and ideas in order to cook the most nourishing and healthiest meals for themselves. In this chapter we summarize the evidence which shows that a diet revolution is needed. We also give practical advice on alternative healthier ways of eating, including fifty-one recipes for summer and winter cooking which demonstrate that healthy eating need not be dull or unimaginative eating.

HEART DISEASE:
THE EVIDENCE AGAINST SATURATED FATS

The first observation suggesting that the rich Western diet is the cause of heart and blood vessel disease came in 1916 from a Dutch physician, C.D. De Langen, who found that the Javanese had much lower quantities of cholesterol in their blood and were much less prone to hardening of the arteries, blood clots, gallstones, and heart disease than were Westerners. These diseases were common among Dutch settlers in Java, the rich Javanese and those Chinese who ate Western food. Dr De Langen recommended a low cholesterol diet. This work was only suggestive, but since then many more detailed studies have been made which have come to essentially the same conclusion.

The Japanese also seldom suffer from heart disease, and this has led to the suggestion that the Eastern races of man may have an inherited resistance to these diseases. However, this has been disproved by the observation that Japanese living in California, who live and eat like other Americans, are more or less equally susceptible to heart disease as other Americans. Japanese living in Japan normally eat little or no dairy produce and relatively little meat. They eat more fish, vegetables and carbohydrate than people do in the West.

Yemenite Jews coming to Israel had much lower quantities of cholesterol in their blood and were much less prone to heart disease than Jews from Europe. However, after a number of years the Yemenite Jews adopted the European diet with large quantities of fat. The cholesterol in their blood went up and they became more vulnerable to heart disease.

Heart disease is most prevalent in Western countries. Finland, Scotland, the United States, Australia, New Zealand and Canada head the list, with England and Wales not far behind. Countries with least heart disease are Bulgaria, Greece, Italy, Poland, Portugal, Romania and Taiwan, with Japan at the bottom of the list. There are, of course, many differences between the diets of these countries. However, sifting the evidence suggests again that the most important difference which accounts for the prevalence of heart disease in Western countries is the amount of saturated animal fat eaten in these countries. Everything points to a Mediterranean or Oriental diet being far healthier than the customary diet of Northern Europe and America.

In many countries, there is a positive correlation bet-

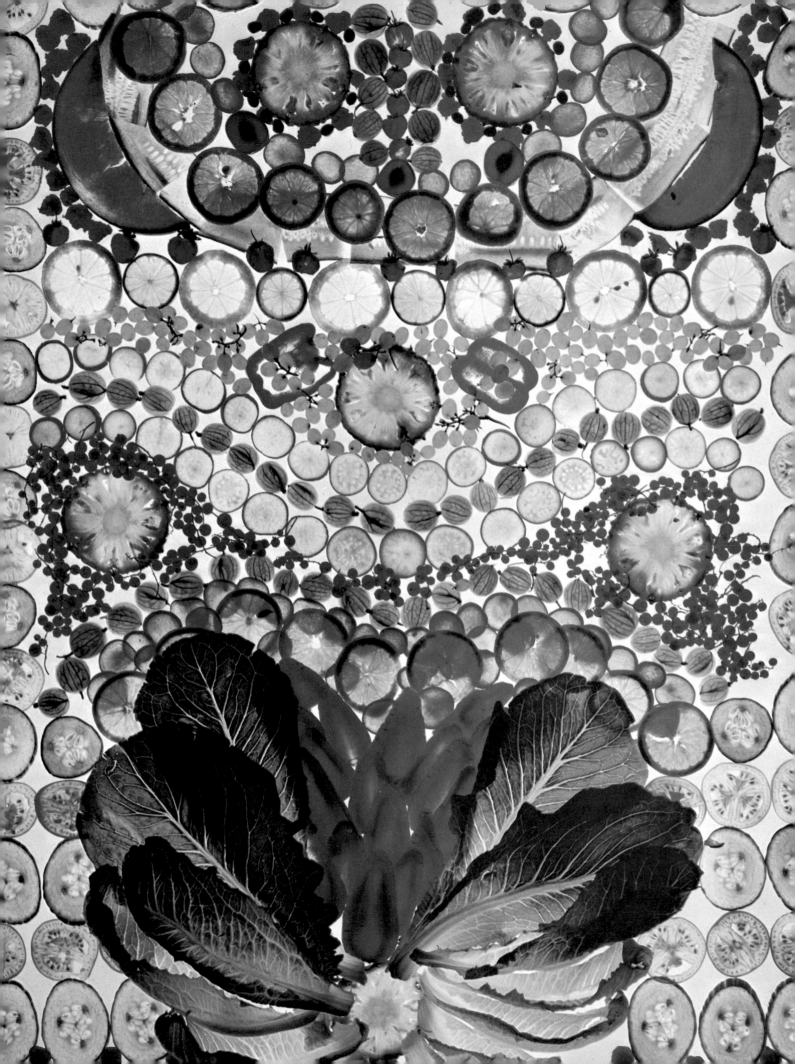

Carbohydrates include sugars, starches and related substances which are chemical compounds of carbon, hydrogen and oxygen. Carbohydrates are made by plants from carbon dioxide and water, using the energy from the sun. Potatoes, pasta (spaghetti etc.), bread, rice, and any grain are rich in carbohydrate. Starch from these foods is broken down into sugars in the body before being used as a source of energy for maintaining the body, for growth and for everyday activities. Cellulose, the main constituent of paper, is also a carbohydrate found in all plants, but it cannot be digested by people, although it can by certain animals such as cows. Nevertheless, cellulose and other undigestible carbohydrates are now thought to be an important part of the diet, as a source of fibre which aids the passage of material through the bowel. However, starchy foods such as potatoes and grains are also important sources of protein (see below).

Cholesterol is a substance resembling fat, although strictly speaking it is not a fat from the chemical standpoint. It is common in most tissues of the body and is probably the starting point for the synthesis of certain hormones. Cholesterol is the main component in atheroma, which accumulates in the body and causes atherosclerosis and coronary artery disease. The only common food to contain high quantities of cholesterol is the egg.

Fats and oils are chemically similar compounds of carbon, hydrogen and oxygen, which is combined in them in a characteristic way different to the carbohydrates. There are many different types of fats and oils. However, the only difference between fats and oils as a whole is that oils are liquid at room temperature. Most animal fats are hard at average room temperatures. Fats contain twice as much energy, weight for weight, as carbohydrates and so it is important to cut down on fats when dieting. However, fats and oils are important in cooking because they carry flavors, and so they should be mixed judiciously with carbohydrate foods.

Proteins are the essential building blocks of the living cell and comprise about 12 per cent of the weight of the human body (water 70 per cent, fat 15 per cent). Proteins are made up from some twenty-two different amino acids. Proteins can be made by the body into an enormous variety of shapes to do various different jobs. Enzymes, the biological catalysts of the body, are all proteins and there are many thousands of them in the body – each one different. Proteins in the food are broken down by digestion into amino acids, which are then rearranged into new proteins needed by the body. If unnecessarily large quantities of protein are eaten, then they are used as a source of energy and broken down into simple substances such as carbon dioxide, water and urea, which is excreted in the urine. Amino acids are composed of carbon, hydrogen, oxygen, nitrogen and sometimes sulphur.

Vitamins are substances needed by the body which the body cannot make for itself from raw materials. Vitamins are only needed in small amounts, mostly as catalysts helping along vital chemical reactions. Shortage of vitamins causes deficiencies such as scurvy (shortage of vitamin C), rickets (shortage of vitamin D), beri-beri (shortage of vitamin B_1) and others. A good mixed diet contains all the necessary vitamins. It is much more important to try to obtain a good mixed diet than to attempt to supplement the diet with vitamins. In fact, too many vitamins A or D can be harmful and excess of the others will serve no purpose. However, there are special circumstances when extra vitamins may be prescribed by a doctor.

---

ween heart disease, or the age at which people die, and their consumption of sugar. However, the amount of sugar people eat and the amount of fat they eat are closely linked. For this reason it is difficult to know whether sugar has a bad effect on the heart. Heart disease is not particularly common in countries such as Venezuela, Mauritius or the Caribbean, where there is a high consumption of sugar, which suggests that there is no need to worry about the effect of sugar on the heart. In the United States a quarter of total calories are on average obtained from sugar which displaces other nutritionally valuable foods in the diet.

Everyone agrees that excessive consumption of sugar, particularly between meals, has a bad effect on the teeth. Excessive consumption of sugar also leads to obesity, which in turn is associated with diabetes and high blood pressure. Therefore it is a good idea to cut down on the use of sugar in cooking, to restrict sweet snacks and drinks between meals and, if overweight, try to cut down on sweet things. Excessive salt in the diet also increases the risk of disease – see High Blood Pressure, page 130.

CANCER: THE EVIDENCE AGAINST FATS

The Japanese have one of the lowest rates of breast cancer in the world. Their chance of contracting it is only a quarter that of English women, and a sixth that of women in Oakland, across the bay from San Francisco. Cancer of the prostate, testis and ovary are also relatively rare in Japan, where they cause about a tenth of the deaths that they do in Western countries. These cancers, together with breast cancers, are the hormone dependent cancers: their growth is apparently controlled by the quantities of several different hormones produced by the sex organs and the pituitary gland in the brain.

Until a few years ago, many scientists thought that the Japanese must have an inherited racial resistance to them. Then it was discovered that Japanese women living in the United States were four times more susceptible to breast cancer than Japanese women living in Japan. Japanese living in the United States also have an increased incidence over native Japanese of cancers of the prostate, testis, ovary and bowel.

Could it be that the change from a rice and fish diet to an American diet rich in meat and fat has made Japanese immigrants more vulnerable? Bowel cancer might obviously be caused by something we eat, but the suggestion that breast – or prostate, testis or ovary – cancer might also have a dietary cause at first seems incredible. However, this is the conclusion that cancer experts are now coming to.

The United States has one of the highest incidences of breast cancer in the world; 33,700 women in the United States died of breast cancer in 1977. Breast cancer is commonest in Europe, Australia, New Zealand, Britain, the

US and Canada – countries which consume most meat, fat and sugar – and is least common in the Far East and South America. Argentina is an exception: breast cancer is almost as common there as in the United States or Britain. Meat consumption is high in Argentina but sugar consumption is low, pointing to meat and perhaps even to beef as a major cause of breast cancer when eaten regularly in large quantities. In Europe, the poorer countries with large peasant populations such as Spain, Greece and Yugoslavia have least breast cancer.

Dr John Berg of the University of Iowa Cancer Research Center says:

One can go so far as to suggest, speculatively, that mankind generally evolved under conditions of prudent – low fat and protein – nutrition, and that the present affluent diet from childhood onward may overstimulate the endocrine (hormone-making) system, producing the same effect that one would obtain running a diesel engine on high octane fuel.

Cancer of the colon and rectum, which kills some 50,000 men and women in the United States each year, may also be caused by a high-fat diet. Countries which have a high incidence of breast cancer and heart disease also tend to have a high incidence of cancer of the colon (large bowel) and the rectum. Scotland, which has a high-fat diet relieved with relatively few fresh vegetables, holds the world record for colon cancer. Deaths from breast cancer in Scotland are also the highest of any in the world, as too are deaths among women from heart disease.

An individual may become ill either with bowel cancer or heart disease, but usually not with both. This at first sight seems odd if both are caused by a high-fat diet. Dr Ernst Wynder of the Naylor Dana Institute for Disease Prevention in New York, one of the pioneers in the field, theorizes that people may fall into two types: those who take cholesterol from the food into the blood and deposit it in the heart and arteries, which leads to arteriosclerosis; and those who do not absorb so much cholesterol, or excrete large quantities of cholesterol products into the intestine and bowel where it causes cancer.

Dr Michael Hill of the Central Public Health Laboratory, Colindale, London, suggests that a high-fat diet causes the production of large quantities of bile acids, which may be changed by bacteria in the bowel into substances which cause cancer. He has found that people who excrete large quantities of bile substances are at greater risk of developing bowel cancer. Dr Hill says that his results imply that cancer of the bowel and rectum is a preventable disease – even though the causal mechanism is not fully understood – and he endorses the low-fat diet.

Seventh Day Adventists have half-to-two-thirds the average incidence of cancer deaths, and almost half the incidence of heart disease, stroke and arteriosclerosis, compared with other Americans. Adventists do not smoke and do not drink alcohol, which accounts for their low frequency of cancer of the lung, mouth, esophagus and bladder. (They also do not drink coffee, but coffee has no proven hazards in animals or man.) However, even if they are compared with non-smokers in the general population, they still have a much lower frequency of cancer of the breast, ovary, prostate and bowel. This is almost certainly the result of the Adventists' vegetarian diet.

All Adventists are strict in not drinking alcohol or eating pork, but a vegetarian diet is not obligatory for them and those who are vegetarian usually eat eggs and milk. On average, the amount of fat in their diet is cut by about a quarter. Dr Roland Phillips of Loma Linda University, California (an Adventist foundation) has discovered that Adventists with heart disease or bowel cancer eat more meat, fish and dairy products than the average Adventist. Adventists who suffered breast or bowel cancer were found to have eaten more fried foods in the past, and to have eaten more refined foods such as white bread, cake and pie. The Adventists who did not get cancer ate more green leafy vegetables, beans and milk.

These studies all point in the same direction. People who eat a low-meat, low saturated-fat diet tend to have a low incidence of cancer as well as heart disease, and it can be safely concluded that someone who eats this diet is likely to be healthier and to live longer than someone on the average Western diet.

FATS AND OILS

Oils are chemically similar to fats; the difference is simply that oils are liquid at room temperature whereas fats are solid. The fats and oils in our diet can be divided up into three categories important for health: saturated, mono-unsaturated, and polyunsaturated. Animal fats, which are usually hard at room temperature, consist mostly of saturated fats (see table) whereas most vegetable and fish oils consist largely of mono-unsaturated and polyunsaturated oils. However, not all vegetable oils are mono- or polyunsaturated. Palm and coconut oil, for example, are relatively highly saturated and hard at room temperature. More authorities agree that the amount of saturated fat in the diet should be restricted, because excessive consumption of saturated fat is associated with heart disease and certain cancers. This can be done by eating less fatty meat and less butter, cream and top-of-the-milk, less hard margarines, fewer eggs and more vegetables – particularly peas and beans – and also by including more fish and poultry rather than beef or lamb in the diet.

Consumption of polyunsaturated fats reduces the amount of cholesterol in the blood. Therefore it is important to replace animal fat as much as possible, by using polyunsaturated fats such as sunflower oil, safflower oil, corn oil, or soya-bean oil for cooking, and by using polyunsaturated margarine (see below) instead of butter. Peanut

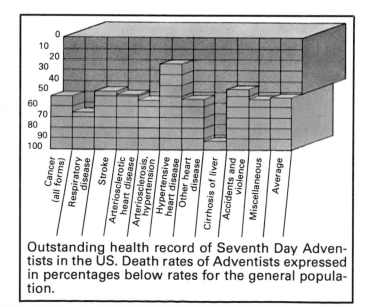

Outstanding health record of Seventh Day Adventists in the US. Death rates of Adventists expressed in percentages below rates for the general population.

(groundnut) oil – *arachide* – is also polyunsaturated, but experiments in monkeys have shown that it causes deposits of atheroma in blood-vessels in the same way as saturated fat, so it cannot be recommended.

Olive oil is mono-unsaturated and is described as neutral from the health point of view. People who live in the Mediterranean region have a remarkably low incidence of heart disease and breast cancer, particularly in those parts of the Mediterranean where most olive oil is consumed. So it can be concluded that olive oil is good for health.

The polyunsaturated margarines are made from oils such as corn oil or sunflower oil, which are rich in polyunsaturates. Eating these margarines instead of butter is a good way of producing a more balanced intake of fat. Eskimos living traditionally have a relatively high fat diet, but the fat is largely polyunsaturated and they have little heart disease.

Margarines are made from various types of vegetable oils often blended together. A liquid oil, such a corn oil, may be blended with a "hard" oil (solid at room temperature) such as palm kernel oil to make a soft easily-spreading mixture. Or more often liquid oils are "hydrogenated" – a chemical process which changes the oils into something nearer fats which solidify at room temperature. This process of hydrogenation destroys some of the polyunsaturated oils which may be beneficial to health if they are substituted for butter. Nearly all margarines contain polyunsaturated oils, but some contain much more than others. For example, Land o' Lakes regular margarine, one of the best tasting brands according to Consumer Reports, contains less polyunsaturates than almost any other margarine, and from this point of view is a poor substitute for butter. However, another brand, Promise (regular), contains 45 per cent polyunsaturates and also has a more agreeable flavour than most margarines according to Consumer Reports. Other brands which contained more than 40 per cent polyunsaturates according to the Consumer Reports survey were: Saffola (regular), Sweet unsalted Chiffon, Soft Chiffon, Empress Soft Corn Oil, Soft Fleischmann's, A&P Soft, Soft Parkay Corn Oil, Mrs Filbert's 100% Corn Oil (soft), Nu-Maid (soft), Squeeze Parkay (liquid). The softness of the margarine is in itself no guide to its composition. Diet margarines contain only about 40 per cent fat – the rest is water and so by law they must be called imitation margarines. The following diet brands had over 40 per cent polyunsaturated fat when surveyed by Consumer Reports: Diet Mazola Corn Oil Imitation, Soft Diet Parkay Imitation, Diet Imperial Imitation, Diet Fleischmann's Imitation.

Eggs contain large amounts of cholesterol, so it is wise to restrict the number of eggs in the diet to a maximum of one a day, or better still, not more than three a week. Vegetarians may safely eat more because they are likely to be eating less fat. However, a vegetarian who eats a lot of dairy produce including eggs may be on just as hazardous a diet as someone eating a lot of meat. Both meat-eaters and vegetarians should aim to get a substantial part of their protein from peas and beans, which are low in fat.

Offal such as liver and kidney contains a lot of cholesterol, but this is compensated for by the fact that these meats contain less fat, and the fat that is in them is more polyunsaturated. Brains contain a great deal of cholesterol but they are eaten too infrequently to worry about. Game such as venison is always very lean and contains little saturated fat, so it is highly recommended. See page 68 for a table giving percentages of fat in food.

Low fat cooking

The healthiest of people are often those peasants who cannot afford to eat meat every day and have learnt to make meat go far when they do have it. In the section which follows, we give some of these recipes which use meat as a flavoring rather than as the main ingredient of dishes: for example, moussaka, page 53; stuffed tomatoes or peppers, page 55; and risotto, page 55. In fact, meat is frequently much more delicious when used in this way, delicately flavored with herbs and vegetables. Neapolitans eat their spaghetti with tomato sauce (page 56) as a daily staple, and they are remarkably free of heart disease. It is no coincidence that the richer meat sauce known in Italy as *ragu* is generally attributed to Bologna, where the incidence of heart disease is much higher.

The way food is cooked can dramatically affect the fat and oil content of what we eat, as the three meals below show. The same ingredients (8oz raw beefsteak, 6oz peeled potatoes, 3oz mushrooms, 2oz onions and 3oz tomatoes per person) are used in the first two meals. In the third, less meat is needed, and so two more vegetables have been added.

FRYING
Lightly fried steak; french fries; fried mushrooms; fried onions and fried tomatoes.
This is the fattiest meal possible with these ingredients. It is high both in calories and fats because the meat, even lean steak, contains a lot of "invisible" fat and the vegetables simply soak up oil or fat. Just by frying the onions and mushrooms, over 21g of fat is added to the meal. French fries have three times as many calories as boiled potatoes. If you must fry food, use sunflower oil, corn oil or other vegetable oil, which are less harmful than animal fat. And even lean meat contains so much fat that if fried in a non-stick pan, it is not necessary to add further fat.
Total: Fat 71g (2.5oz). Calories: 970.

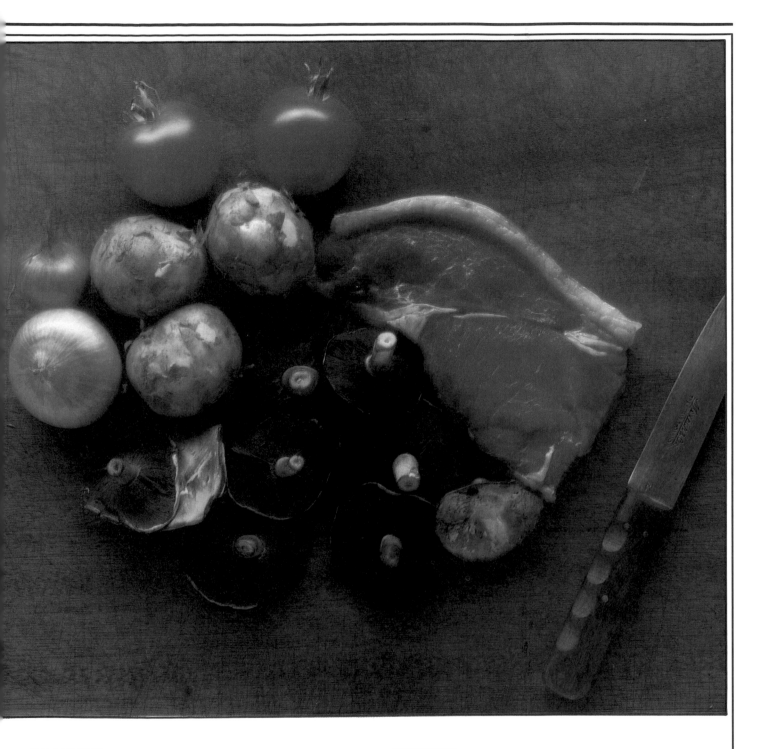

BROILING
Broiled steak; boiled potatoes; tomato, mushroom and onion salad. (Alternatively, broil the tomatoes and mushrooms and boil the onion.)

By broiling the steak, boiling the potatoes and eating the other vegetables raw in a salad, you can halve the fat content of the first meal, even using exactly the same ingredients. Because the vegetables contain only negligible amounts of fat, the only source of fat in the meal is the meat. This should be broiled on a raised wire-mesh rack to allow as much fat as possible to run out. A ¼oz of margarine on the boiled potatoes would add 6g of fat (and 56 calories) to the total below. Similarly, Italian dressing made with ¼oz olive oil on the salad would put the fat content up a further 7g (adding an extra 66 calories).

Total: Fat 36g (1.3oz). Calories: 634.

STEWING
A casserole of steak, onion, mushrooms, tomatoes, potatoes, carrots and peas.

With this kind of meal, meat goes a lot further and so 4oz, half the original amount, is ample for each person. In its place, other vegetables can be added – in this case, 2oz carrots and 2oz fresh or frozen peas, per portion – to make it a lot tastier. The steak is cut into pieces and arranged in layers with the vegetables. Some of the sliced potatoes should be kept aside for the top layer. Water and seasoning are added and the casserole baked in a slow oven for about 2½ hours. The lid of the casserole should be removed for the last half-hour to brown the potatoes. This meal has only one-sixth the fat content of the fried meat, and you could have almost three helpings of it before you would take in the same amount of calories.

Total: Fat 12g (about ½oz). Calories: 362.

Composition of fats and oils. Fats and oils high in polyunsaturated and mono-unsaturated constituents are the best for health.	Saturated	Mono-unsaturated	Poly-unsaturated
Beef	48%	44%	3%
Chicken	32	37	26
Lamb	54	37	4
Pork	36	42	17
Liver	34	27	34
Herring	19	10	66
Milk, butter, cheese	62	30	3
Eggs	33	45	17
Vegetable oils			
Coconut	91	7	2
Corn	17.5	29	56.5
Peanut	13	61	24
Olive	11	74	10
Palm	53	38	9
Palm kernel	85	13	2
Safflower	11.5	13	75.5
Soya bean	17	25	58
Sunflower	12	20	68
Walnut	16	28	51

The total percentage is sometimes less than 100 because of the glycerol present. Chemically, the fat molecule consists of a chain of carbon atoms linked to each other, with each also linked to two hydrogen atoms. In *saturated fats* each carbon atom has the maximum number of hydrogen atoms attached to it. *Mono-unsaturated fats* have one pair of carbon atoms in the chain which each have only one hydrogen atom attached, all the other carbon atoms having two hydrogen atoms. *Polyunsaturated fats* have two or more pairs of hydrogen atoms missing from the chain.

Cooking with polyunsaturated oils

Corn Oil. This is the least satisfactory of the recommended vegetable oils for cooking purposes. The smell as it heats up can be offensive. It fries in a thin and bubbling way, and may leave a poor taste in the food. For salads, the flavor is rather powerful and not entirely agreeable.

Olive Oil. Olive oil is delicious for everything, but is expensive. It has a lovely fruity flavor which varies tremendously from country to country. Some people like the heavy green Greek oil, others the delicate golden Provençal oil, while there are those who swear that the deep yellow Tuscan oil is the pearl. However, it is wasteful to use this oil for frying, since it loses its delicious flavor at high temperatures. Use it for rubbing onto meat or fish before broiling, for marinades, for oiling freshly cooked pasta, and of course for all salads.

Salad Oil. An interesting salad oil can be made by mixing four tablespoons of sunflower oil with two dessertspoons of walnut oil.

Soya Oil. A good oil for frying, but it starts to taste and smell a bit strong at high temperatures. It has the right consistency for salads, but leaves a slight aftertaste which could probably be overcome by putting plenty of crushed garlic in the dressing.

Sunflower Oil. This oil is excellent for frying as it is almost tasteless and does not smell. It gives a very crisp result. As it is so light and thin it makes a rather dull salad dressing, but all things considered it is the best of the recommended polyunsaturated oils.

Walnut Oil. No better than any other vegetable oil for frying, so it is certainly not worth the enormous price except for use on salads, when it gives a sweet, nutty flavor. Try it on a lettuce-and-chicory salad with a few walnuts strewn in. This is a heavy oil which does not keep particularly well so do not hoard it: keep it in the refrigerator.

BREAD AND FLOUR

Before 1870, most people in Europe and America ate bread made from stone-ground flour, which contained appreciable quantities of bran – the fibrous part of the grain. However, mass-production of white refined flour by mills in the 1870s, together with a decline in the amount of bread eaten, has meant that people on average eat about a fifth of the amount of cereal fibre in their diet now than they did a century ago. This change in our diet has been blamed for many of the diseases of civilization which are unknown in people living on an unrefined diet.

The importance of bran in our everyday diet has been pointed out by Dr Denis Burkitt, of the British Medical Research Council, and Surgeon Captain T.L. Cleave, formerly of the Royal Navy, who during the Second World War kept the sailors "regular" aboard his battleship *George V* with the help of bran. Dr Burkitt's interest in fibre was aroused by his work in Africa, where he noticed that native Africans seldom suffered from many diseases common in Western countries.

Appendicitis was rare in Africans until they began to eat the refined Western diet deficient in cereal fibre. Appendicitis also used to be rare in Western countries before the advent of roller milling. When fibre is deficient in the diet, the content of the bowel becomes hard and it is difficult for the bowel to move the content along. The bowel may then become obstructed, causing appendicitis. Another disease called diverticular disease also occurs as a result of the bowel becoming obstructed. In straining to pass the content along the bowel, small "blow outs" – diverticula – may occur in the bowel wall, just as a rubber tire may blow out where there is a weakness. People who have diverticular disease usually improve dramatically when given a diet containing plenty of fibre. Fibre provides bulk in the diet which acts as a natural lubricant, making it easy for the bowel content to move along.

The first and most obvious effect of insufficient fibre in the diet is constipation. People who eat a diet containing plenty of fibre tend to pass large, soft and often unformed stools. If a person regularly needs to strain to move the bowels and the stool is hard, then they probably do not have enough fibre in the diet. Straining to move the bowels increases pressure in the abdomen, and this may damage valves in the veins in the legs, causing varicose veins and hemorrhoids (piles).

Excessive removal of fibre from food also encourages people to eat a diet too rich in highly refined starch and sugar. This leads to overweight, and often to other health problems such as diabetes. Fibre in the diet may also prevent absorption of cholesterol, and so may protect against heart disease. Proponents of the theory suggest that fibre in the diet may also protect against bowel cancer and gallstones. The importance of fibre in the diet is now generally accepted, although *lack* of fibre is not universally accepted as an important cause of bowel cancer and heart disease.

(Sources; *Manual of Nutrition* (HMSO); Van den Berghs; Procter & Gamble.)

It is not difficult to get sufficient fibre in the diet. The easiest way to get more fibre is to eat wholemeal bread and wholemeal breakfast cereals such as All-Bran, whole Puffed Rice, Shredded Wheat or hot oatmeal; vegetables are also a useful source of fibre. Bran itself can also be bought from health stores and, increasingly, from many supermarkets. This can be added to breakfast cereals or put in soups and stews. Wholewheat flour can also be used in a great many ways in cooking. Health food enthusiasts may prefer stone-ground flour but there is no evidence that this is better than ordinary wholewheat flour made in metal-roller mills. It is not necessary to eat wholewheat foods all the time, but try to make them your staple.

Cooking with wholewheat flour

100% wholewheat flour contains the entire wheat grain, including the bran. It is the heaviest and most strongly flavored wheat flour. Some brown flours contain from 80% to 90% of the whole wheat grain, but have some of the coarser particles, mainly the bran, extracted. Brown flour may simply be white flour colored with caramel. White flour contains about 72% of the whole grain, and has all the bran and most of the wheatgerm extracted. All the white flours are given extra vitamins to make up for those which have been extracted, including iron, thiamin and niacin; extra calcium is also added.

100% whole and wheat flours have a warm, nutty and agreeable taste with more character and flavor than white flour, which means that for some dishes, where what is needed is a fairly anonymous pastry crust or delicate basic sauce, they can be a bit much. They are more solid than white flour, so when you want to use wholewheat flour for pastry or bechamel sauce, make sure that the food that it is to be eaten with is robust enough to take it. An onion or leek or cheese quiche or an apple tart would be fine, but if you were using, for instance, smoked salmon or mushrooms, a white crust would perhaps be more suitable. A cheese sauce to go with cauliflower, or a parsley sauce to eat with poached haddock or turbot, would be excellent, but put in lots more cheese or parsley than usual.

Cakes, cookies, muffins, and so forth, can be made very well with wholewheat flour, but are best made with quite a lot of shortening, which should be one of the recommended margarines, or they do become very solid. Noodles can be made with wholewheat flour and be very tasty, whereas pizzas, pancakes, soufflés, éclairs are among the things that do not lend themselves so well to the change. So the best thing to do is to experiment, and where you really like the results, then switch to wholewheat flour for good.

VEGETABLES

Vegetables are useful sources of minerals, vitamins and fibre, and also provide some polyunsaturated fat. Vegetables in the diet may actually protect a person against cancer. A number of surveys have shown that people who eat plenty of fresh vegetables – such as lettuce or celery – are less likely to get stomach cancer. The importance of vegetables in the diet for prevention of cancer has now been demonstrated in animals, and has led to the discovery of a new class of substances which protect against cancer.

Dr Leo Wattenberg of the University of Minnesota School of Medicine discovered that rats which were fed a balanced, *highly purified* diet containing all known vitamins and nutrients, were not able to make certain enzymes (biological catalysts) in the liver which had the vital function of inactivating cancer-causing chemicals. However, when the rats were fed a crude diet containing alfalfa (an animal-fodder plant), they were able to produce the enzymes in their livers. Further experiments showed that rats which are induced to make this enzyme in their livers have increased protection against cancer when chemicals known to cause cancer are added to their diet.

Dr Wattenberg then tested other vegetables, and found that several members of the *Brassica* family, including cabbage, Brussels sprouts, turnips, broccoli and cauliflower, caused the protective enzyme to be made in rats' liver. He found that spinach, dill and celery were effective, but that the vegetables varied in their effect according to their freshness, variety and the soil in which they were grown.

Finally, Dr Wattenberg was able to identify the actual chemicals in the vegetables which cause the protective enzymes to be formed. They turned out to belong to a well-known family of organic chemicals called indoles. Dr Wattenberg also found that citrus fruits (oranges and lemons) contain chemicals called flavones which, like indoles, cause the protective enzymes to be formed in the liver.

Other plant products may protect against cancer. Beans and seeds are rich in plant proteins called lectins which increase movements of the bowel. They have been found to protect animals against cancer in laboratory experiments. Beans also seem to have an important effect in lowering the amount of cholesterol in the blood. Professor Ancel Keys of the University of Minnesota found that Americans given a diet with the same amount of protein, carbohydrate and fat as eaten in Naples had higher amounts of cholesterol in their blood than Neapolitans until they were fed beans. So beans are not only important in being a low-fat substitute for meat; they also seem to have a positive effect in lowering cholesterol, and it does not seem to matter what type of beans are eaten. Beans are best introduced into the diet slowly for people not accustomed to them, because they do cause some people to suffer from a lot of wind – at least at first.

Several different experiments have shown that onions or garlic contain chemical substances which alter the ability of the blood to clot. This has led to the suggestion that onions and garlic are valuable in preventing the formation of blood clots, which are a cause of coronary heart attacks and strokes.

To get maximum benefit from the vitamins in vegetables, cook briefly so that they are still a little crisp to the taste. Overcooking destroys the vitamin C in vegetables and washes other nutrients into cooking water which may be discarded.

A BALANCED DIET

It is essential for a healthy diet to eat a variety of food so that you get all the vitamins, minerals and nutrients you need. Therefore at each meal you should aim to eat as great a variety as you can.

You need carbohydrate or starch, which is present in bread, paste, potatoes, rice and other grains, for energy; these are also good sources of protein, which is necessary for body building. Sugar is also a source of energy but it provides what has been called empty calories: it provides nothing else as well.

Proteins – available in most concentrated form in lean

meat – are made up from chemical building-blocks called amino acids, and are broken down again into amino acids during digestion. Different proteins contain amino acids in different proportions, and plant proteins do not contain amino acids in the ideal proportion for direct use by man, but this does not matter, because the extra amino acids which cannot be used in body building are burnt up as energy. However, protein is scarce in some parts of the world, and then it becomes more important to make the best possible use of the proteins in the diet by providing the different amino acids in the optimum proportions at the same time. This can be done by mixing beans (which are low in the amino acids methionine) and other vegetables, particularly grains (which are low in another amino acid, lysine), in the same dish (see rice and beans, page 49). Beans served by themselves are a good source of both protein and energy too (see pages 58–9).

Fats are also a source of energy; weight for weight, fats provide twice as many calories as protein or carbohydrate. Therefore, by cutting down on fat in the diet, you can eat a little more protein and carbohydrate and so continue to eat the same bulk. A certain quantity of fat in the diet is essential for health, but in practise no one is likely to eat too little fat except under famine conditions, because food without a minimum of fat tastes dry and unpleasant.

If a mixed diet is eaten, then a person is unlikely to run into shortages of vitamins and minerals, except for old people who sometimes eat such small quantities that they may become deficient in some essential nutrients. Vegetarians who eat no meat or dairy produce, as opposed to vegetarians who usually eat eggs and milk products, may be deficient in B vitamins if they do not eat yeast extract or some other source of the essential B vitamins. In pregnancy, special steps should be taken to ensure a good mixed diet (see page 19).

THE NEW DIET: MEAL BY MEAL
Breakfast
The traditional American breakfast with meat and eggs is extremely high in fat. If you want to have a quick, hot breakfast, try baked beans on toast, or a small amount of well-broiled bacon with tomatoes on toast or fish such as poached haddock, fish sticks or fishcake. Try to limit eggs to three a week. If you must have one, poach, scramble or boil it.

Better still, eat a cold breakfast or wholegrain cereal such as whole Puffed Rice, Shredded Wheat, hot oatmeal (without butter), or muesli: they all contain bran which keeps the bowel working smoothly. If you prefer cornflakes (and white bread), make sure you take extra bran or All-Bran. Eat raisins, prunes or chopped banana instead of sugar with the cereal to add interest. Stoke up with wholewheat bread or toast, marmalade and polyunsaturated margarine. Or better still, fill up with fruit such as apples or oranges. You can have as many cups of tea and coffee as you like. Coffee was suspected of having a link with heart disease but has now been cleared, at least for the time being.

Lunch/Dinner
Generally it is wise to eat meat only once a day, for the main meal. Alternatives are fish, poultry or pasta with a light cheese or meat sauce; if you are overweight and find slimming impossible it may be healthier to be fat the Italian way (by eating pasta) rather than the American way (by eating steak and french fries, butter and cream). And try to have at least one vegetarian meal a day.

Broil rather than fry meat. If you must fry, use as little fat as possible – a non-stick pan helps – and pour off excess fat to prevent it being absorbed. Roasting is good because it allows fat to drip off, but do not baste the meat. Use non-fat drippings or stock to baste meat. Cut off excess fat before eating. Alternatively, ask your butcher to prepare the roast without any attached fat and cook in foil; this will take longer to cook than traditional roasting. Use a special sauce boat – *graisse et maigre* – to separate the juices from the fat.

Boiling or pot-roasting meat, or cooking as the French do *en daube*, is a good low-fat method because the fat may be skimmed off. Stews are also good if excess fat is cut off first. If you want to fry the meat first, use polyunsaturated cooking oil. The way you cook meat makes an enormous difference to the fat and calorie content of the whole meal.
Sauces: it is possible to make sauces without using fat, by using cornflour or arrowroot as the thickening agent. Alternatively, use polyunsaturated fat instead of butter, or a vegetable purée (see page 50, chicken with mushroom).
Poultry: most of the fat is in the skin, which should be removed before eating and can often be removed in the preparation, but *not* before roasting.
Salad: if you like olive oil, use it. Or you can dilute it with polyunsaturated oil in dressings. Alternatively, use seasoned natural yoghurt (see page 57), preferably made with skimmed milk, as a dressing: this is delicious with cucumber.

Desserts
Avoid commercially made cakes, pastries, cookies, and ice cream, which are rich in sugar and saturated fat. Serve egg-based desserts only after a vegetarian main course. Never serve cream or fat-based toppings; try natural yoghurt as an alternative. Cut the amount of sugar in most dessert recipes by at least half; it may actually improve the flavor which can be masked in a heavy syrup. Best of all, finish the meal with fresh fruit, or if you like, several fruit and get your vitamin C the natural way.
Cheese: a small portion only, unless you had a vegetarian main course.
Alcohol: only in moderation. Excess increases the flow of fats to the heart and causes you to put on weight. Light wines and beers in moderation may aid digestion and help you relax; spirits are more addictive and so can be a serious threat to health.

Light meals
The biggest mistake most people make is to have two large meals a day. One meal (other than breakfast) should be simple, consisting of, for example: a savory rice or macaroni dish (if these incorporate meat it should be in small quantity, used more as a flavoring); or bread and potatoes; or bread and soup; or baked potato and grated cheese. Always add salad and fruit if you can.

Snacks/supper
Go easy on cakes and cookies; it is better to have a slice of wholewheat bread with polyunsaturated margarine and jam or yeast extract. A milky drink is fine, if you have kept your intake of fats down during the rest of the day; or make it instead with skimmed milk. A banana might be the answer if you are still really hungry.

Twelve rules for healthy eating

1 Eat less meat. Reduce the frequency and the serving-size of beef and lamb. Do not eat meat more than once a day.

2 When you do eat meat, select lean cuts and remove all visible fat before eating. Broil rather than fry.

3 Eat more poultry and fish. Avoid sausage, frankfurters, spam, bologna and other processed meats which are usually high in fat.

4 Reduce severely the amount of cream, butter, cream cheese and ice cream. Restrict the amount of whole milk and cheese.

5 Eat low-fat dairy products such as skimmed milk, cottage cheese, yoghurt. Use margarines high in polyunsaturates.

6 Restrict the number of eggs to not more than one per day and preferably no more than three per week.

7 Reduce consumption of commercial cookies and cakes made with hard fats. Use recommended oils high in polyunsaturates for cooking.

8 Avoid eating highly salted foods such as salted snacks, salted meats e.g., ham, corned beef.

9 For the sake of your teeth, reduce intake of heavily sweetened foods such as sweets and cookies.

10 Eat some fresh fruit every day and, if you can, eat fruit at every meal.

11 Eat more vegetables, particularly peas and beans – fresh or dried – which are a good low-fat source of protein.

12 Eat wholewheat bread as your staple. Eat wholewheat breakfast cereals. Take extra bran if the rest of your daily diet is rather bland.

Recipes Winter

by Caroline Conran

Baked fish with tomato and green
  pepper
Borscht
Boston baked beans
Chilli con carne
Cod Provencal
Coffee or chocolate cake
Dried fruit salad with green ginger
Fish en papillote
Fruit loaf
Gnocchi
Herb bread
Left-over lamb with lentils
Mussels
Noodles
Onion soup
Pork fillet, stuffed with mushrooms
Poulet paysanne with black olives
Rice and beans
Sautéed pork fillet
Scalloped potatoes
Spaghetti sauce Bolognese

Baked fish with tomato and green pepper for four

Fried fish is delicious, but the traditional fried fish and chips is very heavy on fat. More people would bake fish if it did not turn out so tasteless; it is one thing to be healthy, another to eat like an invalid. This recipe is suitable for most white fish, but vary cooking times from short (cod, haddock, hake and soft fleshed fish) to slightly longer for denser fleshed fish like mullet and bream; about 20 minutes for the haddock and 30 minutes for bream, in a moderately low oven (325°F).

about 2lb white fish; ½ small green pepper; 1 small onion; 1 large tomato (or 2 medium); up to a glass of white wine; olive oil; seasoning: thyme, oregano or bay leaf.

With a sharp knife, slit the belly and remove innards if the fish dealer has not done so. Wash under cold tap. Chop off head and tail (good for a quick fish stock, so do not throw it away yet). With your most delicate knife, follow the line of the bone down each side, easing the flesh gently away from the bone. Lay the fish out on its back, two white sides lying uppermost. (The bone can go in your stock with a bit of onion peeling and thyme, the basis of a tasty fish soup.)

Chop the green pepper and the onion very small, and gently fry in a little olive oil until they soften. Cut a chopped, skinned tomato, and blend with green pepper and onion. Butter an oven dish, lay the fish in it, and smother with mixture. Add a scattering of thyme or oregano. Add a tablespoon of olive oil, dripped on, and half a glass of dry white wine.

Cover loosely with foil and bake in moderate to low oven for 20 minutes (haddock, and so on) or about 30 minutes (bream etc.). The wine keeps the fish moist and conveys the flavors of the green pepper and onion.

Borscht for four

A very filling soup, the way it is made in Russia, full of good nourishment. Made as it is in the Ukraine with different kinds of meat it is almost a whole meal. There are almost as many different kinds of borscht in Russia as there are families: with meat, with pork, mutton, beef, duck; or without meat, with vegetables in every quantity and combination. There are two common denominators: beetroot is the main vegetable, and sour cream is added at the end to counter its earthy sweetness. As a concession to the New Diet you can use yoghurt – a Balkan invention – and cottage cheese, mixed in equal parts and sieved, or with plain lemon juice added just before serving.

1lb of uncooked beetroot (or 2lb cooked beetroot); 1lb carrots; ½lb turnips; 1 large onion (optional: two medium tomatoes or two tablespoons tomato purée); 2½ pints chicken stock or meat stock (preferably homemade); salt; pepper; pinch of sugar.

Peel vegetables. Cut into very thin strips (so that the water can extract the maximum flavor). Put in pan with stock, bring gently to boil, and simmer on lowest heat for 45 minutes, with lid on. You may need to add more water if it starts to boil dry. Season with salt, pepper and sugar. Strain, pressing out every bit of juice. Check for seasoning. Serve with blobs of soured yoghurt, or a squeeze of lemon juice.

Boston baked beans for six

Use navy beans for this traditional pioneer dish devised in the days when meat could be scarce in winter. The beans are rich in protein and take on a delicious flavor from the meat. Everybody has a favorite way of making Boston baked beans; purists leave out the tomato, children much prefer them with tomato in. In any case, it makes a very worthwhile lunch on a cold day. Ideally it should be made in a deep earthenware or stoneware bean-pot, but an enamelled iron casserole will do.

1lb navy or pea beans; ½lb fat bacon or fat salt pork in a piece; 1 onion stuck with 3 cloves; 4 teaspoons mustard; 2 tablespoons vinegar; 2 generous tablespoons each of molasses and brown sugar or 4 tablespoons brown sugar; 1 tablespoon tomato purée (optional); 1½ teaspoons salt.

Soak the beans overnight or alternatively put them in a large pan of unsalted water, bring to the boil for five minutes, cover the pan and allow to cool. By the time they are cold they will be as tender as if they had been soaked. Pour this water away. Put the "soaked" beans back into the pan, add the onion stuck with cloves and a *little* salt (remember the salt in the meat) and cover with water. Cook slowly until just tender but not bursting. Put the bacon or salt pork in a small pan, cover with cold water, bring to the boil and drain. Slash the rind in a crisscross pattern. Drain the liquid from the beans and save it. Put the beans in a deep casserole with the salt pork or bacon, rind side up, on top, then mix the mustard, vinegar, molasses or brown sugar, tomato purée and salt with half a pint of the bean cooking liquid and pour it into the cooking pot. (If you don't have half a pint, make it up with more water.) Bake in a very low oven, 300°F, for five hours, checking from time to time and adding more water when it starts to look dry. Remove the lid for the last half hour of cooking, to crisp the rind of the pork.

Chilli con carne for four

Here is another example of stretching a small amount of meat a long way; the meat gives body and flavor to the beans, which are the main and really filling part of the dish.

½lb minced beef; 1lb red kidney beans; 2 onions; 1–2 tablespoons sunflower oil; 1–2 teaspoons chilli powder; 2 cloves garlic; pinch of cumin seeds; 1 teaspoon dried oregano or marjoram, ½ teaspoon dried thyme; 1 can tomatoes; 1 tablespoon tomato purée; about ¼ pint stock; salt; pepper.

First soak the beans in cold water

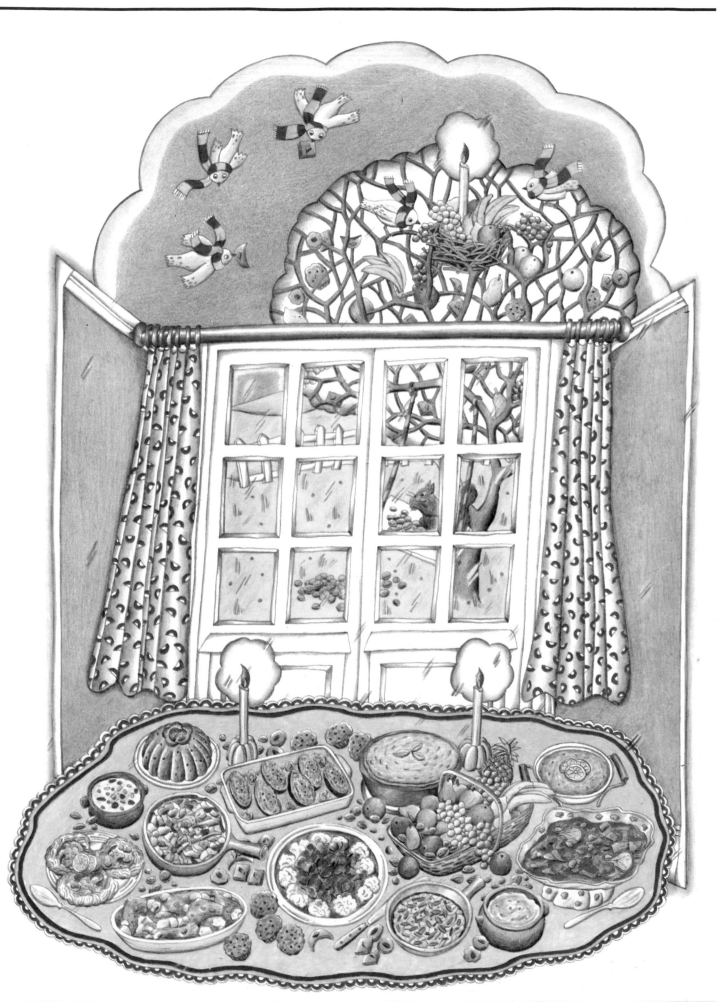

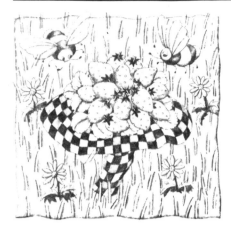

overnight. Put them in a pan of cold water, bring to the boil and simmer until just tender. Chop the onions finely, and fry gently in the sunflower oil until they are becoming translucent, then turn up the heat and add the mince. Stir it round, breaking it up with a wooden fork or spoon. When it is frying well, leave it alone so it can start to brown. Add the garlic, herbs and spices, and fry on. When the meat is browning nicely, add the tomatoes, tomato purée, seasoning and stock. Bring to simmering point, transfer the beans to the meat, and keep their cooking liquid. As the bean and beef mixture becomes somewhat dry, add cooking liquid from the beans in small quantities to keep it just moist. Simmer for 1½ hours. Serve with rice.

Cod Provençal for six
The favorite Southern combination of parsley and garlic is good for many things other than snails, and is perfect for improving the flavor of what can sometimes be rather dull – good, honest cod. This recipe can, in fact, be used for any fresh fish except perhaps the oily varieties such as mackerel.

2½lb fresh cod fillet (or scrod or other white fish); small bunch of parsley; 2 cloves garlic; 2–3 shallots or small onions; 4 tablespoons olive oil; salt and pepper; dried homemade breadcrumbs; 1 lemon.

Put the fish in a buttered flameproof oval dish, skin-side down, and sprinkle it with finely chopped parsley, garlic, and onions or shallots. Season with a little salt and pepper. Sprinkle with dried breadcrumbs and olive oil and cook in a gentle oven, 325°F, for 20–25 minutes, then finish the cooking under the grill. When the top is brown and the fish cooked, sprinkle with lemon juice. Serve with salad and French bread.

Coffee or chocolate cake
This cake – moist, rich and dark – uses high-fibre flour but does not have a lumpy wholewheat quality. It can be eaten hot as a pudding or cold as a cake and can be coffee- or chocolate-flavored. For coffee you need:

6oz 100% wholewheat (or brown) flour; 2oz ground almonds; 3 rounded teaspoons baking powder; 6oz margarine; 6oz brown sugar; 2 eggs; 4 fluid ounces strong black coffee. Strusel topping: 2oz soft margarine; 2oz brown sugar; 1 to 2oz Graham cracker crumbs; 2oz walnuts or hazelnuts.

Grease an 8½-inch loose-bottomed cake pan and line the base with foil or greaseproof paper. Heat the oven to 350°F. Mix flour, ground almonds and baking powder in a bowl. In another bowl, cream brown sugar and margarine and then add the eggs, one at a time, beating them in well. Fold in the flour, moistening the mixture with the coffee. Put the mixture into the cake pan.

For chocolate flavor, use 3oz plain cooking chocolate and 2 tablespoons milk. Where you would add the coffee, instead add milk and chocolate melted over hot water or in a slow oven. Mix thoroughly but lightly before turning the mixture into the pan. Takes 50–60 minutes.

TOPPING. Chop the nuts, crumble the crackers, mix them lightly with the sugar and soft margarine and sprinkle the mixture evenly over the top of the cake. Bake for 35–45 minutes, until set but crumbly.

Dried fruit salad with green ginger for four
Prunes, as we all know, are high on roughage, but what is sometimes overlooked is that they have a really wonderful and luxurious flavor. If you do not want to make custard, mix plain yoghurt with a little honey as an alternative.

1lb prunes; ½lb dried apricots; 2oz sugar; 1oz fresh ginger (or preserved ginger if fresh unavailable).

Make at least 2 days ahead. Soak the prunes and apricots separately in cold water, for about 12 hours or overnight. When they are soft, put them in a saucepan with sugar and the prune water, strained if necessary. Peel and slice the ginger and put it in with the fruits, bring to the boil and simmer until the fruit is tender – about 1 hour. Allow to cool, and transfer to a china bowl. Let it sit and steep for at least a

day, before serving with or without thin custard.

To make an even more exotic dish, replace the ginger with an inch or two of vanilla pod, and add 2oz of walnuts after cooking, but while the fruit is still hot. Just before serving, sharpen the juices with lemon juice. Sprinkle pomegranate seeds over the top and serve very chilled.

Fish en papillote for four
A superb and delicate recipe inspired by a dish invented by Michel Guérard for his well-known book *Cuisine Minceur*. This can also be made with red mullet or with thin fillets of whiting, salmon, cod or haddock.

4 small red mullet; 3 tablespoons sunflower oil; 2 medium carrots; 4oz mushrooms; 2 shallots; 2 tablespoons chopped parsley; 4 tablespoons white wine; salt and freshly ground pepper.

Cut four twelve-inch rounds of aluminum foil. Clean and scrape the red mullet and cut off the fins and tail. Make two diagonal incisions in the sides, cutting almost through to the bone. Sprinkle with salt and pepper. Cut the carrots, mushrooms and shallots into tiny shreds like pine needles, or if you prefer, chop them finely. Heat 2 tablespoons of oil gently in a small frying pan and put in the carrots and shallots. Soften them for 5 minutes over a low heat and then add the mushrooms. Soften, covered, for a further two or three minutes, then add the parsley and stir it into the mixture for a minute or two over a gentle heat, to allow its flavor to permeate the vegetables.

Brush the rounds of foil lightly with oil, make a crease down the middle and fold up the edges a little. You are then ready to make them into half-moon shaped parcels, each one enclosing a fish.

To do this, spread a little of the vegetable mixture on half of each piece of foil, place a fish on top, and cover with the rest of the vegetables divided equally between the four fish. Sprinkle a tablespoon of white wine over each and pleat the edges of the foil together with your fingers, folding them over twice, making hermetically sealed parcels. Serve, if possible, with new potatoes, or with steamed potatoes.

Fruit loaf
1lb stoneground wholewheat flour; ½lb white flour, preferably strong flour; ½ teaspoon salt; 1oz fresh yeast;

2oz soft margarine; 2 tablespoons malt extract; 2 tablespoons molasses; 2oz raisins; 1² fluid oz warm water.

Put the flour, salt and raisins in a large bowl and mix thoroughly. Make a well in the center, pour in the yeast creamed in a little warm water. Add the warm melted margarine, malt, molasses and warm water – enough to make a rather slack, pliable dough. Knead in the bowl until the mixture is even. It thickens up a little and becomes firmer.

Put the bowl in a large plastic bag, oiled lightly inside to prevent it sticking to the dough, and leave to rise for 2 hours, with the mouth of the bag slightly open, or until the dough has doubled in size. Pre-heat the oven to 375°F. Push the mixture down into tins for either two very large 1lb loaves or three smaller ones, and put back in the bag to prove until puffy and swollen – about 45 minutes.

Bake in the pre-heated oven for 50 minutes, turning half way through. Five minutes before the end, paint with a glaze made with 2 tablespoons sugar dissolved in 2 tablespoons of milk and boiled for a minute or two until slightly syrupy. Eat, sliced, like ordinary bread, except that this is sticky, gooey and delicious.

Gnocchi for four
This dish, in which the ham is used to flavor the gnocchi rather than to provide substance, is meltingly light and surprisingly rich considering the restraint of the ingredients. Eat it with a mixed green salad – lettuce, endive fennel and cucumber.

½ or ¾ pint water mixed with ¼ pint milk; onion; 1 bay leaf; nutmeg; 4oz semolina (do not be put off, it is delicious); 1 tablespoon sunflower oil; salt and pepper; 2 slices of ham, chopped finely; few sprigs of parsley, finely chopped; tomato sauce (see page 56); 2oz grated Parmesan.

Bring the pint of water and milk to the boil with the onion, bay leaf, nutmeg, salt and pepper. Let it boil for 5 minutes, then remove onion and bay leaf and sprinkle in the semolina, stirring constantly until it thickens. Cook, stirring, over a very low heat, for 5 minutes. Then remove from heat, add half the grated Parmesan and the chopped ham and parsley. Mix in well.

Oil a large flat plate, and spoon on the mixture, spreading it out to an even thickness of about ½ inch with oiled hands – it is hot, so do it carefully. Let it get cold, cut into squares, and lay them overlapping in an ovenproof dish. Sprinkle with oil and the remaining cheese, and brown under the grill until heated through and crisp – about 10 minutes. Do not allow to boil or they will disintegrate. Serve with tomato sauce and the remaining Parmesan.

Herb bread
The use of herbs with the garlic is so as to provide such a delicious, over-whelming sensation of flavor that you do not notice you are not eating bread drenched in butter. If you prefer, the margarine can be substituted with oil but the paste is pastier and easier to spread if you use margarine.

1 French loaf; 3oz soft margarine; 1 teaspoon of mixed freshly chopped herbs – choose from dill, parsley, marjoram, oregano, basil, tarragon, mint; 1 crushed clove of garlic; 1 tablespoon grated Parmesan.

Cut the bread (not quite right through so that it remains joined together at the base) diagonally into 1-inch slices. Make a paste with the herbs, garlic, margarine and Parmesan. Spread over the insides of the slices, and press the loaf back together. Make a sort of longboat out of kitchen foil to enclose the bottom of the loaf, leaving the top open. Bake in a hot oven, 400°F, for 10 minutes.

Left-over lamb with lentils for six to eight
This dish provides a non-fatty way of stewing lamb, because all the fat is trimmed off before cooking. This trimming actually improves and refines the flavor of the dish, which makes a very good change from shepherd's pie.

1½lb left-over roast lamb – preferably a leg; 2 cloves garlic; salt; pepper; 3 tablespoons oil; 1 small onion; 1 pint stock; 1lb lentils, the greeny-brown or brown variety; 1 bay leaf; a handful of parsley, preferably that "flat" type; 3 spring onions; handful of chopped marjoram.

Pre-heat oven to 350°F. Cut the left-over lamb into pieces of 1 by 2 inches. Season well with fresh-ground pepper, make incisions here and there in the meat and insert finely sliced garlic. Fry in hot oil in a saucepan. Drain thoroughly when well-browned, and keep on one side. Season with salt.

In the same oil, fry the onion, finely chopped, until transparent but not brown. Add the stock and put in lentils, lamb, bay leaf, salt and pepper. Cover the pan and simmer until the lentils are tender and have absorbed the stock. Now stir in the parsley, chopping spring onions and marjoram and, if you like, sprinkle very lightly with olive oil. Serve very hot.

Mussels
Mussels are not only good fat-free protein, but they are also tasty and comparatively inexpensive. Many classic French recipes call for the use of thick cream to carry the flavors of the juices, but the Belgian national dish is a bowl of plainly cooked mussels (accompanied by a heart-rending amount of finely cut crisp french fries. The same style of plain cooking, mopping up the juices with wholewheat bread, is deeply satisfying. For a first course for four (double amounts for a main course) you need:

2lb of mussels, washed (discarding floaters, and broken shells); 1 small onion (or two small shallots); the white of a small leek; sprig of parsley; sprig of thyme; freshly ground black pepper (no salt); glass of dry white wine; tablespoon of olive oil; juice of half a lemon.

Put the washed and bearded mussels in a heavy-bottomed pan, and cover with oil, white wine, the leek, the onion or shallots chopped small, the chopped parsley, and the thyme. Squeeze the lemon juice on top.

Put over a steady heat, with the lid on tightly, and cook till mussels open and are cooked (about 7–10 minutes). You can serve them as they are, shells and soup together, with wholewheat bread, and plenty of black pepper, leaving each person to undo the shells themselves. Dip the bread into the juices.

Noodles for four
In Italy, most families make their own pasta. It can be quicker to make your own than go to a shop to get it. And many times more satisfying. You do use an egg in making noodles, to bind the flour, but it is a very moderate use of egg which is acceptable in the New Diet. The recipe is brief and to the point: skill in rolling out comes with practice. As for cooking, it is as quick as boiling an egg.

1lb strong flour; 1 egg, beaten; salt; water to moisten.

On a pastry board, make a heap of the

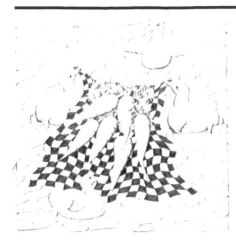

flour. Make a well in the middle, and pour in the beaten egg. Stir with a wooden spoon until it is a pliable mass, then knead it, moistening if necessary with a teaspoon or two of water. Roll into ball. Leave in cool place to settle for half an hour. The refrigerator will do.

Dust the pastry board with flour, flatten ball, and roll out backwards and forwards, and from side to side. Turn pastry over and continue. Keep on rolling and dusting the pastry board, until dough is thin. If your pastry board is not big enough you will have to cut the piece in two and continue rolling.

Cut into long thin strips, and loop them over a string "clothes-line" to dry for 20 minutes or so – longer if you like, but use fresh pasta the same day.

TO COOK: drop them, a handful at a time into a large pan of boiling salted water. Then drop to the bottom. In less than five minutes they come up to the surface, and are done. Serve with one of the sauces for pasta recommended below, or with olive oil, finely chopped garlic and plain tomato sauce. Even though cheese is a doubtful starter in the New Diet, a sprinkling of Parmesan cheese is all right, because one ounce goes such a long way.

Brown noodles for four
Noodles can also be made with brown flour, which is 90 per cent of the whole wheat.

12oz brown flour; 2 eggs; 4 tablespoons cold water; good pinch of salt; 1 tablespoon oil.

The secret of these is to keep the dough very dry. If it is really too dry to be workable, add more water, but only a teaspoon at a time and work it in with your hands. You can knead the dough as much as you like, until it binds together smoothly. Work it well, smooth the oil over the surface, and let

it rest for 20 minutes wrapped in foil.

Now cut off a piece about the size of a large matchbox and roll it into a long strip as thin as you can make it. Roll it up into a cigar shape, and cut it into strips about ¼-inch wide. These will unroll into nice long noodles. Let them dry for a few minutes, or until you need them, and then drop into boiling salted water and cook until tender – about 20 minutes. Serve in the usual way.

Onion soup for two
Here is a traditional dish in which the vegetables themselves, in this case onions, can be made to exude their own juices to replace the usual fat. Although less rich than the usual onion soup, which is cooked with lots of lard, the flavor is equally good.

1 tablespoon oil (sunflower or olive); 1lb large onions; 1 generous pinch of caraway or fennel seeds; 1¼ pint best stock, well skimmed of all fat; 1 teaspoon sugar; 1 teaspoon wine vinegar; 1 small glass of dry white vermouth; 2 large slices French bread; salt and pepper; 2oz Gruyère or Emmental.

Slice onions thinly into rings. Heat the oil just enough to grease the bottom of the pan, put in the onions and stir them round. Add the caraway or fennel seeds, cover the pan and let the onions stew in their own juice for at least fifteen minutes.

Bring the stock to the boil, pour it over the onions, add the vinegar and cook fairly fast for about 15 minutes. Meanwhile, caramelize a teaspoon of sugar by putting it under a hot grill in an old tablespoon and leaving it there until it is a dark chestnut-brown, then stir it into the soup to color it. You will be needing the grill anyway for toasting the French bread. When it is toasted, cover each piece with half the grated Gruyère or Emmental.

Put the soup into bowls, float the toast on top and stick the bowls back under the hot grill until the cheese is bubbling. If you can add a glass of dry white vermouth to the stock it improves the flavor greatly, and a dash of brandy at the end is quite traditional and a great comfort to a tired person.

Pork fillet, stuffed with mushrooms for two
Of all the pieces of a pig, the fillet is probably the leanest and most tender, but does not, alas, go very far. The stuffing makes it go further, and keeps it moist.

1 large pork fillet; 1 tablespoon oil; 2oz chopped mushrooms; 2oz chopped onion; 2oz breadcrumbs, moistened with milk; parsley; a squeeze of lemon juice; grated lemon rind; salt; pepper; nutmeg; half an egg, beaten; 2 teaspoons soft margarine. For the gravy: juices from the pan, skimmed; 2oz small button mushrooms; 1 glass of white wine; ¼ pint good stock; 1–2 tablespoons arrowroot; seasoning.

TO MAKE THE STUFFING:. Pre-heat oven to 375°F. Soak the breadcrumbs in milk and squeeze dry. Half soften the very finely chopped onion in half the oil, then stir in finely chopped mushrooms and cook together gently. Allow to cool. Mix bread, mushrooms, onions and chopped parsley together, bind with half a beaten egg, and flavor with grated lemon rind, parsley, nutmeg and salt and pepper.

Make a cut the length of the fillet and flatten it out. Bang it a little with a rolling pin, season the inside with salt and pepper, and rub it all over with lemon juice. Spread the stuffing over the center and enclose it in the pork fillet. Roll it up and tie with string. Rub the outside with soft margarine and cover the top lightly with foil. Put in a small roasting pan with the remaining oil and roast for 45–60 minutes depending on size, removing foil to baste occasionally, and leaving it off for the last 15 minutes to allow the meat to brown.

TO MAKE THE GRAVY. Put the pork fillet on a dish to keep hot. Skim *all* the fat from the roasting pan. Stir in the white wine and deglaze the pan in the usual way. Dissolve the arrowroot in a little of the stock, add stock and arrowroot, the quartered mushrooms and seasoning, and simmer for five minutes, adding more liquid as needed.

Poulet paysanne with black olives for four
A rather simple combination of chicken, potatoes and black olives makes a very grand dish indeed, and eaten with a green salad it turns into a complete meal.

1 chicken weighing 3lb; 12 small, preferably new, potatoes; ½lb black olives, stoned; 2–3 tablespoons sunflower oil; salt and pepper; 1 tablespoon parsley, finely chopped; 2 cloves garlic, finely chopped; 1 glass white wine or dry white vermouth; ½ pint chicken stock, either homemade or made with stock cubes.

Peel or scrub the potatoes. Dry them in

a cloth. Cut the chicken into six to eight pieces. Heat the oil in a large sauté pan or deep skillet, and put in the potatoes, browning them lightly on all sides. Take them out, draining them well on the side of the pan, and put them on one side.

Now fry the pieces of chicken in the same pan, turning them to brown them evenly on all sides, and letting them cook gently for about 15 minutes. Now put in the potatoes, season with salt and pepper, cover the pan and turn down the heat a little, leaving the chicken to cook for 20 minutes. Add the stoned olives, chopped parsley and garlic and cook on, covered, for about 10 minutes more. At this point the juices in the bottom of the pan will need skimming, so remove the chicken, olives and potatoes to a deep serving dish and skim all the fat from the casserole. Now add the wine or dry white vermouth to the remaining juices, and let it boil for a minute or two. Add the stock, reduce by boiling for 2–3 minutes, taste for seasoning, pour over the chicken on the serving dish and serve with salad.

Rice and beans for six

This is one of those traditional dishes shared by the poor of several countries: Brazil, Turkey and Italy, where this version comes from. The nutritional value of the dish is increased 43 per cent by the complementary effect of the rice and beans in providing essential amino acids (the constituents of proteins) in the most favorable ratio.

½ lb red kidney beans; 2 onions, 2 carrots, 2 cloves of garlic, 2 sticks of celery, all finely chopped; 1 lb canned (or 1 lb fresh) tomatoes; large pinch of thyme; small sprig of rosemary; large pinch of oregano; large pinch of cumin; chopped parsley; 3 tablespoons oil (olive or sunflower); salt; pepper; ¾ lb rice; 4 oz grated Parmesan.

First soak the beans overnight. Next day cook them slowly until tender but not bursting, then drain, reserving the cooking liquid. Cook and drain the rice. Heat the oil in a frying pan and soften the vegetables; then add the tomatoes, herbs and seasoning. Stir the beans into the mixture and cook for at least half an hour, adding bean liquid if it becomes dry. When beans and sauce are nicely married, stir in the rice, heat through and serve sprinkled with parsley and olive oil. Offer the cheese separately.

Sautéed pork fillet for four

This is an excellent way of keeping an otherwise dryish meat, calling out for a rich creamy sauce, juicy and appetizing. It would also work excellently for lean lamb such as you might use for kebabs, or veal. Serve with brown rice and a green salad.

2 small pork fillets; 3 tablespoons olive oil; 1 dried or fresh red chilli; 4 anchovies; 1 sprig of fresh rosemary; ½ lemon; 1 glass of white wine; 2 cloves garlic, crushed; 2 teaspoons wine vinegar.

Trim the fillets and cut into 1-inch pieces. Chop the chilli (seeds removed) and the anchovies. Chop the rosemary very finely and roll the pork pieces in it. Heat the oil, add the chillies, anchovies, garlic and pork, and brown the pork. When it is nicely browned, add the lemon juice and white wine (no salt, anchovies are salty).

Cover the pan and simmer for 10 or 15 minutes until the liquid has lost the fresh taste of the wine. Add the vinegar, and simmer uncovered until the liquid gets syrupy. Serve very hot, with rice or with salad.

Scalloped potatoes for four to six

One of the more demanding vegetables, as far as butter is concerned, is the potato. If it isn't being mashed with loads of butter it is probably being fried in quantities of oil or roasted in lakes of fat. But this dish, a variation on the old Scottish stoved potato when the onions and potatoes are cooked in water and a bit of bacon fat, is nice and creamy although it contains no cream— only milk and a teaspoon of soft margarine.

1½ lb potatoes; 1 medium onion; 1 teaspoon soft margarine; 2 teaspoons flour; salt and pepper; 1 teaspoon fresh chopped rosemary; 1–1¼ pints milk.

Peel the potatoes and onions and slice them thinly. Grease a 3-pint ovenproof dish with margarine. Spread ¼ of the potatoes over the bottom of the dish and put ⅓ of the onions on top. Sprinkle ⅓ of the flour, a pinch of salt, pepper and some of the rosemary over. Repeat the layers, finishing with the final ¼ of potatoes. Pour enough milk over almost to cover the potatoes. Bake at 350°F for 2–2½ hours. Every half-hour, for the first 1½ hours, push the topmost potatoes down under the milk a bit to keep them from browning too much. If the potatoes become dry (there should be juices about an inch

below the top of the dish), add a bit more milk. When cooked, the potatoes should be brown and crusty on top, with creamy juices underneath.

Spaghetti sauce Bolognese for six

The amount of sauce to spaghetti is important. In Italy in a domestic situation, the sauce would be used just to moisten the pasta, and would be mixed into it in the bowl before being served. The huge dollop of sauce in the middle of a small plate of pasta is a restaurant trick. When less sauce is used the pasta itself must be very nicely cooked.

4 oz minced pork; 4 oz minced veal or beef; 2 chicken livers, finely chopped; 2 carrots; 2 sticks of celery; 2 medium onions; at least 1 clove garlic; 1 large sprig of thyme; large pinch of oregano; bay leaf; about 2 tablespoons olive oil; 1 small glass of red wine; salt; pepper; 1 lb can plus 1 small can tomatoes (20 oz); 1 tablespoon tomato purée; about 1¼ pint of stock.

Chop carrots, celery, onions and garlic very finely and soften in oil, stirring occasionally. Turn up heat, add the meats, stir a bit and let the mixture brown over moderate heat. Add chicken livers and wine, and let boil until liquid has all but evaporated. Add tomatoes, herbs, salt and pepper, and purée. Simmer 1½ hours, adding stock as necessary. Cover pan for beginning of cooking.

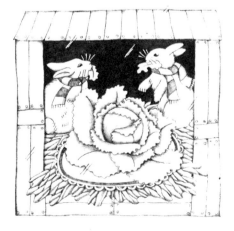

Recipes Summer

by Caroline Conran

Brown rice
Brown rice with ratatouille
Cauliflower and shrimp salad
Chicken with mushrooms
Crudités
Don Luis de Soto's paella
Eggplant purée
Filafel
Houmous
Indonesian soup
Kidneys with mushrooms and sherry
Lamb stew with zucchini
Lemon, grapefruit and orange sorbet
Moussaka
Muesli
Pastry without butter
Pitta bread
Pizza
Pork taraba
Prune soufflé
Risotto alla rustica
Stuffed mushrooms
Stuffed tomatoes
Tapenade
Tomato pie with fresh thyme
Tomato sauce
Tomato toast
Walnut cake
Wholemeal muffins
Yoghurt

Brown rice

The whole secret of cooking brown rice is to soak it for at least half an hour before cooking. This makes it lighter and helps it to cook more quickly.

Soak ½lb brown rice in cold water for about half an hour. Drain and put it into a saucepan with at least 2½ pints of salted water. Bring to the boil and simmer for about 40–45 minutes. Drain and rinse in warm water.

Brown rice with ratatouille for four

This combination of the good and healthy rice flavor and the Southern-tasting vegetables is particularly satisfactory. If any is left over, mix it with a little garlicky oil and vinegar dressing for a very good salad. Brown rice contains natural healthy fibre which is removed from polished white rice.

1 eggplant; 1 onion; 1 green pepper; 2–3 tomatoes; ½ can of tomatoes; ½ brown rice, soaked for 1 hour; 2 cloves garlic; 2–3 tablespoons oil; salt; thyme, oregano, rosemary; 1¼ pint chicken stock; grated Parmesan cheese.

Cut the eggplant in half lengthwise, then slice across into ¼-inch pieces. Sprinkle with salt if you have time, and let the pieces sit in a colander to drain for 30 minutes. Slice the onion and the pepper. Chop the garlic. Skin the tomatoes and chop them coarsely.

Drain the rice, rinse and cook in boiling salted water for 40 minutes. Meanwhile heat 2 tablespoons of oil in a frying pan and fry onions and eggplants for 5 minutes. Add the green peppers, then the garlic and lastly the chopped fresh and the canned tomatoes. Flavor the mixture with herbs – and let it simmer until just cooked, adding stock to prevent the mixture from becoming too dry.

Put the drained rice, steaming hot, in a hot bowl with a tablespoon of olive oil and a tablespoon of freshly chopped herbs. Mix round, then lightly stir in the vegetables. Serve with grated Parmesan.

This can be reheated quite successfully.

Cauliflower and shrimp salad for three or four

Instead of eating a whole plateful of shrimps, it is just as good to make them into a salad with a vegetable, which could be zucchini, potatoes, or in this case cauliflower.

1 cauliflower; ½–¾lb shrimps in shells; 3–4 tablespoons sunflower oil; 1 tablespoon fresh lemon juice; pinch of sugar; crushed clove garlic; salt; red chilli powder or finely crumbled red chilli; 1 tablespoon sprigs of dill weed; 1 tablespoon coarsely chopped spring onions or green onion tops.

Cook and cool the cauliflower, then break into florets. Shell the shrimps, leaving two or three whole to decorate the salad. Make a dressing with sunflower oil, lemon juice, crushed garlic, sugar and salt and red chilli powder or finely crumbled red chilli.

Arrange the cauliflower sprigs in a dish. Cover with shrimps. Sprinkle the dill over the top, and also the green onion tops or spring onions. Now pour on the dressing and stick the whole shrimps on the top. If you have no shrimps, make this dish with eggs – using two eggs cut small for four people. Eat with wholewheat bread.

Chicken with mushrooms and black pepper sauce for four

This chicken dish is for a special occasion, and takes a little trouble; but you will end up with a dish with a succulent sauce which owes nothing to animal fats or cream.

A nice plump chicken; ½ pint very best jellied stock, preferably made from the carcass of a previous chicken; salt; pepper; 1 tablespoon sunflower oil; 3 onions; ½–¾lb young fresh mushrooms (the color of the dish depends on their being pale around the gills); ½ teaspoon at least of black peppercorns, pounded coarsely in a pestle and mortar (mignonette pepper).

Chop the onions fairly finely and put them in a flameproof casserole with a tablespoon of sunflower oil. Put on the lid and let the onions soften over a low heat for 10 or 15 minutes. Then put in the chicken, nicely seasoned, and pour on the stock. Cover the pot and simmer the chicken until the leg will come away but still shows very faintly pink — about 45 minutes. Now tip the pan and skim off all fat from the juices. Add the chopped mushrooms and cook on for a further 15 minutes or until the chicken is done.

Remove the chicken and skim any remaining fat from the juices before reducing the sauce, mushrooms and all, by fast boiling until it is just becoming slightly syrupy. Meanwhile, peel all the skin off the chicken and carve it into joints. Put the pieces on a dish and keep them hot.

Put the sauce in the blender and whizz it to a fine texture, adding a little more chicken stock if necessary to make it light. Stir in half the mignonette pepper, reheat the sauce, pour it over the chicken in its dish and scatter the rest of the pepper over the top.

Crudités (Celery with hot anchovy oil) for four

The French love to offer treats of raw radishes (sometimes with butter and salt), celery and slivers of carrot, served with aioli, which is a lovely garlic-flavored mayonnaise. Unfortunately, this is not so healthy as it sounds, because mayonnaise is an emulsion of cholesterol-rich egg yolks and oil, and it is egg yolks we need to cut down on. But there is no reason why crudités should not be served with an olive oil and vinegar or lemon dressing, or, in the case of celery, with this appetizing hot dressing.

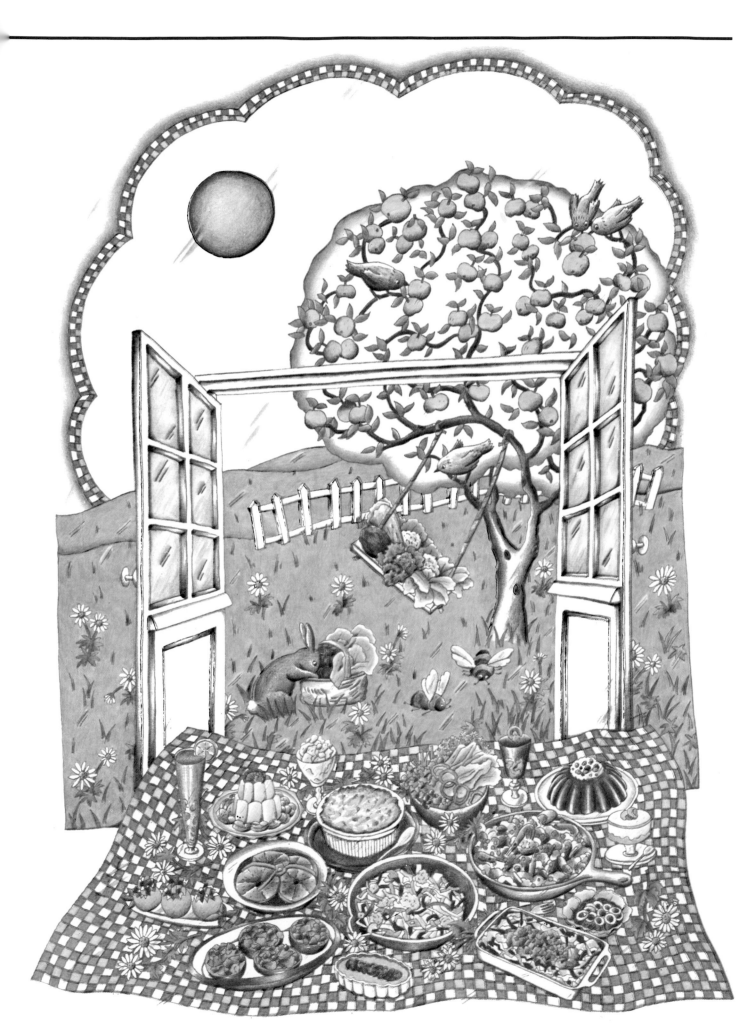

1 small can of anchovies; 1 large head of celery; 3–4 tablespoons of olive oil.

Put the anchovies and their oil in a small saucepan and heat gently; after about 4 or 5 minutes, when they start to dissolve, pound them up. Stir in extra olive oil, beat well together. Keep hot until ready to serve.

Serve the cleaned, cut stalks of celery with the bowl of anchovy dressing, mopping up the juice with plain wholewheat bread.

The mixture is beaten before serving because it will separate. If you like an emulsion, this one stands up to gentle heat without breaking down:

1¾ oz can anchovies; 2 teaspoons Dijon mustard; 2 teaspoons lemon juice; 4 tablespoons olive oil.

Put the anchovies and their oil in a small saucepan and heat gently; after about 4 or 5 minutes, when they start to dissolve, transfer them to a mortar and pound them. The bones stick to the bottom of the pestle and can be removed. Pound in the mustard and lemon juice until well blended, then drip in the olive oil, as though making a mayonnaise. Put back in a saucepan, heat very gently and serve.

Don Luis de Soto's paella for six to eight
This paella is the very complicated and splendid version from the cool kitchen of a Seville olive grower and producer. It should ideally be cooked in a wide, flat paella pan, but an extra large frying pan, or even an oven dish would do.

1lb uncooked pork (shoulder is best) cut into ¾-inch cubes; 1lb uncooked chicken pieces on the bone; 3–4 tablespoons olive oil; 1 onion, chopped; 1 bay leaf; 2 cloves garlic; ½lb raw squid, cut in rings; ½lb tomatoes, skinned, seeded and coarsely chopped; 2 pints of fish or chicken stock; 4 good pinches of saffron; salt (up to 2 level teaspoons); ground black pepper; 1¼lb long-grain rice; 4oz shelled shrimps; 4oz shelled peas (frozen will do); 12 whole shrimps; 1 pint mussels, cooked (use strained liquid for stock); 1 red pepper; 12 Spanish stuffed green olives; slices of lemon.

Brown the pork and chicken in olive oil on all sides in a paella pan, then let the meat cook more gently for about 20 minutes. Add the onion, bay leaf, garlic, squid, tomatoes and the stock in which you have soaked the saffron. Bring to the boil, season with salt and

pepper, then stir in the rice. Add the peas, cover the pan and let the paella cook in the oven at 350°F for 20 minutes.

Place the shrimps and mussels in the half-shell on top, and dot with a few chunks of red pepper and the green olives. Cover the pan again and cook for a further 15–25 minutes until the rice is tender and the stock almost absorbed. Remove the bay leaf. Serve with a slice of lemon on each plate.

Eggplant purée (also known as caviare of eggplants) for four to six
3 eggplants; 1 large onion; juice of 1 lemon; 3 tablespoons olive oil; 2 tomatoes; 2 cloves finely mashed garlic; salt and pepper or chilli powder.

Grill the eggplants until charred on the outside and soft and pulpy inside. (Alternatively, bake them in the oven for half an hour, until they are very soft inside). Cut them in half and scoop out the pulp; mix it with the juice of the onion, obtained somewhat painfully either by grating the onion on the coarse blade of the grater or pulping it in the blender, and then by rubbing it in a wire sieve with the back of a spoon so that the juice is pressed out.

Season the paste with lemon juice, olive oil and garlic, and with salt and pepper. Stir in the tomatoes, skinned and de-seeded and roughly chopped. Serve cold with homemade bread as an hors d'oeuvre.

Filafel for four to six
These little hot cakes from Israel, spiced with cumin and a white sesame sauce, make a wonderful starter for a simple meal, or a very healthy light lunch. In Egypt they are usually made with dried broad beans, rather than chick peas.

8oz chick peas; pinch of baking powder (about ¼ teaspoon); 2 eggs; a handful of parsley, chopped; 1 teaspoon salt; 2 teaspoons cumin seeds; ¼ teaspoon coriander seeds; ½ clove garlic; ¼ onion or 1 shallot.

Soak the chick peas overnight. Grind all the ingredients in a food processor; the texture should be like fine breadcrumbs, but moist. Allow the mixture to stand for about half an hour. Form into small flat or round cakes about the size of a walnut. The mixture is rather crumbly, but it will make cakes if handled carefully. Transfer them to a pan of hot fat with a spatula, and fry to a deep brown. Serve hot with the

following cold sauce. They have a pleasant nutty texture and flavor.

Tahini sauce
2½ oz roasted sesame seeds; ½ clove garlic; 2 tablespoons lemon juice; ¼ teaspoon cayenne pepper; salt, pepper; about ⅛ pint cold water.

Toast the sesame seeds to a light brown by shaking them over a gentle heat in a dry frying pan. Put them with the remaining ingredients except the water into the blender, and blend to a smooth purée. Add enough water to make a light sauce.

Houmous for four
This eastern Mediterranean dish is becoming increasingly popular as Greek restaurants continue to boom. It also happens to be particularly rich in protein, as are all dishes made with pulses; in this case it is chick peas that are the main ingredient.

Although apparently very filling because of the olive oil and sesame-seed oil, it is very safe food. Eaten with plenty of pitta bread and followed by a Greek-style salad it makes a very good lunch. It can be made with canned chick peas, but if you are patient it is very easy to make from dried chick peas.

6oz dried chick peas; 4 tablespoons tahini paste (this is a paste of crushed sesame seeds, and is sold in jars); the juice of 1 lemon; salt; crushed garlic; a sprig or two of parsley; olive oil to taste.

Soak the chick peas overnight. Put them in a pan covered with fresh cold water and bring them gently to the boil. Simmer for about 1½ hours or until tender – it may take as long as three hours. Put the cooked peas through a Moulin Légumes, using the coarse blade first, and then the small blade, to obtain a smooth paste; or mash, pound or beat in a blender or a sieve, whatever method suits you.

Stir in the tahini paste, lemon juice, garlic, salt and chopped parsley, adjusting lemon and garlic to suit your taste. Add enough olive oil to make a smooth moist paste: be generous with everything, you are not trying to run a restaurant. Eat with hot pitta bread (see page 54) or wholewheat bread; you will not need butter.

Indonesian soup for four
This is simply a rich vegetable soup,

nutritious but satisfying in its range of flavors: hot, sweet, sour and spicy. The basic flavor is due to the combination of chicken stock and coconut milk, which is not the liquid from a fresh coconut but an infusion made simply from steeping desiccated coconut in boiling water for 15 minutes, and straining.

1 large onion; 2 large carrots; 2 sticks of celery; 1 small leek; a handful of green beans; 2½ pints of homemade chicken stock; seasoning: clove of garlic, 1–2 chilli peppers (green or dried and pounded), teaspoon of turmeric (optional: a slice of fresh green ginger, the size of a marble); 1 lemon; 2 teaspoons brown sugar; 4 tablespoons desiccated coconut.

Peel vegetables. Cut thinly, but not quite so small as Julienne matchsticks.

Make half a pint of coconut milk by steeping four tablespoons of desiccated coconut in half a pint of boiling water, and straining after 15 minutes.

Gently fry a tablespoon of the onion, very finely chopped, in a very little oil until soft; add crushed garlic, ginger and finely crushed green chillies (or powdered chilli or chilli sauce) and the turmeric. Heat through, without burning, until it is a sticky paste, stirring with a wooden spoon.

Heat the stock with the coconut milk and the spicy paste, add sugar, and add the chopped vegetables, simmering slowly for 30 minutes. Check for seasoning. You can add soya sauce instead of salt for a more characteristic flavor.

Before serving, stir in juice of a lemon.

Kidneys with mushrooms and sherry for four

Offal is free of fat, and as long as you do not use it as part of a hefty mixed grill, which is bad for an overstressed heart, it is economical and nourishing. This particular dish is the recognizable cousin of a French dish, but is cooked with olive oil instead of butter. Sliced liver is none the worse for being cooked in olive oil either, and will not then need the creamy sauces offered in many Italian restaurants, but braised onion instead.

1lb lambs' kidneys (or you can use other kidneys); ½lb mushrooms (tiny button mushrooms are best); 2 medium tomatoes, very ripe and juicy; 1 clove garlic; 1 sherry glass of dry sherry or the same amount of dry white wine; salt and pepper; a little flour; olive oil.

Cook the chopped tomatoes with a crushed clove of garlic in a small pan until they have been reduced to a dryish purée. Sieve.

Skin and quarter the kidneys, removing the core with a sharp knife. Roll them very lightly in a little seasoned flour. Wash the button mushrooms; if large, halve or quarter them, but do not use mushrooms with open black gills as they will darken the sauce too much.

Heat the mushrooms in 2 tablespoons olive oil, tossing them about until they begin to sweat their juices. Remove them with a slotted spoon. In the same fat, sauté the kidneys, adding a little more olive oil if necessary. Combine the mushrooms and kidneys, turn up the heat and pour in the sherry or white wine, stirring well for a minute. Lower the heat, add the tomato sauce, stir, cover the pan and leave to simmer for 3–4 minutes. The texture of the dish will depend on the quality of the mushrooms and tomato sauce, but it should not be too dry. If necessary, moisten with a little stock to give plenty of sauce. Serve with plainly cooked rice.

Lamb stew with zucchini for four

This is one of those well-tempered dishes that can be kept cooking away at an extremely low simmer until people are ready to sit down and eat. A good thick gravy is obtained by using very floury potatoes, while waxy potatoes give a thinner sauce.

large ½ shoulder of lamb; 1lb potatoes; 2 onions; 2 cloves garlic; 3 tablespoons oil; 3 tablespoons tomato purée; salt, pepper; 1lb zucchini.

Peel and slice the potatoes in thick slices and put them in a bowl of cold water. Cut the shoulder of lamb into large cubes, removing the bone and most of the fat. Chop the onions and garlic and soften them in the oil in a large casserole until they are golden, then add the meat and brown it all over.

Add the tomato purée and stir it in well, then add the potato slices and enough water to bathe the meat and potatoes but not to cover them. Season with salt and pepper and cover the pot.

Simmer gently for 1½ hours without disturbing and then add the zucchini, washed and cut into slices about ⅛ inch thick, pushing them well down into the gravy. Half an hour later test the zucchini, and, when they are cooked through, serve hot with a salad and bread.

Lemon, grapefruit and orange sherbet for four to six

Any sherbet which uses fresh fruit as a base, and which is free of eggs and cream, makes a clean refreshing ending to a summer meal. This citrus fruit one can be made in the winter, too. For example, to make a raspberry or blackcurrant sherbet, replace the lemon, grapefruit and orange juice with a pint of fresh fruit purée, having first made the syrup with the lemon peel as before. If the mixture tastes too sweet or bland, sharpen with a little lemon juice.

2 lemons; 1 grapefruit; 2 oranges; 6oz sugar; 1¼ pints water; 1 egg white.

Pare the rind from the lemons. Put it in a pan with the sugar and cold water, and bring to the boil. Boil for five minutes, then allow to cool. Strain the cold syrup. Squeeze the juice of the lemons, grapefruit and oranges and mix it with the cold syrup (thus retaining all the vitamins). Pour the mixture into a container, and freeze to a crystalline mush. Break up the crystals thoroughly in the blender, stir in the white of egg, whisked to a soft snow, and refreeze.

Moussaka for four

If you are going to cook this Balkan delicacy (Romanian-born, though the Greeks are famous for it), you might as well pronounce it right. It is not m'sarka, but mooserka. Cook it the New Diet way, and you will enjoy the nutritious benefits of Mediterranean food (where there is a much lower incidence of heart disease than in America and Northern Europe). A word of warning: many cookbooks take dishes like this and bastardize them, enriching the white sauce with cream and eggs, letting the lamb sizzle in its rich fat, even cooking the eggplants in butter. Wrong, all wrong. The secret of our recipe is in its simplicity; no animal fat, all olive oil.

1 medium eggplant; 1 medium onion; 1lb cheap tomatoes (for sauce) or purée from can; ½lb leg of lamb, cut free of fat, and minced or chopped finely; up to ½ pint chicken stock. For the white sauce: ½ pint milk (or if you are being rigorous, a milk made from dried skimmed milk); if you have not had eggs the same day, you can use one egg yolk with the sauce; 1oz flour; 1oz soft margarine; a little grated cheese; olive oil; salt and pepper; sprig of thyme.

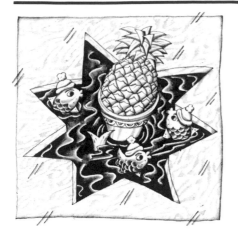

The moussaka is usually cooked in a deep, squarish pan, like a bread pan. It consists of layers of eggplant, meat, onion, tomato and white sauce.

Slice eggplant thinly, leaving skin on. Optional: to remove bitter flavor, sprinkle with salt, stand the slices in a colander with a weighted plate on top, and let them drain for 30 minutes. Then wash free of salt, and mop dry.

In a tablespoon or two of olive oil, lightly fry the onion, finely chopped; remove and fry the lamb, minced or chopped very fine with a sharp knife; finally the eggplant slices, a few at a time.

Make a tomato sauce by simmering the chopped tomatoes for 10 minutes, adding a sprig of thyme and seasoning, and strain through a sieve.

Make a white sauce, melting margarine into a pan, stirring in the flour, and adding as you stir half a pint of boiling milk until it thickens. Leave to cool. (Optional: add a beaten egg yolk to improve texture – it makes it more custardy.)

Line the dish bottom and side with the eggplant slices. Put on the layer of minced lamb. Cover with chicken stock. Smother with the fried onions. Then add a layer of tomato sauce. Finally, pour on the white sauce. Dust with a little grated cheese. Bake in a moderate oven (350°F) for 30–50 minutes, until top is golden.

Muesli

For decades, people have been skeptical about the ideas of the Swiss health-food pioneer Dr Bircher Benner. One of his suggestions was a breakfast of dried and crushed grain, soaked overnight in water or milk, served with dried fruit and fresh fruit. Certainly, if you are trying to cut out fat intake by a quarter, a breakfast of bacon, egg, buttered toast and marmalade, and coffee with cream, is the wrong way to start the day. In fact, many people in this country now eat a cold breakfast, but this usually means one of the store-bought breakfast cereals. These are usually oversweet and over-refined, and the grains may have been cooked in saturated fat. Muesli is one of the many health food ideas being approved by doctors today. It is also an opportunity to take some bran; not only will the roughage help to make you regular, but bran is being found to have other beneficial functions too. Muesli ingredients usually need to be bought from health food stores. Beware of commercial mueslis: many are far too sweet.

YOU NEED: a mixture of any or all of these: *rolled oat flakes, barley flakes, cracked wheat grains*; these may be toasted or not, as you prefer. You can toast your own, tossing them about in a dry frying pan and being careful not to let them burn. And you can soak the grains in milk or water overnight if you wish, which makes them more digestible but rather pulpy to eat.
Bran (allow a tablespoon per serving).
Dried fruit (dried figs and raisins can be chopped up and a tablespoon per serving added).
Hazelnuts or almonds can be added chopped up, a small sprinkling per serving (these can also be toasted for a few minutes).
Peeled or unpeeled apples, or pear can be added, or orange or tangerine.
Honey and wheatgerm are favored by some but although honey tastes good it does not have magical properties; the nutritional value is Lilliputian for our Gulliverish appetites. Wheatgerm oil contains B vitamins, but loses most of its vitamin power in heat-processing, necessary to prevent the oil in the wheatgerm going rancid and bitter. Serve the muesli with milk; or if a purist, with skimmed milk.

Pastry without butter

Even people who have always liked to use butter in their pastry, because of the good flavor it gives, need not be ashamed to offer this pastry to their guests.

4oz plain flour; pinch of salt; a rather generous 2oz soft margarine.

Put everything in a bowl and rub the margarine into the flour until it is like cornflakes – that is to say, nowhere near the fine-breadcrumbs stage reached in making ordinary pastry. Add a couple of tablespoons of water and stir it in with the blade of a knife, then use your fingers briefly to make a coherent mass. Use it straightaway, rolling as lightly and quickly as possible, or keep it in the refrigerator, where it will not become too hard to roll.

Pitta bread (makes 8 breads)

1lb plain white flour; ½oz dried yeast or 1oz fresh yeast; ½oz salt; pinch of sugar; about ½ pint warm water in a measuring cup; olive oil.

Put the flour in a bowl and make a well in the center. Put in a warm place to lose its chill. Mix the yeast to a cream with a pinch of sugar and 1 fluid ounce of the warm water in the cup. Pour olive oil into the cup until it is back to the ½-pint mark, stir in the salt and keep it warm. When the yeast starts to froth, pour it into the center of the flour and then add the water and oil. Knead for 10 minutes. Smooth a little more oil over the outside of the dough and leave it to rise in a warm place for 2 hours, well covered. So far, apart from the addition of olive oil, it is very much like making ordinary bread, but from now you treat the dough more like pastry to achieve flat slippers of bread.

Knock the dough down, cut it into 8 pieces and work each piece into a ball. Cover again and leave to prove for half an hour or so. Preheat the oven to 450°F. Knead each ball of dough a little, put plenty of flour on your board and rolling-pin, and roll each ball gently into an oval shape. Put the shapes on greased and floured baking sheets and let them prove for a further 30 minutes, covered with a cloth.

Brush the tops with water and stick as many breads as you can into the hot oven. Bake 8–10 minutes, turning after the first 5 minutes. Take out of the oven while still pale, and wrap in a cloth to keep them soft. Eat after about ten minutes, cooling, dip into houmous, etc.

Pizza for four

Borrowed from Southern Italy, the pizza is now almost a national dish in America. Usually it is made with too much cheese and a heavy oily sauce. Try this traditional recipe. Be generous with the olives and oregano and you will not need so much cheese. This recipe freezes well. Make a plain bread dough as follows:

1lb plain white flour plus some for kneading; 1oz yeast or ½oz dried yeast; 1½ teaspoons salt; about ½ pint warm water; 2 dessertspoons oil.

Mix the yeast into a couple of tablespoons of warm water. Put the flour in a bowl, pour in the yeast and leave in a warm place to froth up. When it froths, add just under half a pint of warm water to which you have added the salt and oil. Mix to a dough and knead well, adding more flour if needed. Allow to rise in a warm place, covered with an oiled plastic bag, until it has doubled in size.

FOR THE FILLING. While the dough is rising, collect the following together:

A good ½ pint thickish, dryish tomato sauce, flavored with salt, pepper and garlic (make this by simmering two 14-oz cans of tomatoes until thick, and allow to cool); 1 mozzarella cheese; 2 dozen small black olives; 1 can anchovies; plenty of oregano; olive oil.

When the dough has doubled in size, cut it into four pieces. Roll each piece into a ball and flatten it into a flat disc, about 8–10 inches across. Spread the dry tomato sauce over the pizza base. Arrange the olives and anchovies on top. Cut the mozzarella cheese into thick slices and arrange on top of this. Sprinkle well with oregano and olive oil. Allow to sit for 10 minutes or thereabouts. Meanwhile preheat the oven to 450°F. Bake fast for 15–20 minutes. Eat immediately.

Pork taraba for four
These parcels of well-seasoned pork are wrapped in spinach leaves to keep them moist while they cook, and are served in their own simple tomato sauce, flavored with garlic. (They can also be made with lean lamb in the traditional Turkish way.)

1lb absolutely lean pork such as tenderloin, coarsely ground; 1lb spinach; 3 tablespoons olive oil; 2 teaspoons finely chopped parsley or 4–5 sage leaves, finely chopped; 1 small onion, finely chopped; 1 small shallot, finely chopped; salt; generous pinch of cayenne or chilli pepper; 2 whole cloves garlic; 1lb tomatoes, skinned and chopped.

Mix together the coarsely ground pork, one tablespoon of olive oil, chopped parsley or sage, onion and shallot, and one clove of the garlic, finely chopped. Season the mixture with salt and cayenne or chilli pepper. Allow the flavors to develop while you prepare the spinach.
  Bring the large pan of salted water to the boil. Wash the spinach leaves, keeping them whole and drop them

into the pan; allow to cook for 1–2 minutes, then drain and blanch under cold water for a few seconds. Drain well.
  Form the meat into balls about the size of a walnut and wrap each one in two layers of spinach, making neat parcels.
  Put the remaining olive oil in a sauté pan or shallow saucepan, put in the parcels side by side, cover with the skinned, chopped tomatoes, add a whole peeled clove of garlic, and sprinkle with salt and pepper. Cover the pan and simmer very gently for 1¼–1½ hours. Serve with rice.

Prune soufflé for four
½lb prunes; ½ pint cider; 2-inch stick of cinnamon; 4 egg whites; pinch of cream of tartar; 1 teaspoon poppy seeds.

Boil the cider for five minutes with the cinnamon stick. Pour it over the prunes in a bowl and leave to soak overnight. When they are soaked, put them in a pan, cider and all, and simmer until tender. Allow to cool a little, remove the stones and put the pulp through a fine food processor, adding enough liquid to make a nice thick purée.
  Beat the egg whites with the cream of tartar until you have a fairly firm snow. Mix a few tablespoons into the prune purée, then fold the purée into the egg whites with the poppy seeds. Put the mixture lightly into an oiled soufflé dish or charlotte pan and cook in a hot oven, 425°F, for 15–20 minutes. Serve immediately.

Risotto alla rustica for four to six
The amount of meat used for this dish has always depended on the state of the housekeeping money, but in its original Italian days would have been no more than 4oz or so, just a flavoring for the rice. It is still quite healthy to use ¾lb beef for four to six people but it is perhaps preferable to use less, because most of us have more than enough meat.

¾lb minced beef; 1 small slice of ham, chopped; 1 large or 2 small onions, chopped; either 2 carrots and 2 sticks of celery or 4oz mushrooms, cut in quarters; 1oz dried mushrooms (optional); 2 cloves garlic; 1 small glass red wine; 12oz Italian rice; 14-oz can tomatoes; 1 dessertspoon tomato purée; 1¼ pints stock; salt, pepper; thyme; oregano; 2 tablespoons oil – olive or sunflower; grated Parmesan.

Heat the oil and fry the onions, chopped ham and the carrots and celery (if you are using these), cut roughly into small chunks. Add the meat, stir and brown. Add the garlic cloves, peeled and chopped, and the mushrooms if you are using them. Pour in a small glass of red wine to scrape up the brown crust from the bottom of the pan. Let it evaporate.
  Wash the rice thoroughly and add it to the meat. Let it fry for a minute or two, then add the can of tomatoes and tomato purée and half the stock. Season and add the herbs. Simmer until the rice is tender, stirring and adding more stock as it is absorbed. Serve with the grated cheese.
  If you can obtain them, soak 1oz of dried mushrooms in warm water for half an hour. Add them, chopped, with the onions and use the soaking liquid with the stock.

Stuffed mushrooms for two
Mushrooms are particularly good with this stuffing. Serve them with rice and a green salad or with the stuffed tomatoes and a cucumber salad.

½lb large mushrooms (about 10); 2oz ham; 1 large slice brown bread; 1oz pine nuts; 1oz Parmesan, grated; 2 cloves garlic; 4 sprigs parsley; pepper; pinch of thyme; 3 tablespoons olive oil or sunflower oil; ½ lemon.

Stalk the mushrooms, and wipe their outsides with the lemon. Make crumbs of the bread, moisten it well with water and squeeze the water out. Chop the ham, mushroom stalks, parsley and garlic, and mix with the breadcrumbs.
  Heat one teaspoon of the oil and fry the pine nuts in it until they have browned a little. Add the ham mixture and stir it over the heat for a few minutes. Let it cool a bit, then add the Parmesan, thyme and pepper. Put the mushroom caps, top down, in a baking pan, heap the stuffing on top, dribble the remaining oil over them and bake at 350°F for 25 minutes.

Stuffed tomatoes for two to four
These can be stuffed, of course, with almost any mixture, but to make a more filling dish use a combination of rice and meat.

1lb tomatoes; 3oz cooked rice; 3oz raisins; 3oz minced beef or lamb; 1 small onion; pinch of oregano or basil; pinch of coriander and cumin seed; squeeze of lemon; ¼ pint tomato juice; pepper, salt; 2–3 tablespoons sunflower or olive oil.

Cut the tomatoes in half and scoop out the centers. Sprinkle the insides with salt, and leave them upside down to drain for half an hour while you make the stuffing.

Fry the finely chopped onions in half the oil until tender, then add raisins and meat and fry a few minutes more. Now mix this and the tomato juice into the rice, and season well with herbs, spices, salt and a squeeze of lemon juice. Stuff the tomatoes with this mixture, sprinkle with the remaining oil and bake at 320°F for up to an hour in an earthenware dish or baking pan. Serve hot or cold, with a generous green salad or a salad of lettuce, endive, sliced fennel and thinly sliced radishes.

Tapenade for two or three

This blackish, ugly paste is really delicious with fresh homemade wholemeal bread, but is probably best of all, if it is your day for eating an egg, with a hard-boiled egg.

4oz black olives, stoned; 6 anchovies; 1 tablespoon capers; squeeze of lemon juice; 1 tablespoon oil.

Put all the ingredients in the blender and whizz to a slightly rough-textured paste. Serve as a very appetizing and unpretentious starter, with slices of bread and a bowl of the white-tipped radishes called French Breakfast. You can include raw garlic too, but it is quite enough of a relish without it.

Tomato pie with fresh thyme for four to six

By evaporating all the water liquid from fruits or vegetables, you can obtain the very essence of their flavor without adding butter or cream. This kind of cooking should contain lots of concentrated flavors and should never be watery.

2–2½lb ripe red tomatoes; bunch of fresh thyme; dried thyme; salt; dry beans for blind baking; cayenne pepper; pastry made with 4oz flour and 2oz vegetable fat (see page 37).

Line a pie pan with the pastry and bake it "blind" in a hot oven. This means putting foil or beans on greaseproof paper into the uncooked pastry case. After ten minutes or so when the pastry is firm, remove the foil or beans and paper and prick the bottom of the shell. Cook for a further five minutes or until the bottom is done.

Skin the tomatoes. Take 1–1½lb of the ripest of them, cut them in half and squeeze out the pips, giving a shake to remove some of the watery juice. Put the dryish tomato halves in a small pan with plenty of fresh and dried thyme, a pinch of salt and a good sprinkling of cayenne pepper, and cook, stirring occasionally until all the water has evaporated and you are left with a dryish purée. Let this cool. Meanwhile slice the remaining tomatoes carefully with a sharp knife, sprinkle with salt and leave to drain on a tilted board.

When the purée is cool, spread it over the bottom of your pie and lay the sliced tomatoes, well drained, on top, as if you were making an apple pie. Sprinkle with a few drops of oil, and bake in a quick oven for 12–15 minutes or until the tomatoes are *just* cooked through. Serve hot or cold.

Tomato sauce for pasta for four to six

This really is designed to cut down drastically on the amount of oil and butter, which would usually be added both at the beginning and again at the end. It comes from Padua, where certain people are becoming exceedingly health conscious, mainly to the end of looking youthful on the Sardinian beaches. In fact the traditional tomato sauce comes from Southern Italy, where butter would never be used and where there is also very little heart disease. Make this one of your staple meals.

1½lb tomatoes, skinned; 1 onion; 2 cloves garlic; 1 carrot; 1 stick of celery; salt; pepper; basil or marjoram (fresh if possible); 1 tablespoon olive oil.

Chop all ingredients, except the basil, and put them into a pan. Add the salt and pepper. Stew, until carrots and celery are tender. Purée by putting in the blender. Reheat, adding a tablespoon of oil and a handful of basil torn up small.

Tomato toast

This is a lovely, quick, filling outdoor starter for summer, each person making his own toast on the bonfire or over the glowing charcoal. It comes from Spain, where the tomatoes are huge and seem to have a lot of pulp and very few seeds.

Make some thick slices of toast with homemade bread. Cut tomatoes in half. Dribble oil over the toast, then rub the slices with the cut side of half a tomato. Sprinkle with salt and they are ready for eating – they are at their best when eaten immediately.

Walnut cake

Walnuts could be replaced by mixed fruit, poppy seeds, caraway seeds or grated orange peel in this easy basic cake. If you want to eliminate the most branny parts of the flour, sieve it before using or take brown flour instead.

½lb wholewheat flour; 5oz margarine; 5oz Barbados or brown sugar; 2 eggs; 2 teaspoons baking powder; ⅛ pint milk; 4oz walnuts (6–8 left whole for decoration, the rest chopped).

Cream together margarine and sugar until light. Beat in whole eggs, again until light. Mix flour and baking powder together and stir lightly into egg mixture. Add milk, stirring until you have a very soft mixture. Finally, add chopped nuts. Grease and dust with flour a 7-inch-deep pan. Pour mixture in and decorate top with whole nuts.

Cover top of cake pan with a piece of foil pierced at approximately ½-inch intervals with a skewer or sharp knife. Bake at 350°F for 1–1¼ hours. After 45 minutes, remove the foil to allow cake to finish rising and to brown. When done, leave cake in pan for 5–10 minutes, then turn it out on a rack to cool.

Wholewheat muffins

These muffins are made in a very few minutes and should be eaten in a few. When they are hot they are like ambrosia, when cold they become plain muffins.

8oz wholewheat flour; ½ teaspoon salt; 2oz soft margarine; ½ teaspoon bicarbonate of soda; about ¼ pint buttermilk (sour milk or yoghurt will do).

Pre-heat oven to 425°F. Mix together flour, salt and bicarbonate of soda. Rub soft margarine into dry ingredients until finely and evenly distributed. Stir in buttermilk only until all flour is incorporated, and you have a dryish dough. Put on floured board and roll or pat down until ½ inch thick. Cut into circles with 2-inch diameter cutter, or glass. Place on a greased baking sheet. Bake for 10 minutes or until scones are golden brown.

Yoghurt

Since yoghurt can often be used as a substitute for eggs and cream in the thickening of sauces, apart from being an extremely good food in its own right, it is useful to be able to make it at home in quantity. The secret is in nursing the right bacteria at the right temperature, so that they, and they alone, form a culture which sours and thickens the yoghurt to the right flavor and consistency.

To make a pint of yoghurt, the simplest and most primitive method of all is to bring 1 pint of milk to the boil and let it cool until you can keep your finger in it for a count of ten (about 120°F). If the milk is sterilized, however, then this is not necessary, and you may even use such milk straight from the refrigerator, although it may then take longer. Mix it in a bowl with 1 tablespoon of plain yoghurt, either from a store or from a previous batch, and stand the bowl, covered with a folded towel, in a warm place. The place you choose should have a steady temperature – an airing cupboard, warm radiator or over a pilot light will do perfectly.

To get a low-fat yoghurt, choose skimmed milk and, if you like, thicken it by stirring in 2–3 tablespoons of dried milk powder per pint before heating it to make the yoghurt. Vary the amount of added powder and make it as thick as you wish. You can make yoghurt from reconstituted powder. A controlled yoghurt-maker may help but it is not really necessary. If you do not want to keep your yoghurt going constantly, you can deep-freeze two tablespoonfuls in a plastic container and use it to start off the next batch whenever you like.

Rules of Hygiene

Buy only from clean places. Get the food home clean.

Use clean containers in your home. Use your refrigerator properly. If in doubt, find out.

Keep family foods away from food for pets. Use separate utensils and crockery.

Wash your hands always before preparing food, always after using the lavatory. See your children do too.

Cover cuts and sores with waterproof dressings. If you are not well with no one to take your place in the kitchen, then be extra careful about personal cleanliness.

Keep food clean, covered and either cool or piping hot.

Reheated leftovers must be made really hot right through. Do the same with ready packed foods intended to be eaten hot.

Keep working surfaces clean. Use really hot, soapy water. A wipe with a dish cloth is not enough.

Stack washed and rinsed crockery and pans to drain. If you use drying cloths be sure they are clean.

Keep the lid on the trash can.

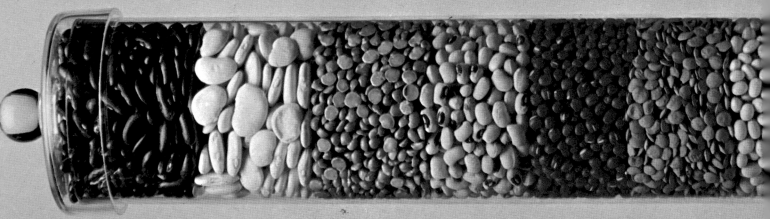

Black beans (frijoles negros).
Handsome, black, shining beans used a great deal in Caribbean cooking. In Cuba they serve them bathed in a mixture of cumin, oregano, onions, red pimentoes and cider vinegar with a hot tomato sauce over the top, or – mixed with rice – as "Moors and Christians." The black beans are the Moors, the Christians the white rice! In China they are equally popular, particularly fermented with salt then cooked with slivers of chicken, ginger, garlic, soy sauce and shallots.

Lima beans can be white or an attractive pale green, and are sometimes smaller than the ones in the photograph. They are greatly prized in American cookery and are used as the British might use haricot beans – for soups, purées and salads – often with sour cream added.

Split green peas. These skinned and split peas are the ones for pease pudding; for dried green pea soup with mint; for purée of peas to serve with a piece of roast pork or glazed ham; or of course for thick Dutch pea soup, afloat with chunks of smoked sausage or frankfurter.

Black-eyed beans (closely related to black-eyed peas) have a delicious, homely, earthy flavor that blends particularly well with spinach, with ham and with garlic. In the Deep South, black-eyed peas are traditionally served with pork and candied sweet potatoes, or with fried ham and red-eyed gravy.

Aduki beans. Known as the Prince of Beans in the Orient, aduki beans are distinctly sweet-flavored and are used in China to make a sweet soup, served in a long glass, like an ice-cream sundae, with grated ice and cream. They are also made into a cream that is something like a chestnut purée, which is used as a filling for wedding cakes.

Brown lentils. These large brown lentils are excellent, robust in flavor, a little floury in texture and a perfect accompaniment to lamb, pork or ham. They soak up oil or butter in large quantities, and are improved by a handful of parsley at the last moment.

Pearl beans or small haricots. These are the original "baked beans," and traditionally cooked with salt pork,

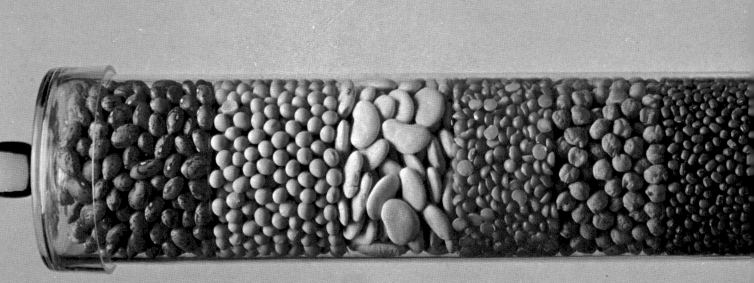

Brown Borlotti beans. Fairly tender beans, useful for making bean soups as they cook to a nice floury, creamy consistency. Can be used to make minestrone or Venetian bean soup – beans cooked with ham bones, onions and cinnamon, with short noodles added towards the end and served with plenty of grated Parmesan. In Piedmont they make a complete meal out of beans cooked all night in the oven, with pieces of bacon and, again, cinnamon. Saluggia beans are very similar but a little smaller.

Soya beans. The most nutritious bean of all, round dried soya beans look more like beans once they have been soaked. ½ cup of soya beans is the protein equivalent of 5oz of steak. They can either be boiled like haricot beans or sprouted like Mung beans. Soya beans provide oil, flour, soya bean curd, soy sauce, and are used extensively in Chinese and Japanese cooking.

Butter beans. These familiar "school" beans have a distinctive flavor and are traditionally served cooked to a soft consistency as a vegetable with roast pork. They are much improved if drained and given a bath of fresh tomato sauce, and flavored with celery towards the end of the cooking.

Split yellow peas are used in Attermed Flask – Swedish yellow-pea soup, flavored with thyme and marjoram, ginger, streaky bacon, onions and cloves. In Sweden it is eaten on Thursdays in memory of King Eric XIV who died on a Thursday in 1577 after his brother had slipped poison into his yellow-pea soup.

Chick peas or garbanzas. Chick peas, which can be as hard as bullets after six hours' cooking, need plenty of soaking (at least 24 hours) and plenty of simmering (at least 3 hours). They are eaten whole as a snack, with beer; made into stews with chicken and saffron; or crushed and mixed with sesame seed paste (tahini), lemon and oil to make houmous.

Mung beans are mainly known as bean sprouts. Soak 6oz of beans overnight in cold water. Drain, and place swollen beans on tray so that air can circulate. Cover beans with wet cloth and keep in a dark place. Rinse beans, tray and cloth with water every morning and evening. In 5 to 6 days you will have

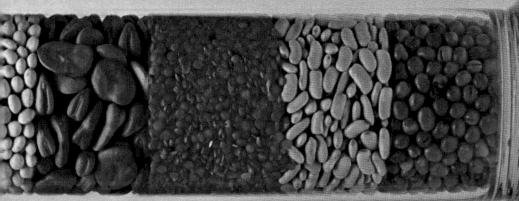

Wonderful world of beans

In Southern India legumes, spiced and fragrant, are an integral part of an essentially meatless diet. In China fermented beans, succulent bean curd and fresh bean sprouts are put on the table at almost every meal. In Brazil, Mexico, Spain and parts of Italy, and all through the Middle East, beans and lentils are a loved and favored food in winter and summer alike, with bean salads a regular feature, while chick peas are daily cooked in stews like meat.

The people of Italy are fond of poor countries add excellent cheap protein and a great deal of variety to their diets when they include these members of the numerous legume family. With a little experimentation, we could add a new dimension to our diet, since legumes provide low-fat protein as well as cutting down on butcher's bills – a little bit of meat goes a long, long way when buried in a large pot of lentils.

Nowadays the legumes we buy, on the whole, are of better quality than they used to be – not so hard, not so dusty, not so full of stones or weevils – and the preparation is very simple. Wash the legumes and put them to soak overnight, then bring slowly to the boil in soft water if it is available, and simmer until tender. Crush one bet-ween finger and thumb, or between the teeth, to test for tenderness. But a quicker way of cooking legumes, saving time all round, is to bring them to the boil slowly, simmer for 5–10 minutes, then remove from the heat and allow to cool for an hour. Now put them back on the stove and cook.

The cooking time will vary greatly according to when the legumes were harvested and how long they have been in store. As a general rule, lentils take an hour, beans one-and-a-half hours or more and chick peas up to three hours or even longer. Legumes need some form of fat – a piece of salt pork or bacon in the pot, a big lump of butter or a generous portion of oil, or even a dollop of cream, which may seem an odd addition to something as homely as lentils or beans, but can make them luxurious and velvety.

The long cooking needed by pulses tends to exhaust the flavorings added at the beginning, so add a little more of the chosen spices and herbs towards the end of the cooking. Most beans are interchangeable, so for any recipe which specifies dried white haricot beans, you can just as easily use red kidney beans, pearl beans or flageolets. The beans or legumes above are among the many now available in America.

---

and are traditionally used in place of white haricots in the making of baked beans. They can be grown and dried successfully in your own garden. Although a dreadful nuisance to shell, they can be kept for months.

Small lentils. These are mauve, but there are also black, white, green, mottled, yellow, pink and orange lentils – over sixty varieties. Lentils are delicious boiled as a vegetable to serve with game or pork. They make a lovely spiced soup with cream and cumin, and take kindly to being curried. They do need fat, though.

Dried white haricot beans (fagioli). These large haricot beans are the sort to eat with a gigot on a Sunday – cook them with garlic and a sprig of rosemary, and crush a few spoonfuls at the end to make a creamy sauce (or add a few spoonfuls of tomato sauce). The juices from the meat provide the necessary moisture.

Red kidney beans. These handsome shiny lacquer-red beans are the ones for chilli con carne and for a hefty Italian bean soup, cooked with garlic and sage. They are also served cooked with tomato sauce, garlic and shredded romaine lettuce, as a vegetable. Mexicans are particularly fond of chillified beans, refried and smothered with grated cheese. In Spain, kidney beans and rice are served in tomato sauce as a filling main course.

Whole green peas. The type used for traditional, mushy green peas, dried peas are a very underestimated food – served with boiled bacon or salt pork they make a most comforting and supportive lunch on a fall day.

---

earthenware pot, sprinkled with brown sugar half an hour before the meal, and allowed to caramelize, uncovered, before serving.

Dried broad beans, either white or brown, are to be found in Greek shops and are probably best bought ready-skinned. They must be well soaked and boiled and can then be served whole, in the Turkish way, as a salad with oil and vinegar, or puréed, sieved and mixed with lemon juice and salt for an *hors d'oeuvre.*

Split lentils. Bright orange or yellowish in color, these are excellent for making dahl to serve with curry, since they cook quickly to a nice, mushy consistency. They are rather dreary, however, without plenty of spice, tasting fairly strongly of sacking. Watch out for small stones, which tend to abound in these lentils to make them weigh more heavily.

Flageolets. Haricots flageolets are a delicate, pale green bean with a more subtle flavor than the ordinary haricot. Cook them to eat with lamb, or make a multi-colored bean salad using red kidney beans, flageolets and ordinary haricots. Flageolets also make a particularly fine, pale green purée which looks very attractive decorated with chopped parsley. Serve it with lamb chops.

Ful Medames (Egyptian brown beans). "Since time immemorial they have faithfully been served in the same manner; seasoned with oil, lemon and garlic, sprinkled with chopped parsley and accompanied by ... hard-boiled eggs, and since time immemorial people have adored them." (Claudia Roden)

Weight Control

ARE YOU TOO FAT?

It is normal for an adult man to have about 10–20 per cent of his bodyweight as fat and for an adult woman to have about 25 per cent fat. To carry a lot more fat than this is unnecessary and is bad for you (see below). Unfortunately, it is impossible for you to measure the actual fat content of your body because this requires expensive equipment, but it is very easy to find out if you are too fat by some indirect methods:

1. Look at yourself naked in a full-length mirror. Can you see large folds of flesh? If so, you are too fat.
2. Use your thumb and first finger to pinch the back of your upper arm, halfway between your shoulder and your elbow. Can you pick up a fold with a total thickness of more than an inch? If so, you are too fat. (Men should also get someone to help them check the skinfold thickness a couple of inches beneath their shoulder blade. A fold thickness of more than an inch here also indicates they are too fat.)

These two methods rely on the fact that a large proportion of your total body fat is found just below your skin. The other methods of deciding whether you are too fat depend on bodyweight. It is unusual for any normal untrained man or woman to change their muscle or bone mass very much during adult life; the only fluctuating component of bodyweight apart from water is body fat. So, provided you have not recently started or stopped intensive sports training, you can assume that a permanent change in your bodyweight reflects a change in your body fat.

The charts printed on page 61 show the best weights for men and women. These are based on the data collected by life insurance companies in America, and represent the weights for each height at which fewest people die. The white line shows the ideal weight for height and the shaded area on each side allows for differences in frame size (there is a 10 per cent allowance from ideal weight on each side). If you find that your weight for your height falls above this shaded area, then you are overweight and, indirectly, you are too fat. Your aim should be to reduce your weight so that it falls within the shaded area.

DOES FATNESS MATTER?

The answer to this question is "yes", for the following reasons:

1. The data collected by life insurance companies has shown that a man or woman who is at least 20 per cent above ideal weight has a greater chance of dying earlier than a normal weight person of the same age. The fatter you are, the likelier you are to die earlier. The same data also shows that if you are fat now, however, you are not necessarily destined for a shorter life. If you reduce your weight to normal, your chances of living longer return to normal too.
2. Fat people are more likely to get certain illnesses, particularly those connected with the heart and blood vessels, and they are particularly prone to diabetes. Also, you might find that the doctor has more difficulty in diagnosing what exactly is wrong with you, because your increased fat hampers a normal examination. Similarly, the

surgeons are not quite as keen to operate on fat people because even an ordinary operation carries a greater than normal risk.
3. Fat people put extra strain on their joints and ligaments, and this often results in them getting arthritis and back pain. They also tend to move more slowly than thin people because of their greater bulk and this means that they get involved in more accidents at home and at work.
4. Fat people suffer, in particular, because of their appearance. They feel less attractive and have difficulty in finding fashionable clothes.

STRATEGIES FOR WEIGHT CONTROL

Diets for reducing weight seem to fall into two categories:

1. Those where you are given lots of information on calorie contents of foods and drinks, and advice on the right calorie limit to set and the right things to choose, and you are then left to devise your own diet. They could be called the *Cut Down* diets.
2. Those where you are given specific advice on what to eat and drink and what *not* to eat and drink. They could be called the *Cut Out* diets.

Research has shown that both types of diet are popular; usually, but not always, the Cut Down diets appeal to women and the Cut Out diets appeal to men. You probably know which appeals to you already. We are going to give you instructions for both types of diet, starting with the Cut Down diet below and then the Cut Out diet on page 66. Even if you know that the Cut Out diet is for you, we advise you to read the Cut Down diet because you should know the basic principles of calorie counting even if you prefer to follow a diet that does not involve any counting or weighing.

THE CUT DOWN METHOD OF WEIGHT CONTROL

Average calorie requirements vary with sex, age and activity, as we show in the diagram on page 65. We must stress here that these figures are only averages and there can be quite a range of calorie requirements even when sex and age are the same. It is very difficult to measure total calorie expenditure directly on a daily basis, and our best estimates come from surveys measuring the energy intake needed to balance output and so maintain a constant weight. This is also your best method of estimating your own calorie output if you are not content to accept the average figure for your age and sex. But you will have to be very careful when you start to work out your calorie input. Everything you eat and drink must be counted, and do not forget that cooking can drastically alter the calorie values of raw foods.

Once you have some idea of your energy output, you must decide on a suitable "energy gap" between your input and output. The size of this gap is your choice, but the chart on page 62 gives you some idea of the rate of weight-loss for different energy gaps. Suppose you consider yourself a fairly inactive 45-year-old woman, and you take the average value of 2,200 calories to be your energy output. If you set yourself an energy gap of 500 calories, this means that your energy input must be 1,700 calories; an energy gap of 700 calories reduces your allowed input to 1,500 calories, and an energy gap of 1,000 calories will limit you to 1,200 calories a day. (Don't ever be tempted to set your calorie limit lower than 800 calories.)

From the chart, you can see that whatever energy gap you set yourself, you will lose more weight in the first week than in any other. This is probably because the first energy reserves that your body calls on when output exceeds input are its starch stores in the muscles. Since these starch stores have quite a lot of water associated with them, you will lose quite a few pounds of water in the first week, as well as a little fat. The amount of water you lose will depend on the size of your starch stores, and this in turn will depend on your previous diet; a diet rich in carbohydrates will fill up the stores. After the first week, it is much easier to predict the rate of weight-loss on a known energy gap because it is known that it takes a total energy gap of 3,500 calories to break down a pound of fat. So seven days on a 500-calorie energy gap will cause a fat-loss of one pound, on a 700-calorie energy gap the fat-loss wil be nearly one-and-a-half pounds, and on a 1,000-calorie energy gap two pounds of fat will be lost.

The lines of weight-loss on the chart are straight because they are based on theoretical calculations and assume that you stick rigidly to your energy gap. Of course, this will certainly not always be the case, but if you try to stick roughly to your energy gap over a matter of weeks you should find that your line of weight-loss will more or less follow the chart line. Gains and losses of water are another thing that will make your actual weight-loss line deviate from the one on the chart. In particular, women might notice a tendency for their weight to "stick" in the week before a period even if they are maintaining their strict energy gap. This is almost certainly due to fluid retention and they will probably get a greater loss than they were expecting in the week after their period.

We have shown the lines on the chart continuing at the same rate of weight loss for twenty weeks. If you need to diet for longer than this, you will probably find that your weight-loss tends to slow up and that your line begins to straighten out. This could be due to the fact that you are being less strict with yourself and that you are now setting a smaller energy gap. If you know that this is the reason, then the remedy is in your own hands. However, there is another reason why your weight-loss rate might slow up, and this is because your body might adapt to the reduced input and automatically reduce its energy output. So the energy gap that you set will get smaller through no fault of your own. By the time this happens (and it won't necessarily happen to you), you should be at least 20 or 30 pounds lighter and, hopefully, you will feel fitter and more active, so that it should be easy to increase your energy output.

If you have a large amount of weight to lose (over fifty pounds, say), it is sometimes a good idea to use the "staircase slimming" method. What you do is to make a definite effort to lose your first ten pounds in a month (by setting a 1,000-calorie energy gap), then aim to maintain this new weight for a month (by eating the number of calories approximately equal to your output), then lose another ten pounds in the next month and so on. This will not only be easier on your nerves (and possibly those around you) but will also allow your skin, which has been stretched by your excess fat, time to shrink back gradually to its original size.

Use the charts on page 61 to help you to decide how much weight you ought to lose. Although it is advisable to get your weight within the shaded portion, it is more impor-

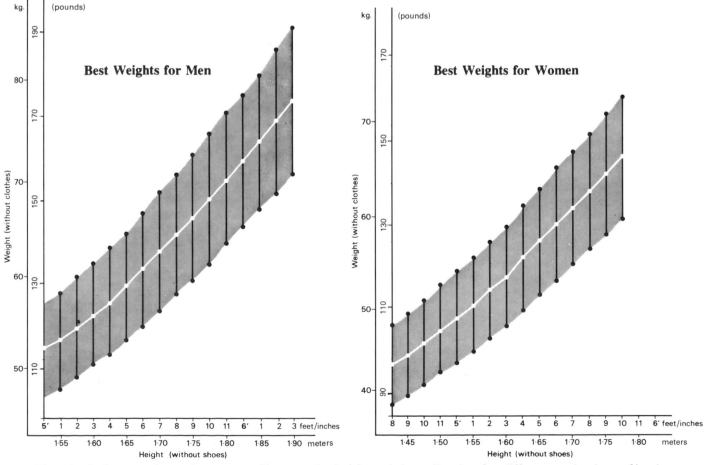

The shaded areas show the range of best or desirable weights, allowing for differences in sizes of body frames – large, average or small – for each height.

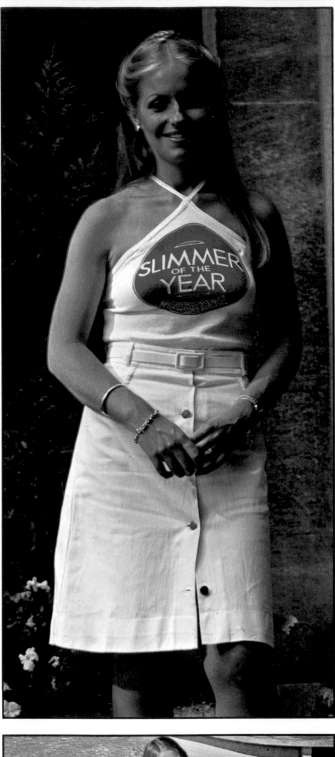

tant that you should maintain whatever weight-loss you achieve. So if you are fifty pounds above your ideal weight, it is far better that you should reduce your weight by twenty-five pounds and keep it there, than lose the complete fifty pounds but not be able to keep it off permanently.

When you have successfully reduced your weight, you will be able to drink and eat more because you will not need to create an energy gap any more. But do not be surprised if you cannot have as much as you could when you were fat: remember that your body needed that much extra fuel in those days when you were expending more energy carrying the extra weight around.

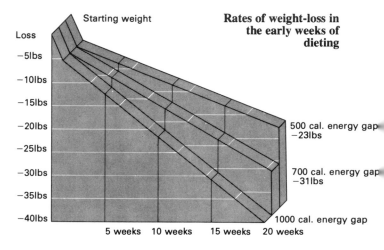

Weight-loss varies according to the 'energy gap' most suitable for you – see text above.

Choosing the Right Calories

As far as calculating fat-losses and gains, all calories are equal and calories from any food or drink which is surplus to your requirements are stored eventually as fat. It follows then that a 1,000-calorie diet of anything will cause a weight-loss because this is bound to create a reasonable energy gap. However, it is particularly important that you should follow the general principles of a healthy diet when you are eating less over-all, and this is why you should try to follow a few rules about the amount of fat, protein and carbohydrate that make up your calorie limit.

For the sake of your long-term health (see pages 34–6) no more than 35 per cent of your total daily calories should come from fat and it is a good idea to apply this principle to your weight-reducing diet. Thus for every 1,000 calories that you allow yourself on your diet, no more than 350 of these calories should come from fat. Since one gram of pure fat contains 9 calories, this restricts the fat in your 1,000-calorie diet to just under 40 grams. To calculate the fat limit in a diet where the calorie limit differs from 1,000 calories, divide your calorie limit by 1,000 and multiply by 40 (e.g., a 1,200-calorie limit will have a fat limit of 48 grams).

In this Cut Down diet we are only going to suggest that you stick to two limits, a calorie limit and a fat limit, because otherwise the counting would get far too complicated. However, do also bear in mind that calories from sugar are "empty calories"; they supply energy and nothing else, and so you should keep your sugar intake low if you want to stay healthy and ward off heart and dental disease.

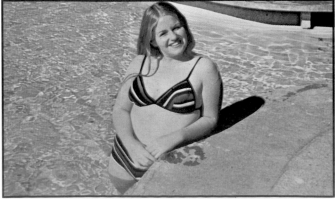

Gail Ingham won a competition after dieting down to 119lb from the 210-lb teenager in the swimming pool.

THE CUT DOWN PLAN – day by day

To show you how the Cut Down plan works out in practice, we have set out plans for seven days which have a 1,000-calorie and a 40-gram fat limit. They have been calculated so that all the breakfasts are about 200 calories, all the snack meals are about 300 calories and all the main meals are about 500 calories. This has been done to allow you to juggle the meals around to suit your fancy: e.g., you can have Day 1 breakfast, followed by Day 4 snack meal, followed by Day 7 main meal. If you are planning your own caloried-counted meals using the chart, then there is no need for you to arrange your calories in this strict fashion. You can have ten small snack meals of 100 calories if you want to: it is up to you to cut down in the way it suits you.

The calorie and fat contents are calculated according to the metric measures and are rounded to the nearest 5 calories and to the nearest 0.1 gram, respectively. All weights are uncooked weights.

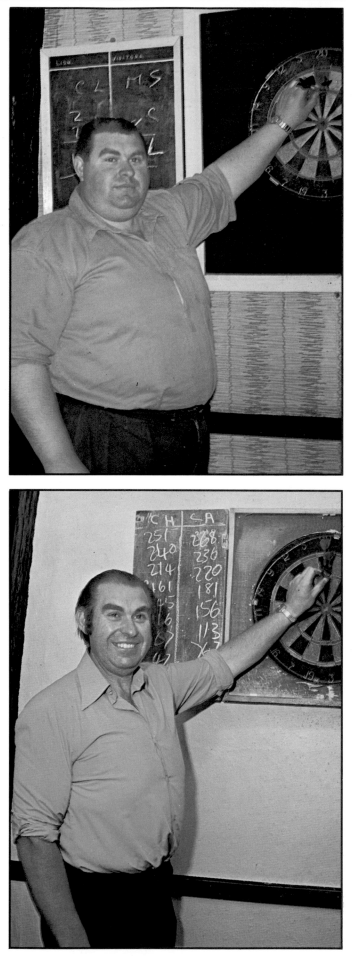

DAY 1

Breakfast	Calories	Fat (g)
25g (1oz) cereal (wholewheat, if possible)	80	1.1
150ml (¼pt) milk	100	5.5
5ml (1 teaspoonful) sweetener (granular)	10	—
	190	6.6
Snack meal		
50g (2oz) wholewheat bread, toasted	115	1.0
10g (½oz) margarine	80	8.5
100g (4oz) baked beans	95	0.4
	290	9.9
Main meal		
100ml (1 glass) of dry wine	70	—
1 portion lamb pie*	360	23.7
100g (4oz) cabbage	10	—
100g (4oz) boiled potatoes	75	—
	505	23.7
Totals	995	40.2

Day 2	Calories	Fat (g)
Breakfast		
1 egg (boiled)	90	6.6
25g (1oz) wholewheat bread	55	0.5
5g (¼oz) margarine	40	4.3
	185	11.4
Snack meal		
50g (2oz) Edam cheese	160	11.5
2 apples (200g)	90	—
	250	11.5
Main meal		
100ml (1 glass) of dry wine	70	—
100g (4oz) chicken piece, broiled	205	10.3
150g (6oz) boiled rice (brown, if possible)	185	0.5
100g (4oz) peas	50	—
125g (5oz) yoghurt, low fat	70	2.3
	580	13.1
Totals	1015	36.0

Handyman Claude Halls at play: from 462lb to 180lb in just 14 months

Day 3	Calories	Fat (g)
Breakfast		
1 grapefruit	30	—
150g (6oz) poached haddock	145	1.2
	175	1.2
Snack meal		
300ml (½pt) beer or cider	95	—
150g (6oz) liver, broiled	215	12.2
100g (4oz) tomatoes, broiled	15	—
100g (4oz) small baked potato	105	—
	430	12.2
Main meal		
300ml (½pt) soup, e.g. tomato	210	9.3
1 portion cauliflower cheese	205	8.9
	415	18.2
Totals	1020	31.6

Day 4	Calories	Fat (g)
Breakfast		
1 egg, poached	90	6.6
25g (1oz) wholewheat bread	55	0.5
5g (¼oz) margarine	40	4.3
	185	11.4
Snack meal		
50g (2oz) shrimps	50	0.9
100g (4oz) cottage cheese	120	0.5
100g (4oz) lettuce	10	—
25g (1oz) whole grain bread	55	0.5
1 orange (100g, 4oz)	40	—
	275	1.9
Main meal		
100ml (1 glass) dry wine	70	—
100g (4oz) small steak, broiled	305	21.6
100g (4oz) sprouts	15	—
1 portion jello with	95	—
1 chopped (100g, 4oz) banana	60	—
	545	21.6
Totals	1030	34.7

Day 5	Calories	Fat (g)
Breakfast		
100g (4oz) baked beans	95	0.4
50g (2oz) wholewheat bread (toasted)	110	1.0
	205	1.4
Snack meal		
75g (3oz) cold lean pork	245	17.8
50g (2oz) boiled potatoes	40	—
	285	17.8
Main meal		
300ml (½pt) beer or cider	95	—
1 portion tomato casserole	165	5.3
100g (4oz) boiled pasta	115	0.6
150g (6oz) stewed apples, sweetened artificially	70	—
125g (5oz) natural yoghurt	70	2.3
	515	8.2
Totals	1005	27.4

Day 6	Calories	Fat (g)
Breakfast		
50g (2oz) wholewheat bread	115	1.0
10g (½oz) margarine	80	8.5
10g (½oz) jam or marmalade	25	—
	220	9.5
Snack meal		
50g (2oz) sardines, drained	150	11.3
25g (1oz) wholewheat bread, toasted	55	0.5
	205	11.8
Main meal		
100ml (1 glass) dry wine	70	—
1 portion kidney casserole*	215	10.6
150g (6oz) cooked rice	180	0.4
1 banana	60	—
1 orange (100g, 4oz)	40	—
	565	11.0
Totals	990	32.3

Day 7	Calories	Fat (g)
Breakfast		
1 portion plain omelette (1 egg)	90	9.3
50g (2oz) wholewheat bread	110	1.0
	200	10.3
Snack meal		
300ml (½pt) soup, e.g. tomato	210	9.3
25g (1oz) wholewheat bread	55	0.5
1 apple (100g, 4oz)	45	—
	310	9.8
Main meal		
1 portion baked, stuffed haddock*	370	5.8
100g (4oz) peas	50	—
100g (4oz) boiled potatoes	75	—
	495	5.8
Totals	1005	25.9

DIETING RECIPES

There is no shortage of detailed recipes for dieters, and we list some of the best books in Appendix 2. But often it is just a question of using common sense in adapting well-known dishes to the slimmer's particular needs. For instance, we kept the calorie count down to 205 per portion in the cauliflower cheese (Day 3) by using skimmed milk or milk made from low-fat milk powder. The stewed apples (Day 5) were sweetened with artificial sweetener – saccharin.

The calorie counts of some other dishes – notably tomato casserole, kidney casserole and lamb pie – could have been reduced further by using a low-calorie margarine rather than a low-saturated-fat margarine which only reduces saturated fat, not calories. We print below detailed recipes for three of the dishes. Do not think that these are the only ways to cook diet versions of these meals. Build upon the principles of diet cookery and use the food fact finder on pages 68–70 to develop your own favorites.

*See recipe opposite

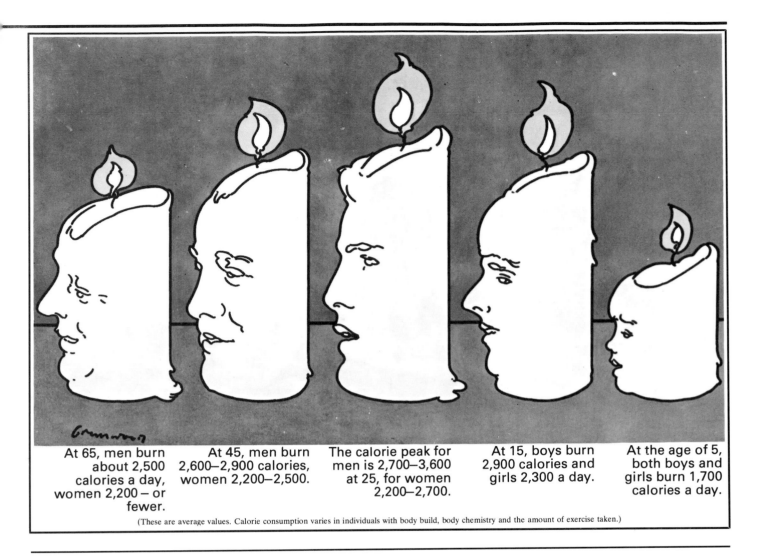

| | | At 65, men burn about 2,500 calories a day, women 2,200 – or fewer. | At 45, men burn 2,600–2,900 calories, women 2,200–2,500. | The calorie peak for men is 2,700–3,600 at 25, for women 2,200–2,700. | At 15, boys burn 2,900 calories and girls 2,300 a day. | At the age of 5, both boys and girls burn 1,700 calories a day. |

(These are average values. Calorie consumption varies in individuals with body build, body chemistry and the amount of exercise taken.)

Lamb pie for four

	Calories	Fat (g)
1 large onion	25	—
1 large carrot	20	—
10g (½oz) margarine	80	8.5
400g (1lb) minced cooked lean lamb	1085	70.0
2 egg yolks	150	13.1
150ml (¼pt) stock	15	—
2 egg whites	30	—
pinch of mixed herbs	—	—
seasoning	—	—
10g (½oz) Parmesan cheese	40	3.0
	1445	94.6

1. Chop onion and carrot finely.
2. Melt the fat and fry meat, onion and carrot in it.
3. Separate the eggs and add the yolks plus stock and herbs to the meat and vegetables.
4. Mix well and cook for a few minutes. Transfer to ovenproof dish.
5. Whisk up egg whites until they are stiff. Add seasoning and spread meringue over meat mixture.
6. Sprinkle Parmesan cheese over top of meringue.
7. Cook in a fairly hot oven (375°F) for about 15 minutes or put under a broiler until the meringue is golden brown.
Calories per portion 360
Fat per portion 23.7g

Kidney casserole for four

	Calories	Fat (g)
25g (1oz) margarine	200	21.3
400g (1lb) of kidney	475	21.2
4 large onions	100	—
300ml (½pt) tomato soup	80	—
seasoning	—	—
chopped parsley	—	—
	855	42.5

1. Melt the fat in a frying pan or large saucepan.
2. Cut the kidneys into bite-sized pieces. Chop onions finely.
3. Toss kidneys very quickly in the melted fat. Add onions.
4. Add soup to pan, bring to boil stirring. Add seasoning to taste.
5. Reduce heat to a simmer, cover pan and continue cooking for 15 minutes.
6. Add the chopped parsley just before serving.
Calories per portion 215
Fat per portion 10.6g

Baked stuffed haddock for four

	Calories	Fat (g)
2 large haddocks (about 1200g or 3lb total)	1165	9.6
200g (½lb) chopped mushrooms	15	—
2 tomatoes, skinned and sliced	20	—
4 small onions, chopped	40	—
25g (1oz) breadcrumbs	60	0.5
1 clove of garlic, crushed	—	—
2 eggs	180	13.1
	1480	23.2

1. Prepare the fish: remove scales, fin, tail and gut the fish if this has not been done already. Wash in cold water and dry on kitchen paper.
2. Prepare the stuffing. Mix mushrooms, tomatoes, onions, breadcrumbs and garlic and bind with the beaten eggs.
3. Fill the cavity of the fish with stuffing and secure with skewers or with needle and thread.
4. Put the fish in an ovenproof dish or wrap in foil, and bake for 30 minutes. (350°F).
5. Garnish with lemon slices and parsley.
Calories per portion 370
Fat per portion 5.8g

THE CUT OUT METHOD OF REDUCING

Unrestricted
Liver, kidney, heart, brain, poultry (not duck), game
White fish and seafood
All green and root vegetables (but see below for potatoes)
All fresh fruit
Cottage or pot cheese
Consommé, and low-calorie soups
Water, black tea and coffee, low-calorie drinks

Go carefully (No more than the indicated helping each day, and no more than 4 items from this category)

Milk	300ml (½pt)
Eggs	1
Margarine	25g (1oz)
Meat	100g (4oz)
Oily fish, (e.g., herring, mackerel, sardines, tuna, salmon)	100g (4oz)
Cheese	100g (4oz)
Breakfast cereals (wholegrain, if possible)	100g (4oz)
Bread (wholewheat, if possible)	2 slices (50g, 2oz)
Alcohol	1 normal measure of beer, wine or spirits
Soups	300ml (½pt)
Rice (brown if possible)	100g (4oz)
Spaghetti or pasta	100g (4oz)
Potatoes	100g (4oz)

Cut out completely
Butter, fats and oils
Cream
Cream cheese
Patés and fatty meats, like salami
Sugar, candy, chocolate
Cakes, pies, pastry, cookies, heavy puddings
Honey, syrup, molasses, jam, marmalade
Fruit canned in syrup, dried fruit
Chips, nuts
Salad cream, mayonnaise, rich creamy soups

Not everybody likes to count calories when they are dieting because it involves quite a lot of accurate weighing and measuring, at least at the beginning. Some dieters would rather sacrifice the flexibility that calorie-counting allows for the simplicity of a system where they divide various foods and drinks into certain categories, and have specific rules which tell them how to treat the items in these categories.

There are three categories in our Cut Out plan, and we have placed items of food and drink into these following the general principles for a healthy diet that we have already outlined in this chapter, i.e., a diet which is low in fat and cholesterol and sugar but which provides sufficient proteins, vitamins, minerals and roughage.

The first category is the one containing the unrestricted foods and drinks. All of them have a low fat and sugar content and contain relatively few calories.

The second category is called "go carefully," because you must limit your over-all intake of these foods as suggested. These foods and drinks are not alarmingly high in fat or sugar when taken in reasonable quantities and they will ensure that you do not go without any important vitamins, minerals or roughage.

The foods and drinks in the third category are the ones you must *cut out* completely. They are the foods which are either very high in fat, or very high in sugar content, or sometimes high in both. Cutting out these items from your diet will do no harm whatsoever, in fact it should improve your health considerably.

It would be very surprising if this diet did not involve a considerable reduction in your calorie intake if you follow it carefully. You should lose weight at roughly one or two pounds a week (more in the first week), and your health will certainly benefit in many ways.

AIDS TO HELP YOU DIET
Appetite-reducing pills. Those you can buy without a prescription from a chemist are useless; those you get on prescription – fenfluramine (Pondimin), phentermine (Fastin), diethyl propion (Tenuate, Tepanil), and mazindol (Sanorex) – can be quite helpful to some people but others find that their side effects reduce their use. The side effects vary from sleepiness to tenseness. It depends on the pill and it depends on the individual; but the side effects are quite minor compared to those of amphetamines such as Dexedrine which may cause dependence and which doctors are increasingly reluctant to prescribe. Doctors vary in their readiness to prescribe appetite-reducing pills because they are relatively ineffective, and useless without dieting.

Burning Up Calories

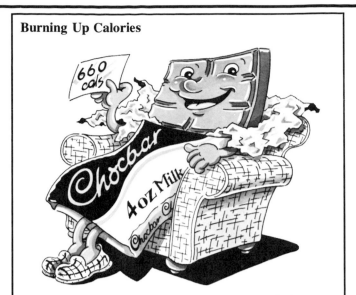

By eating a 4oz. bar of milk chocolate about 660 calories are added to your daily total. If these are in excess of daily requirements, the length of time it takes to burn them off may make you think twice before indulging. If you don't burn off the calories they become body fat – 3oz. per chocolate bar. Exercise will burn off calories – but it takes longer than you think to do so. To indulge in a bar of chocolate and excess calories without gaining extra weight, one of the following activities should be performed for the duration indicated.

Activity	Duration
Walking at 4mph	2 hours 10 minutes
Cycling at 13mph	1 hour
Driving a car	4 hours
Digging the garden	1 hour 20 minutes
Swimming 20 yards a minute	50 minutes
Ironing clothes	2 hours 40 minutes

Substitute meals. You can buy these in cookie form, drink form, or complete meal form. The principle of them all is that they tell you exactly how many calories are in the product, and you count this in your calorie-controlled diet. They can be quite useful to some people, especially those who want a quick snack which does not involve too much cooking. However, there are plenty of other snacks that can be made or bought for the average 300 calories in these products, and you will find that you pay quite a lot extra for the convenience of having a calorie-counted product. Remember that they are meal *substitutes* and not meal *supplements*.

Sweeteners and low-calorie alternatives. The general principle behind these products is that a low-calorie substance is substituted for a high-calorie one. In general, saccharin substitutes for sugar, water substitutes for fat, and air substitutes for starch.

There is a wide range of drinks (mixers, squashes, colas) sweetened with saccharin instead of sugar reducing the calorie content to virtually zero. If you like your tea or coffee sweetened, you can get sweeteners in pellet, powder or granular form. The pellets are calorie-free but the powder and granual sweeteners contain sugar and saccharin so that they are not completely calorie-free (usually one-quarter of the normal value). Eating sweet things is an acquired habit, and it is possible to change your tastes slowly and learn to take your food and drink less sweet. This is a better strategy than using sweeteners because saccharin is under increasing suspicion of being a cause of cancer, albeit a weak one. It is probably quite safe to use it

down, but in the long run you should aim to re-educate your palate to take food and drink which is less sweet.

In low-fat spreads, low-calorie sauces and low-calorie soups, some of the fat content of the parent product has been replaced by water, thus reducing the total calorie content of the product by about half.

Dieters' breads and rolls contain the same number of calories on a weight basis as ordinary bread. However, they are lighter (i.e. contain more air) and so an average slice of dieters' bread contains about half the calories.

The products in the last two categories will appeal to you if you eat bread, butter, etc. by volume. They enable you to eat your normal volume of food for half the calories. Of course, these special low-calorie alternatives might cost you more and you might not like them as much as the real thing. But if you do not have the will power to cut your volume by half, then you will find them useful.

DIET MYTHS

The information and instructions we give you in this chapter should be all you need to lose weight successfully and keep it off. But you are bound to come across other diets in newspapers and magazines or be told about them by your well-meaning friends. Beware of these myths.

Diets which restrict fluids. There are no calories in water and virtually none in artificially sweetened drinks, black tea and coffee. Provided you have normally functioning kidneys, your body will get rid of all the surplus fluid, so you can drink as much of these as you like. Severe fluid restriction could lead to chronic dehydration with some serious consequences.

Diets which tell you to overdrink. It is true that one of the reasons for an adequate water intake is to help remove waste products from the body. But it is *not* true that drinking a lot of water will actively cause breakdown of fat and speed its removal from the body. And drinking water before or after meals will make no difference to the calories you absorb from the meal.

Grapefruit and lemon diets. Grapefruit and lemon are low-calorie fruits and are therefore useful for dieters. But there is no scientific evidence to suggest that they can speed up the conversion of fat to energy.

Diets where you can eat as much as you like. Some low-carbohydrate diets are worded very badly and give the impression that any food not containing carbohydrate can be eaten *ad lib* without making you fat. See page 66 for the Cut Out plan, which is a low-fat, low-carbohydrate plan which *will* work.

Diets which claim that eating fat burns up fat. The only way in which fat is burnt up is when your diet creates a calorie deficit and body fat is needed as a fuel. Dietary fat has no magical, direct effect on body fat. If you eat more fat, you will get fatter unless you eat a lot less of other things.

YOU ARE WHAT YOU EAT:
The Low-Down on High-Risk Food

On the following pages we give the all-important percentages of fat in various foods, as well as protein, calories and carbohydrate; the remaining percentage is usually water. You can calculate the *type* of fat you are eating by referring to the table on page 40. Check your daily calorie intake against the recommended totals on pages 63–5 and measure the precise proportions of fat, protein and carbohydrate in your diet.

Food	Food energy (cals)	Protein (g)	Fat (g)	Carbohydrate (g)
Almonds, dried	598	18.6	54.2	19.5
Apples, fresh, not pared	56	0.2	0.6	14.1
Apple juice, canned or bottled	47	0.1	trace	11.9
Apricots, raw	51	1.0	0.2	12.8
Avocados, raw, average all varieties	167	2.1	16.4	6.3
Bacon, cured, raw	665	8.4	69.3	1.0
cured, cooked and drained	611	30.4	52.0	3.2
Bananas, fresh	85	1.1	0.2	22.2
Barley, pearled, light	349	8.2	1.0	78.8
Bass, black sea, raw	93	19.2	1.2	0.0
Beans, common, mature, white, raw	340	22.3	1.6	61.3
common, mature, white, cooked	118	7.8	0.6	21.2
common, mature, red, raw	343	22.5	1.5	61.9
common, mature, red, cooked	118	7.8	0.5	21.4
Pinto, calico, and red Mexican, raw	349	22.9	1.2	63.7
lima, raw	123	8.4	0.5	22.1
mung, sprouted seeds, uncooked	35	3.8	0.2	6.6
Beef:				
Carcass, total edible, trimmed to retail level, raw:				
Choice grade (75% lean, 25% fat)	301	17.4	25.1	0.0
Good grade (78% lean, 22% fat)	263	18.5	20.4	0.0
Standard grade (82% lean, 18% fat)	225	19.4	15.8	0.0
Retail cuts, trimmed:				
Chuck, choice grade, total edible, raw	257	18.7	19.6	0.0
Chuck, choice grade, total edible, cooked	327	26.0	23.9	0.0
Chuck, choice, separable lean, raw	158	21.3	7.4	0.0
Chuck, choice, separable lean, cooked	214	30.0	9.5	0.0
Hindshank, choice, separable lean, raw	134	21.7	4.6	0.0
Loin, Porterhouse, choice, separable lean, raw	162	21.1	8.2	0.0
Loin, T-bone, choice, separable lean, raw	164	21.2	8.1	0.0
Loin, Club, choice, separable lean, raw	182	20.8	10.3	0.0
Sirloin, round-bone, choice, separable lean, raw	143	21.5	5.7	0.0
Rib, choice, separable lean, raw	193	20.7	11.6	0.0
Round, choice, separable lean, raw	135	21.6	4.7	0.0
Rump, choice, separable lean, raw	158	21.2	7.5	0.0
Hamburger (ground beef), lean raw	179	20.7	10.0	0.0
Hamburger (ground beef), regular, raw	268	17.9	21.2	0.0
Beef, corned, medium fat, canned	216	25.3	12.0	0.0
Beets, common, red, raw	43	1.6	0.1	9.9
Beverages:				
Alcoholic				
Beer (3.6% alcohol by weight)	42	0.3	0.0	3.8
Gin, rum, vodka, whisky:				
80-proof (33.4% alcohol by weight)	231	—	—	trace
90-proof (37.9% alcohol by weight)	263	—	—	trace
100-proof (42.5% alcohol by weight)	295	—	—	trace
Wines				
Dessert (15.3% alcohol by weight)	137	0.1	0.0	7.7
Table (9.9% alcohol by weight)	85	0.1	0.	4.2
Carbonated, sweetened sodas	31	0.0	0.0	8.0
Cola type	39	0.0	0.0	10.0
Cream sodas	43	0.0	0.0	11.0
Fruit flavored sodas	46	0.0	0.0	12.0
Ginger ale	31	0.0	0.0	8.0
Root beer	41	0.0	0.0	10.5
Biscuits, from home recipe	369	7.4	17.0	45.8
Blueberries, raw	62	0.7	0.5	15.3
Bouillon, cubes or powder	120	20	3.0	5.0
Brains, all kinds, raw	125	10.4	8.6	0.8
Bran flakes (40% bran)	303	10.2	1.8	80.6
Breads:				
Cracked wheat	263	8.7	2.2	52.1
French or vienna	290	9.1	3.0	55.4
Italian	276	9.1	3.0	55.4
Rye, American ($\frac{1}{3}$ rye, $\frac{2}{3}$ clear flour)	293	9.1	1.1	52.1
White made with 3–4% non-fat dry milk	270	8.7	3.2	50.5
Wholewheat made with 2% non-fat dry milk	243	10.5	3.0	47.7
Wholewheat made with water	241	9.1	2.6	49.3
Broad beans, raw, mature seeds, dry	338	25.1	1.7	58.2
Broccoli, raw spears	32	3.6	0.3	5.9
Brussels sprouts, raw	45	4.9	0.4	8.3
Buckwheat, whole grain	335	11.7	2.4	72.9
Butter, salted	716	0.6	81.0	0.4
Buttermilk, fluid, cultured from skim milk	36	3.6	0.1	5.1
Cabbage, raw	24	1.3	0.2	5.4
Cakes, baked from home recipes:				
Angel food	269	7.1	0.2	60.2
Chocolate (devil's food). without icing	366	4.8	17.2	52.0
Plain cake or cupcake, without icing	364	4.5	13.9	55.9
Sponge	297	7.6	5.7	54.1
Candy:				
Caramels, plain or chocolate	399	4.0	10.2	76.6
Chocolate, milk	520	7.7	32.3	56.9
Hard	386	0.0	1.1	97.2
Peanut bars	515	17.5	32.2	47.2
Carrots, raw	42	1.1	0.2	9.7
Cauliflower, raw	27	2.7	0.2	5.2
Celery, raw	17	0.9	0.1	3.9
Cheeses:				
Blue or Roquefort type	368	21.5	30.5	2.0
Camembert (domestic)	299	17.5	24.7	1.8
Cheddar (commonly called American)	398	25.0	32.2	2.1
Cottage, uncreamed	86	17.0	0.3	2.7
Cream	374	8.0	37.7	2.1
Parmesan	393	36.0	26.0	2.9
Pasteurized processed, American	370	23.2	30.0	1.9
Cherries, raw, sweet	70	1.3	0.3	17.4
Chestnuts, fresh	194	2.9	1.5	42.1
Chicken:				
Light meat without skin, raw	117	23.4	1.9	0.0
Light meat without skin, roasted	166	31.6	3.4	0.0
Dark meat without skin, raw	130	20.6	4.7	0.0

COMPOSITION OF FOODS taken from Agriculture Handbook Number 8, US Department of Agriculture 1975.
Table gives the quantity of food energy in calories, protein, fat, and carbohydrate in a 100 gram (3.5oz approx.) edible portion.

Food	Food energy (cals)	Protein (g)	Fat (g)	Carbohydrate (g)
Dark meat without skin, roasted	176	28.0	6.3	0.0
Chick peas (garbanzas), mature seeds, dry, raw	360	20.5	4.8	61.0
Clams, raw, soft, meat only	82	14.0	1.9	1.3
Cocoa, dry power, low medium fat	220	19.2	12.7	53.8
Cod, raw	78	17.6	0.3	0.0
Coffee, beverage	1	trace	trace	trace
Coleslaw made with French dressing	129	1.1	12.3	5.1
Coleslaw with mayonnaise	144	1.3	14.0	4.8
Cookies:				
Assorted, packaged, commercial	480	5.1	20.2	71.0
Brownies with nuts, home recipe	485	6.5	31.3	50.9
Chocolate chip, commercial type	471	5.4	21.0	69.7
Fig bars	358	3.9	5.6	75.4
Corn, sweet, raw, white and yellow	96	3.5	1.0	22.1
kernels cooked on cob	91	3.3	1.0	21.0
Corn flour	368	7.8	2.6	76.8
Corn fritters	377	7.8	21.5	39.7
Corn grits, cooked	51	1.2	0.1	11.0
Corn flakes	386	7.9	0.4	85.3
Corn flakes, sugar-covered	386	4.4	0.2	91.3
Cornbread from home recipes:				
Corn pone made with white, wholeground meal	204	4.5	5.3	36.2
Southern style made with wholeground meal	207	7.4	7.2	29.1
Spoonbread made with white, wholeground meal	195	6.7	11.4	16.9
Cornmeal, wholeground	355	9.2	3.9	73.7
degermed, dry	364	7.9	1.2	78.4
Cornstarch	362	0.3	trace	87.6
Cowpeas (blackeye peas), mature seeds, dry, raw	343	22.8	1.5	61.7
Crab, steamed	93	17.3	1.9	0.5
Crackers, butter	458	7.0	17.8	67.3
saltines	433	9.0	12.0	71.5
soda	439	9.2	13.1	70.6
wholewheat	403	8.4	13.8	68.2
Cream, half-and-half	134	3.2	11.7	4.6
light, coffee, or table	211	3.0	20.6	4.3
light whipping	300	2.5	31.3	3.6
Cucumbers, raw, not pared	15	0.9	0.1	3.4
Dates, domestic, natural and dry	274	2.2	0.5	72.9
Doughnuts, cake type	391	4.6	18.6	51.4
yeast-leavened	414	6.3	26.7	37.7
Duck, domesticated, raw, flesh only	165	21.4	8.2	0.0
domesticated, raw, total, edible	326	16.0	28.6	0.0
Eggs, raw, whole	163	12.9	11.5	0.9
raw, whites	51	10.9	trace	0.8
raw, yolks	348	16.0	30.6	0.6
Eggplant, raw	25	1.2	0.2	5.6
Farina, regular, dry	371	11.4	0.9	77.0
regular, cooked	42	1.3	0.1	8.7
Fats, cooking (vegetable)	884	0.0	100.0	0.0
Figs, raw	80	1.2	0.3	20.3
sirup pack, light	65	0.5	0.2	16.8
Fish cakes, fried	172	14.7	8.0	9.3
Flatfishes (flounders, soles, and sanddabs), raw	79	16.7	0.8	0.0
Grapefruit, all varieties	41	0.5	0.1	10.6
Grapes, raw, American type	69	1.3	1.0	15.7
Haddock, raw	79	18.3	0.1	0.0
Halibut, Atlantic and Pacific, raw	100	20.9	1.2	0.0
Heart, beef, lean, raw	108	17.1	3.6	0.7
Ice cream and frozen custard, regular, approx. 12% fat	207	4.0	12.5	20.6
Jams and preserves	272	0.6	0.1	70.0
Kidneys, beef, raw	130	15.4	6.7	0.9
Lake trout (siscowet), raw, less than 6.5lb, round weight	241	14.3	19.9	0.0
Lamb:				
Composite of cuts trimmed to retail level:				
Prime grade (72% lean, 28% fat), raw	310	15.4	27.1	0.0
Choice grade (77% lean, 23% fat), raw	263	16.5	21.3	0.0
Good grade (79% lean, 21% fat), raw	247	16.8	19.4	0.0
Retail cuts, trimmed:				
Leg, choice, separable lean, raw	130	19.9	5.0	0.0
Rib, choice, separable lean, raw	158	19.3	8.4	0.0
Shoulder, choice, separable lean, raw	148	18.5	7.7	0.0
Lemons, raw, peeled fruit	27	1.1	0.3	8.2
Lentils, mature seeds, dry, raw	340	24.7	1.1	60.1
Lettuce, raw, Cos or romaine	18	1.3	0.3	3.5
raw, crispbread varieties such as Iceberg	13	0.9	0.1	2.9
Liver, beef, raw	140	19.9	3.8	5.3
beef, fried	229	26.4	10.6	5.3
Lobster, northern, canned or cooked	95	18.7	1.5	0.3
Macaroni, dry	369	12.5	1.2	75.2
cooked, firm stage (8–10 mins)	148	5.0	0.5	30.1
Mackerel, raw	191	19.0	12.2	0.0
Margarine	720	0.6	81.0	0.4
Milk, cow, 3.7% fat	66	3.5	3.7	4.9
cow, skim	36	3.6	0.1	5.1
human, US samples	77	1.1	4.0	9.5
Molasses, cane, medium	232	—	—	60.0
Muffins from home recipes, plain	294	7.8	10.1	42.3
Mushrooms (agaricus campestris, commercial) raw	28	2.7	0.3	4.4
Muskmelons, raw	30	0.7	0.1	7.5
Mussels, Atlantic and Pacific, raw, meat only	95	14.4	2.2	3.3
Noodles, egg, dry	388	12.8	4.6	72.0
egg, cooked	125	4.1	1.5	23.3
Oatmeal breakfast cereal, dry	390	14.2	7.4	68.2
cooked	55	2.0	1.0	9.7
Oils, salad or cooking	884	0.0	100.0	0.0
Onions, mature, raw	38	1.5	0.1	8.7
Oranges, raw, peeled fruit, all varieties	49	0.1	0.2	12.2
Orange juice, raw, all varieties	45	0.7	0.2	10.4
Oysters, raw, meat only, Eastern	66	8.4	1.8	3.4
Pancakes from home recipe	231	7.1	7.0	34.1
Parsnips, raw	76	1.7	0.5	17.5
Peaches, raw	38	0.6	0.1	9.7
Peanuts, raw with skins	564	26.0	47.5	18.6
roasted and salted	585	26.0	49.8	18.8

	Food energy (cals)	Protein (g)	Fat (g)	Carbohydrate (g)
Peanut butter made with small amount of added fat, sweetener	582	25.5	49.5	19.5
Pears, raw, including skin	61	0.7	0.4	15.3
Peas, green, immature, raw	84	6.3	0.4	14.4
mature seeds, dry, raw	340	24.1	1.3	60.3
mature, split, cooked	115	8.0	0.3	20.8
Peppers, sweet, raw	22	1.2	0.2	4.8
Pies, baked, apple	256	2.2	11.1	38.1
baked, butterscotch	267	4.4	11.0	38.3
baked, cherry	261	2.6	11.3	38.4
baked, lemon meringue	255	3.7	10.2	37.7
Piecrust, plain pastry, baked	500	6.1	33.4	43.8
Pineapple, raw	52	0.4	0.2	13.7
Pizza with cheese from home recipe, baked	236	12.0	8.3	28.3
Plums, raw, Japanese and hybrid	48	0.5	0.2	12.3
raw, prune type	75	0.8	0.2	19.7
Popcorn, sugar-coated	383	6.1	3.5	85.4
Pork:				
Composite cuts, medium fat, separable lean, raw	174	19.1	10.2	0.0
Composite cuts, medium fat, separable lean, roasted	236	28.0	12.9	0.0
Ham cut, medium fat, separable lean, raw	153	20.0	7.5	0.0
Ham cut, medium fat, separable lean, roasted	217	29.7	10.0	0.0
Loin, medium fat, separable lean, raw	189	20.1	11.4	0.0
Loin, medium fat, separable lean, roasted	254	29.4	14.2	0.0
Spareribs, medium fat, total edible, raw	361	14.5	33.2	0.0
Spareribs, medium fat, total edible, braised	440	20.8	38.9	0.0
Cured ham, separable lean, raw	168	21.5	8.5	0.0
Cured ham, separable lean, roasted	187	25.3	8.8	0.0
Potatoes, raw	76	2.1	0.1	17.1
pared, boiled	65	1.9	0.1	14.5
French-fried	274	4.3	13.2	36.0
hash-browned held overnight	229	3.1	11.7	29.1
Potato chips	568	5.3	39.8	50.0
Potato salad, from home recipe made with mayonnaise, French dressing, eggs	145	3.0	9.2	13.4
Pretzels	390	9.8	4.5	75.9
Prunes, cooked without added sugar	119	1.0	0.3	31.4
Pumpkin, raw	26	1.0	0.1	6.5
Raisins, uncooked	289	2.5	0.2	77.4
Rice, brown, raw	360	7.5	1.9	77.4
brown, cooked	119	2.5	0.6	25.5
white, common varieties, raw	363	6.7	0.4	80.4
white, common varieties, cooked	109	2.0	0.1	24.2
Rice, puffed	399	6.0	0.4	89.5
Rolls, hard	312	9.8	3.2	59.5
sweet	316	8.5	9.1	49.3
Rye flour, medium	350	11.4	1.7	74.8
Salad dressing:				
French, regular	410	0.6	38.9	17.5
Italian, regular	552	0.2	60.0	6.9
mayonnaise	718	1.1	79.9	2.2
mayonnaise type	435	1.0	42.3	14.4
Roquefort type, regular	504	4.8	52.3	7.4
Russian	494	1.6	50.8	10.4
Thousand Island, regular	502	0.8	50.2	15.4
Salmon (Atlantic), raw	217	22.5	13.4	0.0
canned	203	21.7	12.2	0.0
Sardines, drained solids	203	24.0	11.1	—
Sauerkraut, canned, solids and liquid	18	1.0	0.2	4.0
Sausage:				
Blood types	394	14.1	36.9	0.3
Bockwurst	264	11.3	23.7	0.6
Bologna (average type)	304	12.1	27.5	1.1
Braunschweiger	319	14.8	27.4	2.3
Brown and serve, browned	422	16.5	37.8	2.8
Frankfurters, cooked	304	12.4	27.2	1.6
Luncheon meat (boiled ham)	234	19.0	17.0	0.0
Mortadella	315	20.4	25.0	0.6
Pork, cooked	476	18.1	44.2	trace
Salami, dry	450	23.8	38.1	1.2
Sesame seeds, dry, whole	563	18.6	49.1	21.6
Sherbet, orange	134	0.9	1.2	30.8
Shrimp, raw	91	18.1	0.8	1.5
Sirup, cane	263	0.0	0.0	68.0
Sirup, Maple	252	—	—	65.0
Soup, canned, cream of chicken	39	1.2	2.4	3.3
canned, tomato	36	0.8	1.0	6.4
Soybeans, mature seeds, dry, raw	403	34.1	17.7	33.5
Soybeans, mature seeds, cooked	130	11.0	5.7	10.8
Spaghetti, dry	369	12.5	1.2	75.2
cooked "al dente"	148	5.0	0.5	30.1
Spinach, cooked, boiled, drained	23	3.0	0.3	3.6
Squash, summer, all varieties, raw	19	1.1	0.1	4.2
all varieties, boiled, drained	14	0.9	0.1	3.1
Sweet potatoes, all varieties, raw	114	1.7	0.4	26.3
Sweet potatoes, boiled in skin	114	1.7	0.4	26.3
Tapioca, dry	352	0.6	0.2	86.4
Tea, beverage	2	—	trace	0.4
Tomatoes, ripe, raw	22	1.1	0.2	4.7
Tomato juice, canned or bottled, regular	19	0.9	0.1	4.3
Tongue, beef, raw	207	16.4	15.0	0.4
braised	244	21.5	16.7	0.4
Tuna, canned in oil, drained solids	197	28.8	8.2	0.0
canned in water, solids and liquid	127	28.0	0.8	0.0
Turkey flesh without skin, raw	162	24.0	6.6	0.0
flesh without skin, roasted	190	31.5	6.1	0.0
Turnips, raw	30	1.0	0.2	6.6
boiled, drained	23	0.8	0.2	4.9
Venison, lean meat only, raw	126	21	4.0	0.0
Waffles from home recipe	279	9.3	9.8	37.5
Watermelon, raw	26	0.5	0.2	6.4
Wheat flour, whole (from hard wheats)	333	13.3	2.0	71.0
80% extraction, hard wheat	365	12.0	1.3	74.1
patent bread flour	365	11.8	1.1	74.7
patent cake or pastry flour	364	7.5	0.8	79.4
Wheat bran, commercially milled	213	16.0	4.6	61.9
Wheat and malted barley breakfast cereal instant cooking, dry	382	14.0	1.6	76.2
Wheat flakes, breakfast cereal	354	10.2	1.6	80.5
Wheat, puffed, breakfast cereal	363	15.0	1.5	78.5
Wild rice, raw	353	14.1	0.7	75.3
Yoghurt made from whole milk	62	3.0	3.4	4.9
made from partially skimmed milk	50	3.4	1.7	5.2

THE COMMON EXCUSES FOR FATNESS: HOW MUCH WEIGHT DO THEY CARRY?

Glands, metabolism and inheritance. Some of the common excuses made by a fat person run along the lines of "it's my glands", "it's my metabolism" or "it runs in my family". These excuses can all be considered together because they might all contribute partly to the fatness of some people (but not necessarily those who use them as an excuse).

Obesity due solely to the malfunctioning of one particular endocrine gland is very rare, probably accounting for one only in ten thousand cases. It has been said that the only glands which are not working properly in a fat person are the salivary glands, which work too well! This is probably a little unfair because some studies of over-all eating patterns have shown that fat people eat no more than thin people.

"Metabolism" is a very general term to describe the way in which food is turned into energy by the body, and studies of metabolic rate have indeed revealed vast differences between individuals, so that the amount of food they can eat without getting fat will also vary greatly. It has also been shown that individuals vary in their response to over eating. Some (the "easy-gainers") will gain the theoretically calculated amount of weight when they are overfed while others (the "hard-gainers") will gain less than predicted. Exactly why this happens is not known yet.

The fact that obesity runs in families is a well-documented one. However, it is so difficult to separate nature from nurture that it is difficult to say how valid an excuse it is. The studies of twins and adopted children which are usually undertaken to resolve this nature-nurture conflict give confusing results, although there is a definite indication that some genetic factor plays a part.

In summary, it seems that some people do have a genetically inherited tendency to fatness which manifests itself in metabolic changes. However, there is nothing to stop those with a tendency to fatness overcoming it, even though the task for them might be harder than it is for others.

Childhood obesity. Recently, scientists have been particularly interested in classifying fat people according to the age of onset of their obesity. This followed some reports in the early 1970s that the child-onset obese had more fat cells than the adult-onset obese, and it was inferred by others that the child-onset obese would have greater problems with slimming as adults. The publicity given to their theory, while being useful in the prevention of infantile and childhood obesity, has been harmful in another way: being fat as a child has become quite a common excuse for adults who cannot lose weight easily. There is now doubt if this excuse is valid because (a) it has never been shown that the child-onset obese cannot lose weight and (b) further research has cast doubts on the original fat-cell theory.

Baby fat. The term "baby fat" is used by some teenagers and their parents to describe increased fatness during adolescent years. It is true that the changes in sex hormones during these years will lead to an increase in body fat in girls in particular, but any overeating during this time will lead to surplus body fat and this cannot be blamed on the hormones.

Getting fat on the pill. Some women complain that they managed to maintain a reasonable weight until they went on the pill. Unfortunately, there is no large-scale survey which can validate this claim: usually, average weight changes on different pills are given as zero because an equal number of women lose weight on the pill as those that gain it. However, it is known that certain pills cause some fluid retention in some women and this could cause a weight-gain of up to 7lb (3kg). If a weight-gain on the pill is due to fluid retention it will be fairly obvious as soon as the pill is withdrawn because the weight will drop very quickly. A change to a pill with a different hormonal composition will often be the solution to the problem.

Getting fat during pregnancy. A lot of women will say that having children was their downfall as far as weight was concerned. Here again, it is impossible to separate the physiological factors associated with pregnancy with the changes in lifestyle that usually accompany pregnancy and the subsequent caring for children. A sensible weight-gain during pregnancy is between 22 and 28lb (9.5 and 12.5kg). A weight-gain above the maximum limit will almost certainly mean that the mother has added too much of her own fat-stores. Although it has never been shown that extra fat gained during pregnancy is different from normal fat, or that the mother's metabolism alters appreciably, some women find that they never lose this extra fat. Mothers who have a second child soon after the first might find it particularly difficult to lose the fat without a positive effort, because they lose track of what it was like to have a normal figure (see Chapter 1 for advice on diet during pregnancy).

Giving up smoking. It is true that a lot of people do put on weight when they stop smoking. A recent American survey showed that men who had given up smoking during a certain five-year period had gained much more weight on average than men who continued to smoke. However, this only shows an average trend and does not indicate that a weight-gain is a biological certainty. There is no evidence that smoking alters your metabolism by an appreciable amount, and those who do gain weight are often very willing to admit that they do eat more when they stop smoking, probably because they feel the need to have something in their mouth all the time. If this is your problem, try chewing low-calorie gum. It is generally agreed that smoking is a greater health risk than obesity, so it is worth making the effort to give up smoking.

Middle-aged spread. The average weight of both men and women increases with age although there is no physiological reason why it should do so. More often than not, surplus fat accumulates gradually with age because of a gradual decline in physical activity coupled perhaps with an increase in food and drink consumption. Small changes in your lifestyle, such as taking the elevator instead of walking up the stairs each time, can make quite a difference in the long term.

LOSING WEIGHT WITHOUT DIETING

It is the eternal hope of every fat person that someone, someday, will invent a method of reducing which does not involve a diet. Unfortunately, this has not happened yet although some clever ads would have you believe it! Real weight-loss means the breakdown of fat and this is only achieved physiologically by creating an energy gap between your input and your output. No amount of mechanical rubbing with massages and creams or vibrator belts will do any good whatsoever.

If you include the loss of water in your definition of weight-loss, then you could say that sauna baths, Turkish baths and sweat garments are effective. But water loss is only temporary and any weight-loss you might see will disappear as soon as you eat and drink.

It is possible to improve your shape without losing fat if you do something to tighten up certain muscles. You can buy expensive electric muscle stimulators to do this (or go to clinics to use them) but they are really only effective with long-term continual use. A better way of losing inches in certain areas (as opposed to losing fat) is to do some exercises which are specific to certain muscle groups in your body.

EXERCISE AND WEIGHT-LOSS

We have already stressed how you must create an energy gap for yourself if you want to get rid of fat, and so far we have concentrated on telling you how to decrease your energy input. You can also create this energy gap by increasing your energy output, i.e., doing more exercise. This alone is rather a slow way of losing weight but if you combine it with dieting, you will not only get slim quicker but you will feel much fitter as you do it, and you will end up with a better figure. See the next chapter for a full discussion of exercise, but whichever method you decide to use, remember that for any exercise to be effective in weight reduction it must be:

1. *reasonably vigorous*, so that it uses up more energy than just resting.
2. *sensible for your age and ability*, so that you don't overdo things and injure yourself.
3. *enjoyable*, so you don't resent it.
4. *regular*, so that it makes a worthwhile contribution to your energy gap.

There are two main ways in which you can increase your energy output:

A. You can arrange to get more natural exercise, e.g. walking rather than driving, or climbing stairs rather than using the elevator. Just ten minutes a day of walking or climbing stairs will increase your energy output by about 300 calories in a week and this could get rid of 3lb of fat in a year.

B. You can increase the amount of specific exercise that you do. This does not have to involve other people and organized sports. You can see from the chart that an hour's standard walking by yourself will do you as much good as an hour spent playing hockey or tennis. The chart gives you a rough idea of the energy values associated with different types of exercise. They cannot be more accurate because people vary in the amount of energy they use for the same task according to their sex, their size, their physical fitness and the effort they use. The values given are for an hour's activity in each case to make comparison easy, but this does not mean that you must do an hour of the activity – as little as half an hour's exercise is helpful if you do it regularly.

DO BE SENSIBLE

It is possible to become obsessive about dieting. The condition known as anorexia nervosa is becoming increasingly common in teenage girls and young women. Sufferers from this condition go to all lengths to avoid eating and endanger their health in so doing. Do make certain that you know not only when to start but also when to stop! If you have a child who is seriously underweight and does not eat normally, take the child to your doctor.

HOW EXERCISE CAN HELP

Level*	Walking	Running	Sports and Games
Level A			
(about 175 cals per hr)	Ambling, strolling (1½–2½ mph)	—	archery, pool, lawn bowling, croquet, golf, rifle-shooting, sailing, table tennis
Level B			
(about 270 cals per hr)	Slow, easy walking (2½–3½ mph)	—	badminton, bowling, canoeing, dancing, diving, rowing, softball/baseball, surfing
Level C			
(about 355 cals per hr)	Standard walking (3½–4 mph)	gentle jogging (3–5 mph)	basketball, bowling (cricket), cycling, fencing, gymnastics, hockey, judo, karate, lacrosse, orienteering, hiking, skating, sub aqua swimming, tennis, trampolining
Level D			
(about 435 cals per hr)	Brisk striding walk (4–5 mph)	Slow running (5–6 mph)	climbing, soccer, skiing, swimming
Level E			
(about 740 cals per hr)	Sprint walking (6–7 mph)	Standard running (7–8 mph)	boxing, handball, football, squash, water polo, wrestling

*NB: Remember that you would use up approximately 60 calories if you rest for an hour. All these figures include this value for resting metabolism.

The human hump

It is not only the weight of the body that changes as we accumulate or lose fat. The shape of our body changes too — as the diagrams below illustrate. The numbers indicate the danger points where excess fat first reveals itself.

Accumulation of fat is the result of eating more food than the body needs for its daily expenditure of energy. Thus fat represents the body's main reserve of available energy. The body of a healthy adult man varies between 10 and 20 per cent of his total bodyweight. It tends to increase with age. Healthy adult women carry more fat — about 25 per cent — although this also increases with age. Not only do women have a thicker layer of fat under the skin than men, it tends to be concentrated around certain areas, notably the breasts, buttocks and legs.

The body's fat pads are numbered on the pair of figures on the left. The "middle-age spread" on the pair on the right results from an increase in the thickness of the fat layers in these pads.

This table gives, in millimeters, the desirable average thickness of fat for each pad.

Fat pad	Man	Woman
1 Shoulder	18	18
2 Outside arm	4	6
3 Inside arm	4	7
4 Hip	19	19
5 Top of thigh	16	28
6 Outside leg	5	7
7 Inside leg	6	11
8 Front of leg	3	4
9 Back of leg	7	13

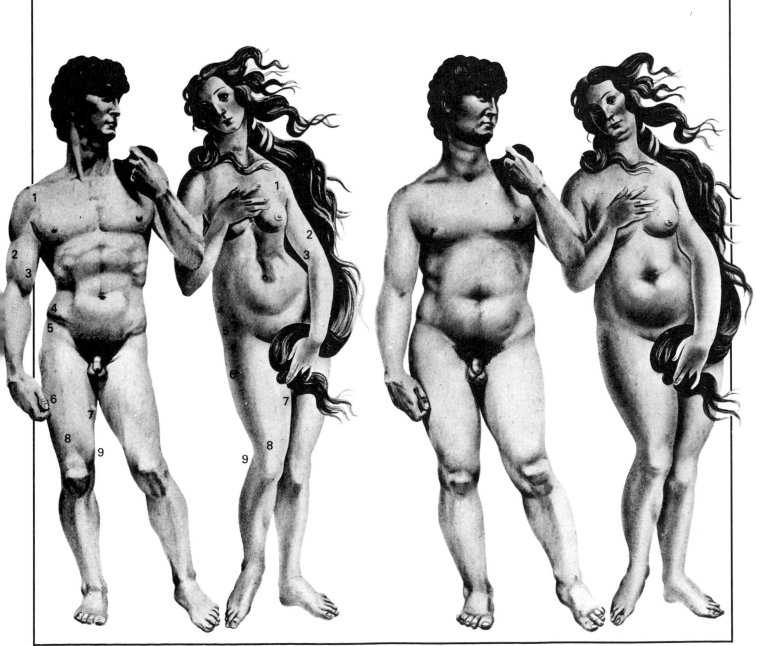

FITNESS

The Joys of Exercise

Fitness is good for you. There are few other statements about our health which can be made with equal certainty. So why is unfitness an increasing problem in Western countries? To a considerable degree it is a direct result of our way of life. We ride to work in cars, buses or trains; we use elevators rather than stairs; we sit down most of the day not only in offices but on many factory production-lines; we rely more and more on mechanization and automation; most of us cease to play any sport when we leave school; we spend more time watching television than on any other leisure activity; and too often the walking, gardening and do-it-yourself work around the house that we do cannot make up for it. No wonder so many of us are so unfit.

Unfitness is easier to recognize than fitness to define. However *organic fitness* is generally taken to mean a body free from disease and infirmity – in other words, basic health – while *dynamic fitness* is the ability to move vigorously and live energetically. Dynamic fitness, to which this chapter is devoted, has several components: the efficiency of the heart and lungs, muscular strength and endurance, balance, flexibility, co-ordination and agility.

WHY FITNESS MATTERS:
10 BENEFITS OF REGULAR AND ADEQUATE EXERCISE

The people most in need of exercise tend to be those who least feel like taking it. Yet there are clear physiological benefits to strengthen the resolve.

We list below ten benefits of regular and adequate exercise that have been observed and established with various degrees of certainty, although individuals differ in response within each category of benefit. They illustrate the message that exercise should be taken for its own sake because it is beneficial and makes sense in itself, quite apart from any possibility of the prevention of a heart attack. "Regular adequate exercise" is described in detail below.

1. The first thing to mention is that exercise enhances well-being, is enjoyable and reduces boredom. Sports and recreation are ideal family activities.

2. The training effects of vigorous or aerobic exercise (also known as large-muscle, dynamic activity) are greater efficiency of circulation and respiration, including peripheral circulation, and of oxygen transport around the body. Less effort is required of heart and lungs to provide the body with energy. Exercise improves blood supply of the heart muscle itself and of the peripheral muscles. There is greater physical endurance and less fatigue; individuals are better able to tolerate physical effort.

3. More generally, physical activity increases muscle strength, the strength of joints, their flexibility and mobility, the strength of tendons and muscle attachments. Strengthening of the lower back may protect against injury and other trouble.

4. These all contribute to increased physical working capacity.

5. Exercise – expenditure of calories – counteracts obesity.

6. Exercise improves a wide range of physiological functions, e.g., lowering the level of blood fats, of triglycerides, and more doubtfully of cholesterol; it raises the level of protective high-density lipoproteins.

7. Physical activity may counteract stress and channel aggressive drives. For many people it helps with sleep.

8. Exercise improves posture, appearance, self-image.

9. It is also a constructive preparation for an active and happy old age.

10. So general is the effect of exercise on bodily processes that innumerable benefits have been claimed at one time or another. Much remains speculative, and much interesting and important research is under way – for example, on the contribution of exercise to maintaining youthfulness, and to mental functioning in old age.

LIVING LONGER

Exercise is no elixir of life. Fitness can guarantee neither good health nor a long life, but it does make both more likely. Life is prolonged primarily through the effect of dynamic exercise, such as sport or brisk walking, on the heart. There is the secondary effect of reducing weight and this, too, ultimately benefits the heart. The consequences of inactivity are that the body deteriorates as the key organs weaken. It is *unfitness*, therefore, that shortens life.

Farrah Fawcett-Majors and husband Lee Majors, stars of TV's *Charlie's Angels* and *The Six Million Dollar Man*, jogging for fitness and beauty if not necessarily bionic powers.

This section does not cover exercise for children or the elderly, since this is discussed in Chapters 1 and 10.

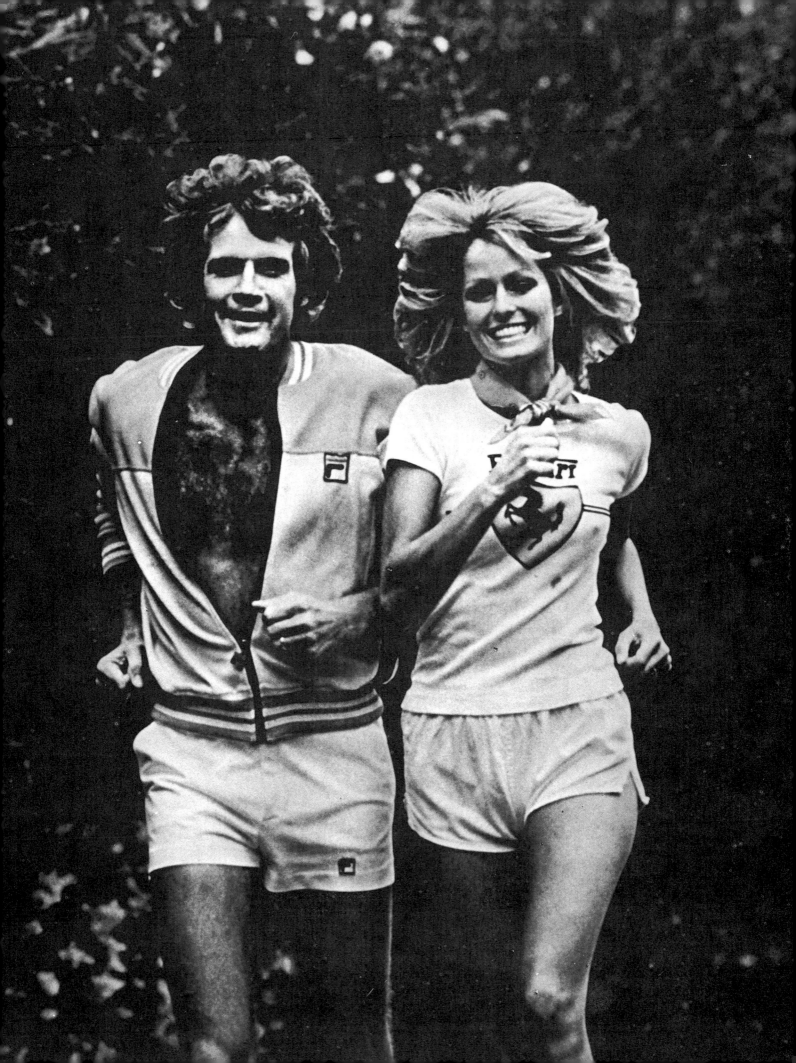

Heart disease is the biggest single killer illness in the Western world. In America it is responsible for a third of all deaths in men aged 40–59. Anything that can lessen the chance of such heart failure, therefore, has a dramatic effect on the prospects for life and health. Numerous research projects have now shown that people in light or sedentary jobs are more likely to suffer and die from coronary heart disease than people in jobs involving substantial physical activity. For instance, in a study of San Francisco longshoremen, whose health was followed for twenty-two years, men classified as being in jobs requiring repeated bursts of "high energy output" had a death rate from coronary heart disease only half that of the men in jobs requiring a medium or low energy output. Other surveys have since indicated similar benefits from exercise in leisure time.

One of the most significant surveys has been undertaken by Professor J.N.Morris, of the University of London and Britain's Medical Research Council. This studied the daily lives of almost 18,000 British civil servants engaged in sedentary or very light work between the years 1968 and 1970. The survey sampled the physical activity undertaken in their spare time, and the results clearly show that people taking vigorous exercise are significantly less likely to suffer from coronary heart disease. By "vigorous exercise" Professor Morris meant high-energy exercise equivalent potentially to heavy industrial work. The form of the exercise in practice varied from swimming and hill-climbing to brisk walking and heavy gardening.

LIVING BETTER

For many people the fact that they enjoy exercise and feel the better for it, plus (if they think of it) the possibility of a longer life, will be reason enough for exercise. But for many people in their twenties or even in middle age the statistics of life and death may be an insufficient spur. There are other benefits than longevity, however.

Losing weight. Most people calculate how far you have to walk to lose ten pounds and conclude that exercise cannot help much in slimming. But nobody becomes fat overnight, so it is unrealistic to expect to become slim overnight. In fact recent research which has included exercise as well as dietary measures in weight-control programs, plus the results of studies of metabolic consequences of exercise for overweight people, suggests that exercise should now be regarded as an integral part of programs to counter obesity. The increased energy expended during a two-mile walk, for instance, may be small, but in the long-term it is highly significant if it becomes a daily habit. The effect of exercise on the metabolism may be even greater, since it now seems that exercise raises the metabolic rate and leads to the loss of far more weight than would have been predicted for the actual exercise undertaken. Thus a previously inactive person walking an extra four miles a day, even at the slow pace of two miles per hour, would lose twenty pounds over the year assuming no change in diet. Combining exercise with dieting is even more effective.

Gaining vigor. The effects of exercise on the heart, lungs and blood means that you will have more vigor. If you have to run for a bus, or walk briskly, or climb some stairs, you are not so likely to get out of breath. You will be less tired at the end of a normal day. You will have energy left over to undertake fresh activities. You will be more lively, and life will seem more fun. These are subjective feelings, but they are none the less real for many people, and thus the greatest incentive of all for physical fitness. The improved flow of blood to the skin tones it up, so that you may *look* better, too.

Coping with stress. Healthiness in body traditionally has been associated with healthiness in mind. It sounds like puritan propaganda but greater vigor does enable people to accomplish their daily tasks with less strain. Many people also report sleeping better at night if exercising regularly. This contributes to a calmness or psychological resilience in the face of stress which is difficult to measure but which is generally reckoned by doctors to be one of the greatest benefits of physical fitness. It is also possible that physical activity is a way of channeling aggressive drives.

Types of exercise
The two broad types of exercise are *isometric* and *dynamic* exercise. Isometric exercise involves concentrated muscle contraction without any body movement; related to it is isotonic exercise which creates muscle contractions through movement, usually involving the use of weights. Both isometric and isotonic exercise are useful for developing the strength of particular muscle groups, although they are not recommended by the American Heart Association for people suffering from heart disease or high blood pressure. It is dynamic exercise which most improves general physical fitness and health.

Dynamic exercise offers many routes to fitness. We will look at three broad categories of dynamic exercise: the limbering-up exercises or calisthenics (page 78), aerobic exercise and sport. What they have in common is that each involves some degree of body movement. Each type of exercise has its advantages, but aerobic exercise is the most important component in any fitness program. This is because it improves the efficiency of the body's most important muscle – the heart. Aerobic or cardiovascular exercise means sustained rhythmic activity that involves large muscle groups (particularly the legs) and increases the amount of oxygen processed by the body in a given time. Thus the lungs are made more efficient, the pulse rate lowered and a heart attack less likely. (Nutrition, smoking and stress are also associated with heart disease, however, as we discuss elsewhere in this book.)

While it is therefore important to incorporate some form of aerobic activity in any exercise program, it is also essential to find an activity that you enjoy. Otherwise you are unlikely to practice it sufficiently regularly to achieve its potential benefits. Whatever activity is pursued, do not neglect the possibilities for improved fitness through simple changes in your everyday life. Putting more effort into your gardening, using stairs rather than elevators and, above all, walking can significantly improve overall fitness. Increased walking often provides the essential first step in any fitness program for a previously inactive person and is particularly suitable for older people.

Who can exercise?
Pretty well anyone can get fitter. Neither a late start nor a low starting-point will completely deny the benefits of physical fitness. Indeed, a low base offers most individuals a greater potential for improvement. You may never run a four- or five-minute mile, but what matters is coming close to your own body's potential. Exercise is necessary to prevent physical atrophy. In other words, the long-term health hazard of *not* exercising is far more acute than the short-

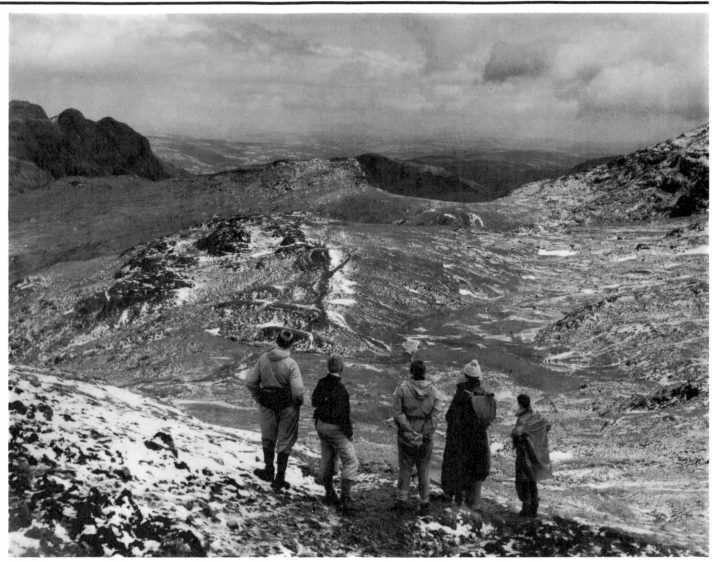

Walking – one of the most satisfying of the many routes to physical fitness and health.

term risks associated with unaccustomed exercise. But before undertaking any major program of increased physical activity, see your doctor or public health clinic physician. If you are under thirty and have had a check-up within a year, even this may be unnecessary: for most people there are no risks in regular dynamic exercise as long as the program begins gently and only gradually increases in vigor. However, most American doctors recommend a thorough examination for anyone over thirty with people over forty subjected to an electrocardiogram (ECG) test on the heart during an exercise program. You should also see your doctor *regardless of age* if you have any history of cardiovascular problems (or suspect their existence) or if during exercise you develop unexpected symptoms such as dizziness, palpitations or getting too easily out of breath. Physicians will be able to recommend particular exercise programs to suit individual circumstances.

Elaborate "self-testing" methods have also been devised which involve either monitoring the pulse rate after exercise or measuring the distance covered in set times. These have come under increasing criticism, particularly from European physiologists, who argue that they are not only too discouraging but too demanding for people who have not taken any physical exercise for twenty years or more. However, one simple test is suggested by the President's Council on Physical Fitness and Sports in *One Step at a*

Time, an introduction to running:
The "walk test" will help you determine where to begin. If you can comfortably walk three miles in forty-five minutes, it's OK to start running. Or, more precisely, alternately running and walking. If you can't pass the test, walk three miles a day until you can.

And what applies to running applies also to other vigorous activities. The truth is that the average middle-aged American took many years to achieve his or her present state of unfitness, so it will take awhile to repair those years of neglect. But even ailing bodies can be strengthened by careful progressive exercise. Be patient: do not expect miracles overnight. Aching limbs will precede radiant health, but if you persist you will soon feel better. Some people like to set themselves targets, but unfit people should beware of pushing themselves too hard. You should, for instance, be able to talk comfortably when taking exercise such as jogging.

When to exercise.
Sometimes the form of the exercise dictates the time you can practice it. But the only time not to exercise vigorously is in the hour or so after a meal. Whatever generations of army physical instructors may say, there is no medical merit in the early dawn. Exercise at the time of day that best suits you.

Calisthenics

The convenience of these exercises has always been among their strongest attractions. No special clothing or equipment is required. They are usually done indoors, so the weather outside is irrelevant. You do not need to rely on other people turning up as in most competitive sports. You do not waste time traveling to the sports center. Nobody (other than your family, perhaps) will laugh at your early puffing efforts. They can be done at any time of the day (or indeed night) except in the hour after a meal.

The advantages of keep-fit exercises are their concentration and variety. You not only waste no time traveling or dressing but you are also benefiting every minute you are exercising. Yet that is also the drawback of calisthenics: you benefit *only* when you are doing a particular exercise. Activity is not normally sufficiently sustained in order to have the optimum beneficial effect on the heart and lungs. Make the most of these limbering-up exercises by moving quickly from one activity to another, with running in place the only "rest" permitted. Calisthenics are perhaps best deployed as an addition to a general exercise program. They certainly develop greater mobility than, say, running, which otherwise is "good" cardiovascular exercise. Another attraction of this form of exercise is that it is programmed to incorporate a complete range of physical activities for not only different muscle groups but also all levels of fitness – or unfitness.

The *Body Maintenance* Exercises fulfil these objectives. There is a less demanding *Grade 1* which is essentially to get you up and down stairs without all that huffing and puffing; *Grade 2* will at least make it possible for you to run for a bus without feeling that what you need instead is an ambulance; and *Grade 3*, if you keep it up for any length of time, should get you back to near the fitness of your youth. Whatever your grade, the exercises only take a few minutes. What matters is to practice them *every day*.

These exercises were first devised for the average man or woman by Captain Simon Cook and Sergeant Tony Toms of Britain's Royal Marine Commandos. Such origins should remind us that although the exercises may be a speedy way towards fitness, they will not necessarily be easy – especially for the very unfit. But do not be scared: the exercises were devised for ordinary mortals who want to climb stairs rather than scale cliffs.

Be sure to follow the instructions for each exercise carefully. People who suffer from back pain should take particular care, and perhaps consider alternative forms of exercise. The number of repeats specified is only a guide. You can do more or less, according to what level of fitness you are aiming for or indeed to what you can manage. Stick to one grade if you like, or graduate from one to another. Aim to improve your performance in terms of skill and speed as well as number. Forgetting it "just for one day" makes it easier to forget for another day as well. The more you demand of yourself, the more you will benefit and the more enjoyable the exercises themselves will become.

Grade 1: A Loosening-Up Course to Start

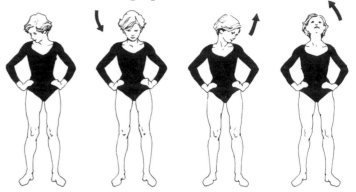

1. *Head-circling.* Stand erect, feet comfortably apart, hands on hips. Pull chin in, circle head 10 times in one direction, then 10 times in the other direction.

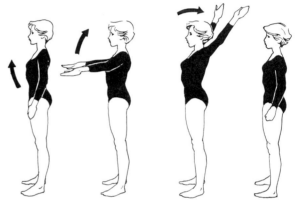

2. *Arm-circling.* Stand erect, feet apart. Circle both arms simultaneously like propellers 10 times, then 10 times in reverse direction.

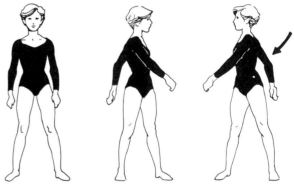

3. *Trunk-twisting.* Stand erect, feet apart, arms loosely by sides. Turn trunk and head to left and then to right. Repeat this whole movement left and right 10 times.

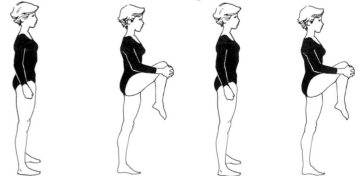

4. *Knee-clasping.* Stand erect, feet apart. Bend one knee upwards and pull it vigorously into your chest with both hands. Same with other knee, and repeat 10 times with each knee.

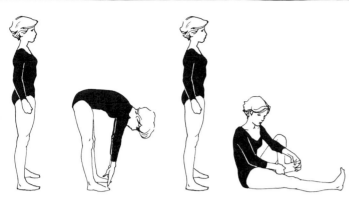

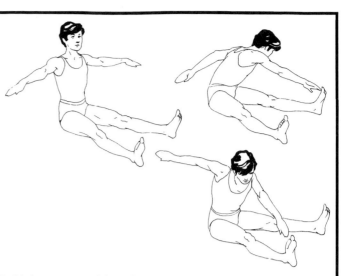

5: *Toe-touching.* Stand erect, feet apart. Bend down to touch toes, keeping legs straight if possible. Return to upright position, repeat 10 times.

6. *Ankle-rotating.* Sit on floor with one leg straight. Bend other leg over the straight leg, hold the foot of the bent leg, and turn ankle full circle. 10 times each ankle.

Grade 2: Getting in Trim the Easy Way

For men. This is for bodies fit enough for stronger exercises. Warm up first with thirty seconds on each of the Grade 1 exercises.

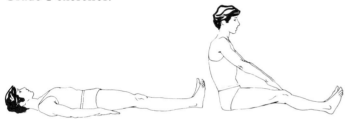

1. *Sit-ups.* Lie on back with a comfortable cushion for the head. Rise without use of arms to near-sitting position. Hands must touch knee-caps. Return to lying position. Repeat 15 times.

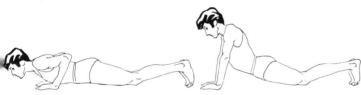

2. *Half push-ups.* Lie facing floor. With palms flat, push up till arms are straight, lower trunk remaining on floor. Return to lying flat and repeat 10 times. (This may be uncomfortable for anyone with back pain. An alternative is to do a few push-ups using knees as the fulcrum — starting with the knees bent.)

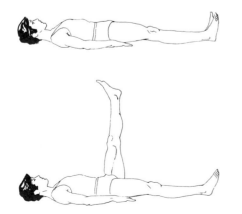

3. *Leg-raising.* Lie on back and raise each leg alternately to the vertical. 20 times each leg.

4. *Sitting toe-touching.* Sit with legs straight and apart, stretch right hand to touch left toe then left hand to right toe. Repeat whole movement 30 times rhythmically.

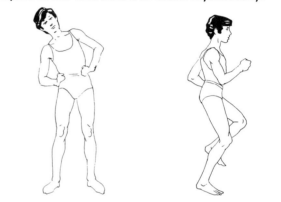

5. *Side-bending.* Stand with feet comfortably apart, hands on hips. Bend body from waist, reaching down as far as you can, first on left side, then on right. 20 times each side.

6. *Spot-running.* Run on spot counting a pace each time the right foot touches the floor. 100 paces or one minute.

For women. These exercises can help posture and to some extent flatten the tummy and reduce the waist, but they are not an alternative to a diet for the overweight. Warm up first with 30 seconds of each Grade 1 exercise.

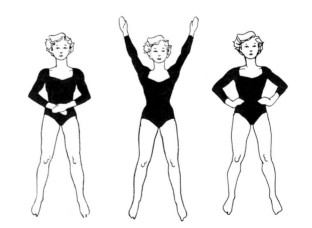

1. *Arm-raising.* Stand with feet comfortably apart, cross wrists over stomach. Keeping arms straight, swing them upwards and outwards and return. 20 times.

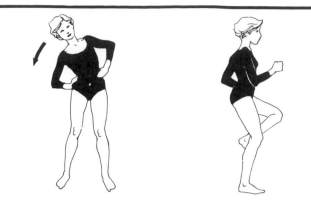

2. *Side-bending.* Stand with feet comfortably apart, hands on hips. Bend body from waist, reaching down as far as you can, first on left side, then on right. 15 times each side.

3. *Spot-running.* Run on spot, counting as right foot touches floor. 40 paces.

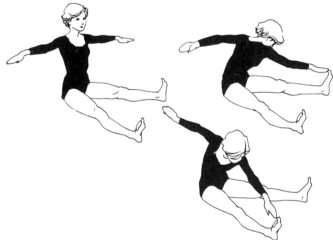

4. *Sit-ups.* Lie on back with a comfortable cushion for the head. Rise without use of arms to near-sitting position. Hands must touch knee-caps. Return to lying. Repeat 15 times.

5. *Sitting toe-touching.* Sit with legs straight and apart, stretch right hand to touch left toe, then left hand to right toe. Repeat whole movement 10 times rhythmically.

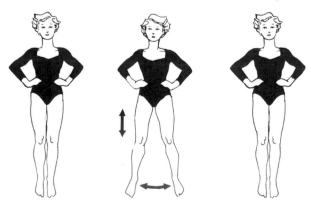

6. *Astride-jumps.* With hands on hips, jump feet apart and then together again, repeating whole movement 30 times rhythmically.

Grade 3: Bursting with Health

For men. Once you have attained this level without too much discomfort you can say you are giving your body a thorough servicing. Warm up first with thirty seconds of each Grade 1 exercise.

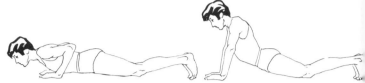

1. *Half push-ups.* Lie facing floor. With palms flat, push up till arms are straight, lower trunk remaining on floor. Return to lying flat. Do as many as you can up to 20 times. NB: back-pain sufferers should see the cautionary note under the first exercise in Grade 2 for men.

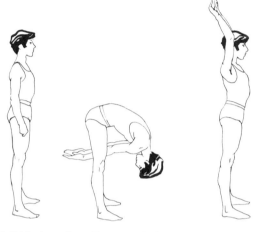

2. *Side-bending.* Stand with feet comfortably apart, hands on hips. Bend body from waist, reaching down as far as you can, first on left side, then on right. 15 times each side.

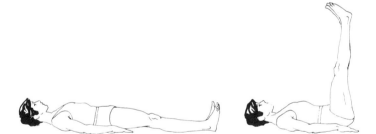

3. *Leg-raising.* Lie on back. Raise both legs to the vertical, then lower them slowly to floor. 15 times.

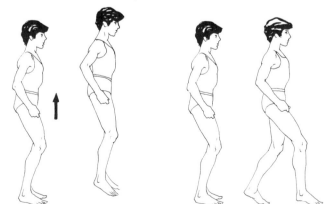

4. *Skip-jumps.* Stand with feet together, hands by sides. Spring up and down off the balls of your feet, 30 times. Repeat 30 times more, skipping with one foot forwards, other backwards alternately.

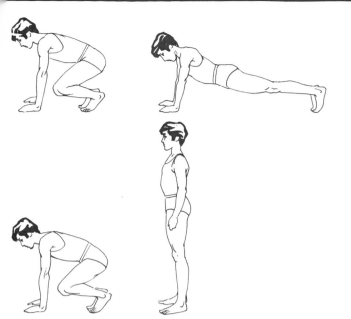

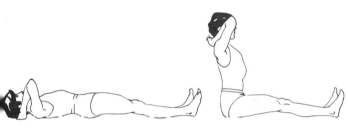

5. *Burpees.* From standing, crouch with hands on floor, then shoot legs backwards to the push-up position. Return to crouch and then stand up. This is one burpee. Repeat 15 times.

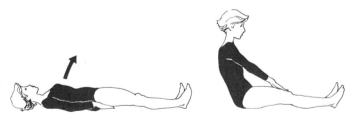

6. *Sit-ups.* Lie on back. Sit up to vertical position, bending knees if necessary. 30 times.

For women: This grade should be attempted only after six weeks of daily Grade 2 exercises. Warm up first with twenty seconds of each Grade 1 exercise.

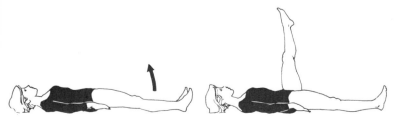

1. *Sit-ups.* Lie on back, rise without use of arms to near-sitting position. Hands must touch knee-caps. Return to lying. 20 times.

2. *Leg-raising.* Lie on back. Raise both legs to the vertical, then lower them slowly (to count of ten) to floor. 10 times.

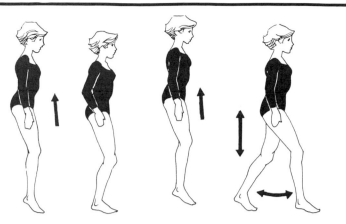

3. *Skip-jumps.* Stand with feet together, arms by sides. Spring up and down off the balls of your feet, 30 times. Repeat 30 times more, skipping with one foot forwards other backwards alternately.

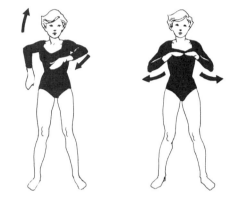

4. *Free-standing swim.* Stand with feet comfortably apart and with your arms "swim" the crawl, breast-stroke and back-stroke. 20 of each stroke.

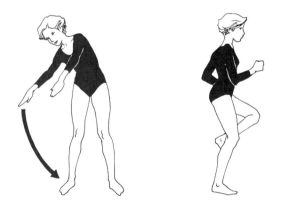

5. *Trunk-rotating.* Stand with feet comfortably apart, arms stretched up above head. Make a circle with arms and trunk, brushing floor with hands in front at lowest point of movement. 10 times to left, 10 times to right.

6. *Spot-running.* Run on spot for one minute.

Health Checks

If everyone was observant about changes in their health and did not hesitate to ask their own doctor when they were worried about something, health screening checks would not be necessary. As it is, there is a steady demand for annual screening tests. People who have their health screened are often worried about some change in health which they would find difficult to pinpoint and explain to their own doctor. Usually nothing can be found to be wrong, and after screening a person can go away with relief of their immediate anxiety. Nevertheless, among those who are screened there is more undiagnosed disease than might be expected, although most of it is minor. Screening services can also identify those people who are at high risk of developing certain diseases, particularly those caused by smoking and excessive drinking, and give precautionary advice.

Screening has however been criticized because disease often cannot be detected by scientific tests before a person has noticed symptoms themselves. And even when disease is detected in the early stages it is not always possible to do anything to prevent it from worsening.

The most important part of a check-up, when you talk to the doctor about your health and he asks you questions, is your previous history. More than 50 per cent of internal illnesses are picked up by doctors on the basis of the history alone, 20 per cent are picked up by physical examination and the remainder by laboratory tests. So it is no use choosing an outfit which only does a series of lab tests on blood and urine.

Choose a doctor or clinic which is prepared to spend time with you. A thorough check-up should take about an hour. Some of the tests may be done by nurse practitioners, but the final physical examination and interview should be with a doctor. Tell the doctor anything which is worrying you, even if you are afraid he may think it is silly.

The most valuable tests are for high blood pressure, certain hearing and vision defects and perhaps cancer of the cervix or breast (see pages 132–4). Testing of older people (over 60) for hearing and vision, poor nutrition and difficulty in walking is specially worthwhile. Old people can often be given immediate practical help with problems which they may have accepted as an inevitable part of life.

Ears.

Almost 50 per cent of men and women over 65 are deaf to some degree. In a proportion, this can be cured by simply syringeing the ears to remove wax. For others, specialist advice, an operation or hearing aids can improve hearing and bring a new interest in life. The screening of old people, and of people in noisy jobs, for deafness is badly needed; in older people deafness is as common as poor sight.

Heart.

Electrocardiograms (ECGs) sensitively record every beat of the heart and if it misses a beat, or a beat is irregular, then the machine records it. Even so, between 25 and 50 per cent of those who suffer from angina – an early symptom of heart disease – have normal ECGs. Although some heart disease can be detected it is not possible even with the most elaborate tests to be certain that someone's heart is in good condition. And it is not until heart disease has progressed a long way that it can be detected by screening tests. This is still in time for diet, exercise and giving up smoking to be

Eyes.

If you cannot read a license plate at twenty-five yards, or a telephone directory at nineteen inches, you may need glasses. Anyone who has reached the age of forty-five without needing glasses should get their eyes checked, because sight fails increasingly with age. Check-ups every two or three years afterwards are advisable.

One in ten blind people have lost their vision as a result of *glaucoma*, a disease which causes a rise of pressure in the eyeball. The increased pressure flattens the small blood vessels in the back of the eye, cutting off the blood supply to the light-sensitive retina which then dies. People who have a relative who has suffered from glaucoma, and people over fifty are most at risk of getting the disease. Routine tests are useful for over-40s.

Glaucoma can be treated effectively if caught early before too much damage is done. Danger symptoms include the following: pain in the eye, occasional bouts of blurred vision occurring in dull light, large rainbow rings round a clear bright light, and loss of the ability to see an object, at the edge of the field of vision, which is not being looked at directly. If you have these symptoms seek an early eye examination.

Lungs.

Mass radiography has proved useful in detecting tuberculosis, but so far has not proved useful in detecting lung cancer. By the time a lung cancer is detectable on an X-ray it is usually so large that the chances of effective treatment are no better than they are for people whose cancers are picked up in the normal way by their own doctor. Dr Victor Hawthorne of Glasgow University picked up about 200 lung cancers out of nearly a million people X-rayed. Despite being picked up early they did no better than other lung cancer patients.

Early lung damage which is the first stage in the development of chronic bronchitis can be detected by a test of lung volume. This test could be used as part of a campaign to persuade people not to smoke. However, identifying the people at risk – smokers – is not the problem. The problem is to persuade them to give the habit up.

Liver.

Blood tests may detect early liver disease. The most frequent cause is drinking too much alcohol; a new test can pick up early damage to the liver and indicate those people who are drinking more than they should.

Rectum.

Bleeding from the rectum is often neglected because people blame it on piles. Bleeding from the rectum should always be investigated because it can also be a sign of rectal cancer. Rectal cancer has excellent prospects of cure if caught early. Piles should in any case be treated, because if neglected they can cause anemia simply through persistent loss of blood. Tests are also available for hidden blood in the stools, which may be a sign of cancer higher up the bowel. However, these tests are not yet considered sufficiently reliable for use on people who have no symptoms. In older people any major changes in bowel habit should be reported to the doctor. Sigmoidoscopy – examination of the sigmoid colon through a fibre-optic tube inserted into the bowel – is useful in over-50s.

Weight.

Being overweight is the easiest condition to screen for since it simply means weighing someone. It is associated with an increased risk of death from diabetes, blood vessel disease, stroke, pneumonia and diseases of the digestive system.

More details on all these problems can be found elsewhere in this book. Executive health checks are generally regarded as a largely male preserve. This is not in fact so. Most private organizations offering such services welcome female as well as male customers. And there are some tests which are only applicable for women, of course, most notably the highly desirable checks for cancer of the cervix and breast, subjects covered in Chapter 6.

Blood-pressure.

A few people who suffer high blood pressure complain of headaches, dizziness or palpitations but most complain of no symptoms, so the condition is not likely to be discovered unless someone has their blood pressure measured. High blood pressure has serious consequences if left untreated, and so screening for blood pressure is the most rewarding of all the standard health checks. (See Chapter 6 for further details of how to avoid and treat high blood pressure.) An annual check-up is wise for adults.

Urine.

Tests may detect kidney disease, diabetes or infection. However, kidney disease is not commonly enough detected to make the test useful for health screening. A test for sugar in the urine may provide a useful early warning of diabetes, but the disease cannot always be treated effectively until it progresses to the point where the patient begins to be bothered by other symptoms which would bring him to consult a doctor.

AEROBIC EXERCISE

The term aerobics was invented by an American fitness expert called Dr Kenneth Cooper, who as much as anyone else is responsible for the jogging craze. It is christened "aerobic" because it is exercise which needs a lot of air, or rather oxygen. Not only needs it, as indeed one needs oxygen all the time, but demands it as a matter of urgency, requiring possibly more than it can get. It might have been better to call it Heart-Lung or cardiovascular exercise since this is the area of its effect, but aerobic is the name which caught the public imagination.

Aerobic exercise is the jogger running one or two miles at sustained speed, rather than the sprinter who runs 100 meters – a task achieved on his body's store of oxygen and energy. Aerobic exercise has three characteristics:
1. It must involve large muscle groups of the body, such as the legs.
2. It must be performed continuously for at least 20 minutes.
3. It must be vigorous enough to engage the whole body. During such rhythmic, sustained and vigorous exercise your pulse rate and breathing will be more rapid, because you are using oxygen as fast as you can to fuel the hard-working muscles.

The ultimate consequence of this training effect is to improve the efficiency of the cardio-respiratory system, thus strengthening the heart and improving the circulation.

To achieve this training effect it is generally agreed that "regular and adequate exercise" means exercise at least three times a week for between 20 and 30 minutes. It also raises the heartbeat or pulse rate to around 70 per cent of its maximum.

The easiest place to count your pulse or heart rate is the radial artery in the wrist. Turn your palm to face you, move your second and third finger along the thumb side of your wrist until you feel a steady pulsation, then count the number of pulsations.

It is also simple enough to work out your "pulse rate goal". The maximum individual heart rate declines steadily with age from about 200 at twenty years of age to 160 at sixty – sex differences are less important. The much-respected Stanford Heart Disease Prevention Program thus suggests these pulse rate goals for aerobic exercise:

Age 20–29: 138–142 beats per minute
Age 30–39: 130–134 beats per minute
Age 40–49: 122–126 beats per minute
Age 50–59: 113–117 beats per minute
Age 60–69: 105–109 beats per minute

But pulse rate goals or targets should not be interpreted so zealously that exercise loses its sense of enjoyment. Similarly the amount of exercise needed by individuals will vary. If obesity is a problem, as well as general unfitness, it is likely that some form of exercise will be required more frequently than three times a week.

As an example of how ordinary people can take up "vigorous" or aerobic exercise and as a demonstration of improved efficiency and well-being, we offer two case histories from a dozen middle-aged people whom we tested over a nine-month period which began and ended with tests on a treadmill ECG (electrocardiogram).

Sylvia Baynham

Aged 57 when tested, housewife and part-time library assistant. After raising a family she "had taken no real

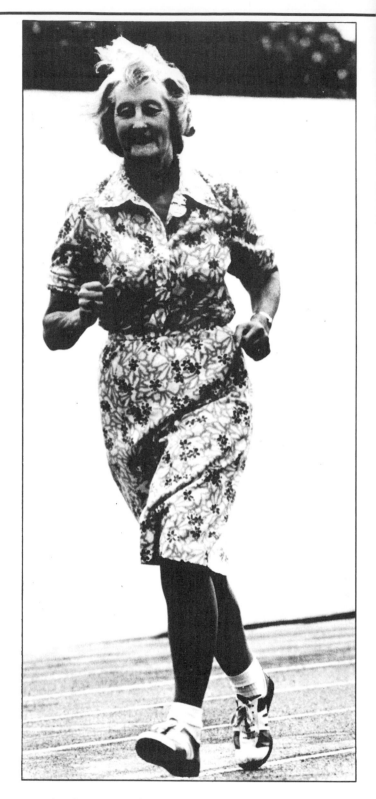

exercise for twenty-five years. I had never felt *un*-fit," but walking up stairs was hard work and she was aware that flab meant she was a bit overweight. On the initial treadmill ECG test she accomplished the fourth of a maximum seven stages. The ECG showed some irregularity, so she started a modified fitness program. Within three months, the irregularity of the ECG pattern had been abolished and her exercise no longer needed to be restricted:

I'll always remember that first time on the treadmill, the last couple of minutes were agony – and I only got to stage four! So I was delighted that on my second session I reached the same stage without too much effort, and this accomplished just by running up and down stairs each day. I chose this method of exercise because I hate the cold, and the thought of going for a walk or run in the winter just meant I would never exercise. Now, I can exercise whenever I have fifteen minutes to spare without changing into special clothes.

The stair-climbing routine consists of choosing a flight of ten stairs (in her case, ten of a flight of thirteen) and going up them five times to a minute, i.e., five times up, five times down. A doddle, perhaps, for just one minute, but fairly demanding when it involves – as it soon did for Mrs Baynham – fifty flights in ten minutes:

People have asked me if I get bored, and ask what I think about. In fact I don't really have much time to think, I'm too busy counting my trips, and as to being bored – well, surely if it is boring, it's worth it for such a short time to get fit. I'm glad I started exercising, for I am now fitter, I walk better and I don't get out of breath so quickly. Psychologically it has also done me good; I was the oldest of the group by about six years and, having stayed the course, this has done wonders for my morale.

Alan Thurgood

Aged 42 when tested, businessman. Until five years previously, he had taken regular exercise and was once "ridiculously fit". As a competitor in orienteering, he remembered that "when fresh, one found the check-points more easily". For a business executive like himself, he reasoned, this must indicate that physical fitness enhances mental efficiency. Mr Thurgood, described by the officiating doctor as "well-motivated" – despite being overweight at nearly 200 pounds – did well in the treadmill test to accomplish the maximum stage, number seven.

Running became his principal form of exercise. At his holiday cottage near the coast, a round of golf was either preceded or followed by some running. Other people might not wish to chain themselves to time-and-distance goals, but Alan Thurgood is evidently one of the variety for whom this is the only way to take exercise:

I need motivation and incentive. Initially it was very encouraging to see the medical results, which were good, but than I had to set other incentives. This I did by planning a new circuit each month, immediately running it very hard and setting a time; then having as my objective to run it in the same time with reasonable ease by the end of the month. New circuits are one way to avoid boredom. Another way is to have company, and chat. Or to have a race with the other fellow, with handicaps. Above all, to make it enjoyable you have to make it a habit; if you're doing it regularly it's enjoyable, less often and it's hard work.

By the end of the program Alan Thurgood was, he says, enjoying his cigars and his beer more: and he had lost weight (ten pounds) and was once again taking up orienteering and squash. His test figures indicated, according to the doctor, "the unmasking of a true athletic heart which had been starting to go to seed".

The figures overleaf show the generally improved performance of these two candidates when, nine months after the first test, they exercised on the ECG treadmill to the same level they had initially achieved.

Improvement was achieved by all the twelve people whom we tested. Amongst all of them, heart rate at the highest exercise load averaged out at 160 in the first test, and in the second the average was 142. And the figures after one minute's recovery showed a drop from an average of 123 to an average of 94.

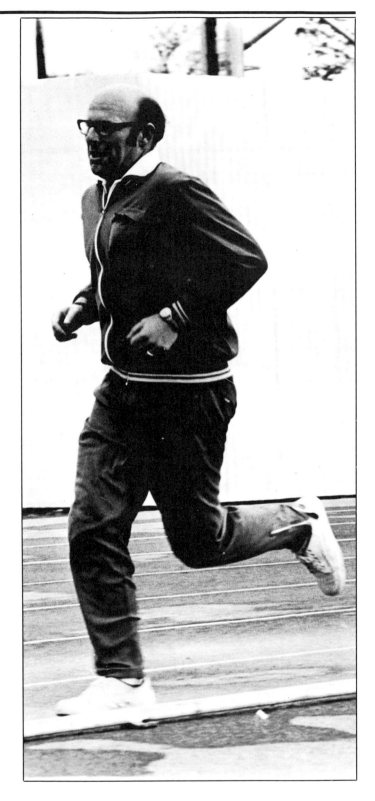

What this means is that all 12 people were, as a result of the program, doing the same exercise more economically at less stress. But this was not all. There were also interesting results in tests for the level of cholesterol, the substance which, in increased amounts, is associated with coronary thrombosis. Some evidence for the effect of exercise seems to be indicated when all the candidates showed an obvious decrease in cholesterol level, almost invariably *without* any alteration to diet.

Additionally, there were of course the less tangible benefits connected with a sense of well-being, which all the subjects said they experienced. For example: "I'm getting more value from sleep – even with less sleep, there's more

Heart-Rate:Beats/min	Sylvia Baynham		Alan Thurgood	
	Before	After	Before	After
At rest	77	82	64	40
During Exercise				
Stage 1	110	95	78	48
Stage 2	125	105	87	62
Stage 3	138	123	100	75
Stage 4	155	148	112	86
Stage 5	—	—	132	110
Stage 6	—	—	160	120
Stage 7	—	—	168	140
Recovery after Exercise				
Minutes 1	130	100	123	78
Minutes 3	92	80	98	55
Minutes 5	95	84	87	45
Weight (Kilos)	68.5	67.5	89.1	81.7

benefit . . . I am at a period in my life which does tend to cause depression, and I've been feeling much less depressed, much more cheerful. . . . At the end of a long flight, I no longer suffer from the pilot's chronic complaint of backache. . . ."

The attractions of vigorous or aerobic exercise are that (a) improvements in fitness can be monitored; (b) activities can be pursued by individuals, unlike most competitive sports; (c) activities are intensive and therefore improve fitness quickly.

Simply taking your own pulse rate one and five minutes after exercise will give you an indication of improvement. Many people like or need this encouragement; people such as Alan Thurgood like to set themselves goals. And many like elaborately structured fitness programs such as those offered by Dr Kenneth Cooper in his various aerobics books (see Appendix 2). Dr Cooper took the basic activities for individuals such as walking, running, swimming and cycling, and worked out point-scores according to the distance covered in different times. Choose whatever activity you like, do it as often or as little as you like, says Dr Cooper, just so long as you score 30 points a week for men or 24 points for women. This will mean that you will have exercised at sufficient intensity to have raised your pulse or heart rate to beneficial levels.

Running and brisk walking are the most obvious aerobic activities. **Jogging** is running at a slow pace or trot – slightly quicker than a brisk walk, and very roughly about 9–10 minutes-a-mile pace. But even the slowest jog is ideal aerobic exercise. To run, no matter how slowly, and not to raise the pulse rate to a decent level is virtually impossible. By comparison, **walking** and **cycling** do not require so much effort: it is up to you to make a positive effort, to push yourself. Thus, in these activities especially setting your own time-and-distance target will probably help.

Running my also prove to be the most demanding of activities, requiring will power to overcome discomfort. The new jogger can suffer especially from soreness in the Achilles' tendon (at the back of the ankle), and all runners are liable, in rough ground especially, to minor muscle, tendon and joint injuries, which take a long time to mend and are generally a nuisance. Such injuries can be eased or forestalled by wearing "training" shoes with underfoot support (as opposed to sneakers) and an adequate heel height. Remember that your leg mechanism is conditioned by the higher heels or street shoes, so help it to adjust. Slight strains or soreness need not prevent continued training, if the running is done on soft grass. Stretching exercises before and after running lessen the chances of injury and increase flexibility.

Swimming is another excellent aerobic activity – so long as it is done actively. Paddling between swimming and sunbathing will achieve nothing more than a feeling of pleasant relaxation. But swimming actively at around thirty yards a minute or more will increase the efficiency of the heart and lungs by achieving the target heart rates described earlier. Legs, arms, back and abdominal muscles are also strengthened. And one particular plus for swimming is that it is a non weight-bearing sport, so that it is good exercise for people suffering from joints problems. The overweight, too, can often benefit more – and more quickly – from swimming than running.

Some people may have no fluency and will benefit enormously from a little coaching. One man in our middle-aged fitness experiment, a comparatively new swimmer, found incentive and pleasure in the following graduated program. He started by swimming six lengths, breast-stroke, with a pause every two lengths. Then he managed to connect up the lengths, doing six without pause; he next increased the lengths to ten, with pauses; then connected up again. Then he followed the same progression with the more difficult crawl-stroke.

Gardening and **do-it-yourself** are very common forms of recreation among adults. Both include a whole range of activity, from the gentlest pruning of the roses and mending a fuse to heavy digging and sawing wood. Both also offer more than enough scope for anyone who wishes to take vigorous exercise during their recreation without the trouble of making expeditions to, say, the swimming pool or the hills.

Indoor exercise, like skipping rope, stair-climbing or running on the spot, is more disciplined. It should be undertaken for at least five minutes, non-stop, once you become accustomed to the exercise. Stair-climbing is, in fact, excellent exercise.

Books offering detailed fitness programs are listed in Appendix 2. But generally you can make your exercise tougher and more beneficial, either by increasing the distance or the speed, or both. Aim in general to exercise longer before you exercise faster. Start by achieving as much distance as you can, even if this means doing it with brief rests – in the case of running, with short stretches of walking. Aim to do this distance – say, two miles – slowly, without stopping, at least two and preferably three times a week until you have done it with reasonable comfort several times, or at least for two weeks. Then, perhaps, run just one mile at a faster pace. Then, run further than two miles, slowly. And so on.

You may also achieve a better training effect by increasing the frequency although this is also likely to make you feel more tired. Certainly to begin with, it is best to allow at least one day's rest in between each session.

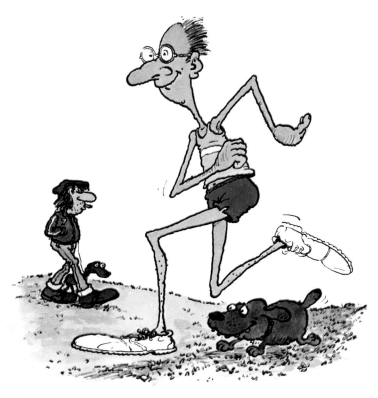

FITNESS THROUGH SPORT

All exercise may be good for you but different types of exercise affect the body in different ways. The jogger who pounds round the local park, for instance, will have more stamina than the gymnast – who has flexibility and suppleness of body. Can sport be the perfect exercise, offering enjoyment and fitness?

Some people will use exercises or jogging simply to achieve sufficient fitness to take part in their favorite sports; others will hope that sport itself will get and keep them fit. It all depends, of course, on the sport they wish to pursue, and on their own state of fitness. In the table on the right, we have rated sixty-four sports and other activities for their differing physical effects on the human body. An individual's benefit from any sport will also depend on his or her degree of skill, fitness and competitiveness.

The tables are adapted from the findings of an International Committee on the Standardization of Physical Fitness Tests. Medical experts from thirty-seven countries were represented on this committee, whose research provided the basis of a minutely detailed textbook, *International Guide to Fitness and Health*, published by Crown Publishers Inc. of New York. Some doctors believe that the fitness potential of many everyday activities such as do-it-yourself and gardening are generally underestimated. We have therefore included a few of the domestic and non-sporting activities contained in the *International Guide*'s tables in order to provide a comparison of their fitness potential with some of the most popular sports.

The fitness ratings of sport

A. General Endurance
B. Muscular Strength
C. Mobility of Joints
The potential effect of each activity in each category is indicated by three ratings:
1. Great effect (***)
2. Moderate effect (**)
3. Little or no effect (*)

	General Endurance	Muscular Strength	Mobility
1. Archery	*	**	*
2. Badminton	**	**	**
3. Baseball	*	*	**
4. Basketball	***	**	**
5. Billiards	*	*	*
6. Bowling	*	*	*
7. Boxing	***	***	*
8. Canoeing	**	***	*
9. Climbing stairs	**	**	***
10. Cricket	*	*	**
11. Croquet	*	*	*
12. Curling	*	*	**
13. Cycling (Speed)	***	**	*
14. Dancing	**	*	*
15. Darts	*	*	*
16. Digging in garden	**	***	**
17. Driving	*	*	*
18. Fencing	*	**	***
19. Fishing	*	*	*
20. Football	**	**	**
21. Golf	*	*	**
22. Gymnastics	*	*	**
23. Hiking	**	**	*
24. Hockey	**	**	*
25. Horse riding	**	*	*
26. Housework	*	*	**
27. Hunting	**	*	*
28. Ice-hockey	**	**	*
30. Jogging in place	**	*	*
30. Judo	*	**	**
31. Jumping (Ski)	*	**	**
32. Karate	*	**	**
34. Kayaking	**	***	**
34. Lacrosse	**	**	**
35. Mountain climbing	***	**	**
36. Mowing lawn	*	**	*
37. Orienteering	**	**	*
38. Rowing	***	***	*
39. Rugby	**	**	**
40. Running (Sub-maximal)	***	**	*
41. Sailing	*	**	**
42. Sawing	**	***	*
43. Scuba diving	**	*	**
44. Sculling	***	***	**
45. Shooting	*	*	*
46. Skating (Ice)	**	**	*
47. Skating (Roller)	**	**	*
48. Skin-diving	***	*	**
59. Skiing (Cross-country)	***	***	**
50. Skiing (Downhill)	**	**	**
51. Snooker (Pool)	*	*	*
52. Soccer	**	**	**
53. Squash	**	**	***
54. Surfing	*	**	**
55. Swimming (Sub-maximal)	***	***	***
56. Table tennis	*	*	**
57. Tennis	**	**	**
58. Volleyball	*	*	**
59. Walking briskly (over 1 hr)	**	*	*
60. Washing/polishing car	*	**	**
61. Water polo	***	**	**
62. Water skiing	**	**	**
63. Weight lifting	*	***	*
64. Wrestling	**	**	***

(Adapted from *International Guide to Fitness and Health*, by Leonard A. Larson and Herbert Mickelman. (c) 1973 by Leonard A. Larson and Herbert Mickelman; used by permission of Crown Publishers Inc. The full guide contains additional activities and categories such as "Skills" and "Neuro-Muscular Relaxation" which we felt were more subjective.)

The table shows the differences between sports. The common denominator, though, is pleasure. And because sports are a social pleasure, and doing well at them is part of this pleasure, there is a greater chance that you will not only keep at them but also train for them. This makes it far more likely that you will reach and maintain a healthy level of fitness. You can get fit through sport, therefore, but do not expect to do so with one weekly game of squash or tennis. Nor should you expect much pleasure if you are too unfit to enjoy a sport. Some sports demand a reasonable level of fitness *before* you take them up – basketball, for instance. Even hill-walking needs a rudimentary fitness. If you are unfit, then choose a sport where you can select your own level of exertion – solo canoeing or swimming, for instance – and can thereby do more to improve your own level of physical fitness.

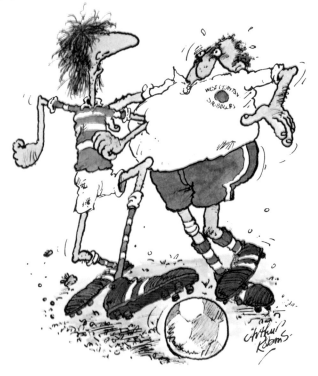

Team games. Rarely the best way to get fit, although, sadly, often all that is learned at school. The unfit are left lagging far behind their fitter colleagues or the ball or both. Even the fittest individuals only participate in many team games for short periods of time. Stop-watch checks on soccer players, for instance, have shown that the very best players in the most "active" midfield positions rarely possess the ball for more than three minutes of a 90-minute match. But at least they will be running for most of the remaining 87 minutes, unlike baseball players, few of whom are usually actively participating in the game at any one time. Some people, however, like the camaraderie of teams, which may give them their incentive to keep participating. The desire not to let their colleagues down may also encourage them to go on training-runs between the weekly matches.

Competitive sports. Some people need the spur of competition to provide the motivation for their exercise. But if competition implies the desire to win, they should prepare themselves for disappointments as they grow older, or at least seek their opponents solely from their contemporaries. Otherwise the inevitable decline in strength and speed as you grow older becomes increasingly the difference between success and failure. Ball games between individuals are generally better for fitness than team games, but they still depend on the ability of *both* players to sustain the action. Squash is perhaps the best ball game for keeping less good but moderately fit players on the move. The spasmodically explosive nature of these sports, however, can lead to strains on muscles and joints.

Middle-aged sports. There are only two special rules for the middle-aged and they apply whether the seeker-after-fitness is bent on sport, jogging or morning exercises:

1. Do take things cautiously. You cannot erase years of neglect with a sudden bout of furious activity. Running too fast too soon can lead at the least to strained muscles and joints, as we have noted.
2. Exercise within the heartbeat range described earlier is harmless enough, but the main thing is to be sensible about yourself. Use your common sense, therefore, but do also read the general Safety Check outlined earlier in this section.

Many sports and clubs have special classes, competitions or sections for the over-40s, -50s and even over-60s. Choosing a sport is very much a matter of individual preference; there is no universal best-buy offering the maximum health benefit for the minimum exertion. But generally the best sports for middle-aged people are those where the level of activity is determined by themselves rather than by opponents who may be much better (or much worse) than them. Likely sports in this category include swimming and solo rowing or canoeing. Golf, lawn bowling or hiking offer gentler exercise but good recreation. Badminton, tennis and – for fitter middle-aged people – squash are the most popular competitive sports.

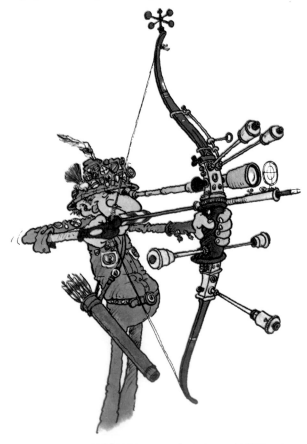

Sports for the family. Sport is often regarded as an enemy of family life. The husband and the father who spends the week days at work disappears for long stretches of the week end to play tennis or golf. Some sports, however, are ideal for all the family. Swimming in the local pool or leisure center, country walking, cycling, tennis, badminton, canoeing and orienteering, for instance, offer opportunities for families to play together at week ends or during their holidays. The children, and perhaps their parents, will learn new skills; the parents will certainly improve their fitness.

Sports for women. Most of the sports featured in our tables can be played by men and women. But women have far fewer "active recreations" than men and have traditionally been more reluctant than men to take up organized sport in their middle age. There is no reason why this should be so and many sports report increasing female participation. The popularity of running, for instance, has not been confined to men and there are now many specialist books on fitness for women. If women do still feel shy or ungainly, they should consider calisthenic exercises or keep-fit classes. Yoga, too, has considerable attractions, and dancing, especially country, folk and square dancing, is also fine exercise.

OTHER ROUTES TO FITNESS

Newspapers and magazines regularly advertise other aids to fitness. "Ten minutes daily," the advertisements say, "is all you need to get fit" – provided the ten minutes is spent using the advertised rowing machine or indoor bicycle or bar-bell and weights, or chest expander.

There are times when indoor exercise *is* an attraction. And although ten minutes a day will not make you fit, half an hour's vigorous cycling on a machine would train your heart and lungs to much the same extent as thirty minutes spent cycling in the open air. But no equipment can ever be a substitute for human effort – especially for really unfit people. Exercise bikes still have to be pedaled, rowing machines still have to be rowed.

The disadvantages of exercise machines is that they are rarely cheap and more likely to be boring. Pedaling an exercise bike on a winter's day may seem more attractive than going outside in the cold, but cycling along a country lane is more likely to tempt people into exercise on warmer days. Indoor exercise on machines is exercise for its own sake, undiluted by any other pleasure. It generally requires greater will-power for it to be maintained.

Yet Mrs Baynham achieved fitness by trotting up and down the stairs; Mr Thurgood by running set distances as fast as he could. The only thing that matters is that people maintain their exercise. If exercise bikes or rowing machines help people to do this, then good luck to them. Possibly the money spent on a "home gymnasium" may influence their determination. All they should beware of is thinking that machines will make anything easy, and be especially wary of all claims for the magical slimming-properties of any machines.

Exercise equipment, in fact, can fulfil a valuable role in *maintaining* fitness. If you are a keen cyclist, for instance, an exercise bicycle is valuable when bad weather or dark evenings make it difficult to achieve your usual hour or so's cycling. Similarly with rowing machines. If you do use an indoor bike, try to set it so that your riding position is similar to that which you use when cycling and adjust the

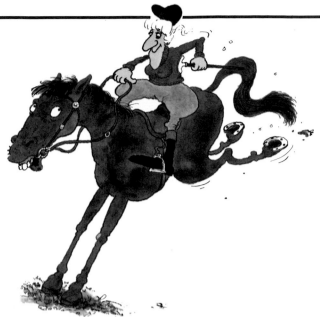

resistance to a realistic value. You can train, or keep in training, for riding on the road with a program that includes bursts of speed and shortish recovery periods of more gentle pedaling. Rowing machines cannot approximate so closely to real rowing.

Exercise bikes and rowing machines are both forms of the dynamic exercise to which we have devoted most of this section. They both use rhythmic large-muscular movements; the heart and lungs work in the same way as they would in a sport so that there is the same benefit.

Only buy chest expanders, bar-bells and other forms of isometric equipment if you want to develop your strength or improve particular muscles. They will help you look more like Mr Universe but they will not bring the benefits to general health offered by dynamic exercise. If you must pursue a program of isometric exercise, take care not to overtax your strength. Dynamic exercise can lead to strains but in general it is self-limiting. With a bar-bell, you can easily hurt yourself. Always start with small weights and only gradually increase the weights.

Sometimes the most difficult part of any fitness program is summoning the initial will-power to start each day. Our middle-aged aerobic guinea-pigs conquered this temptation generally by remembering that they *always* felt better afterwards. But on a cold winter's day it can be especially difficult. This is one reason why money spent on warm clothing, such as track suits, is money well spent. Another is that if you look smart, you will be less self-conscious about venturing outside. Many people, however, find they need more motivation than they can themselves provide. For them, regular keep-fit classes may be the answer. Private health clubs are booming in the US, but most put more emphasis on weight-training and body-building than dynamic exercise. They are also quite expensive, so check out clubs carefully before signing any contracts. In general the nonprofit-making YMCA is a better bet than private clubs.

Special keep-fit classes are often run for people over sixty. Exercise remains just as important for the elderly as the middle-aged (see Chapter 10). The extraordinary potential of the human body is demonstrated every year in veterans' athletic championships. Most people will have humbler ambitions. But if they find life more enjoyable, as well as healthier, they are likely to be well satisfied by the fruits of their fitness.

Relaxation and Stress

Everybody is under stress. Adam and Eve in the Garden of Eden were under stress. Yet most medical experts agree that there is more stress in our lives today than ever before. Driving a car, for instance, or traveling by plane produces a stress that our ancestors did not have to cope with. More than ever before, we need a strategy to deal with the hidden strains and pressures of life.

Every week most of us face stress in our daily lives. We run for and miss that bus or train that will take us to work. We face worrying tax demands and bills; the mortgage, the bank overdraft, the rent or some other financial anxiety nags at us. We work with people we don't really like, or we have an occasional quarrel with husband, wife, boss or colleague. All these experiences, which are the normal wear and tear of living, are stressful.

Then there are the more serious strains. If a parent, a partner or a close friend dies, the bereavement takes its toll of our mental and physical health. Divorces, court cases, accidents, or an illness in the family are all major strains. Oddly enough, success can be stressful, too. Promotion, starting a new job, more responsibility, all take their toll.

For some people these stresses will be relatively easy to live through. We all know people whose response rate is low. They are able to deal with panics without getting upset. Their attitude to life is easygoing, relaxed and, indeed, they are often very enjoyable people to have around. For others, stress piles up. Under the strain of events, they feel nervous, anxious, or always on the go.

When we are upset by the strains and stresses of life, most of us suffer minor disorders, like headaches, insomnia, indigestion, diarrhea, or just general aches and pains. Stress, indeed, has been linked with conditions like migraine, asthma and ulcers. Even more serious disorders like hypertension or high blood pressure, and coronary heart disease, many doctors believe, are more likely to occur to people under a great deal of stress. Proving this link is extraordinarily difficult. But what has been proved is that a stressful event definitely has its effect on the health of human beings. Dr Richard Rahe did a careful study of some 2,500 naval officers and men in America. He looked at their lives, and in particular whether there had been any major changes in the last six months. Then he checked their health in the following six months.

He found that those men who had experienced events that changed their life pattern were more likely to become ill – possibly just minor illnesses like flu or colds, but nevertheless illnesses. In a way his findings echoed what folk wisdom has always said: if you are run down or got down by events, you catch whatever germs are around.

Dr Rahe then went further. He decided that it was too vague just to say that life events which required change made a human being more likely to develop some kind of illness. So he tried to draw up a scale of events, which gave a numerical value to each event so that the effect of an event

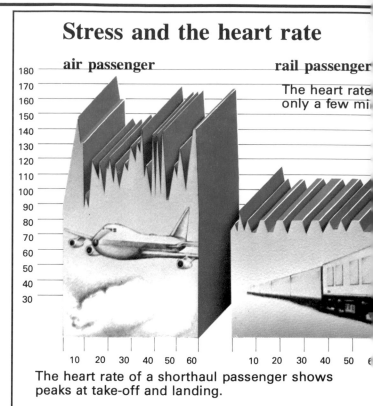

Stress and the heart rate

The heart rate of a shorthaul passenger shows peaks at take-off and landing.

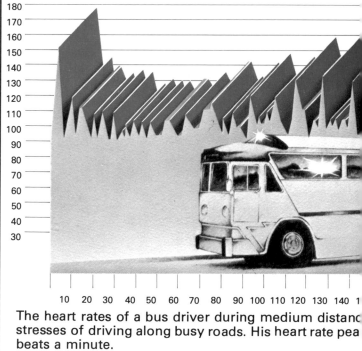

The heart rates of a bus driver during medium distance stresses of driving along busy roads. His heart rate peaks beats a minute.

on the average person could be measured. Four hundred Americans helped him work out the relative stressfulness of such events as divorce, the sack, mortgage difficulties and even Christmas (see Stress Quiz, page 94).

This way of measuring stress is extremely useful, but it cannot allow for individual differences. There is no doubt that personality, and the way we react to stress, makes a great deal of difference. It is interesting to note, for instance, that migraine sufferers tend to be people who are not only ambitious but perfectionists, intolerant of unpredictability, indecisiveness and uncertainty, and reluctant to sacrifice standards.

In the same way, heart disease has been associated with a particular – and not dissimilar – collection of personality

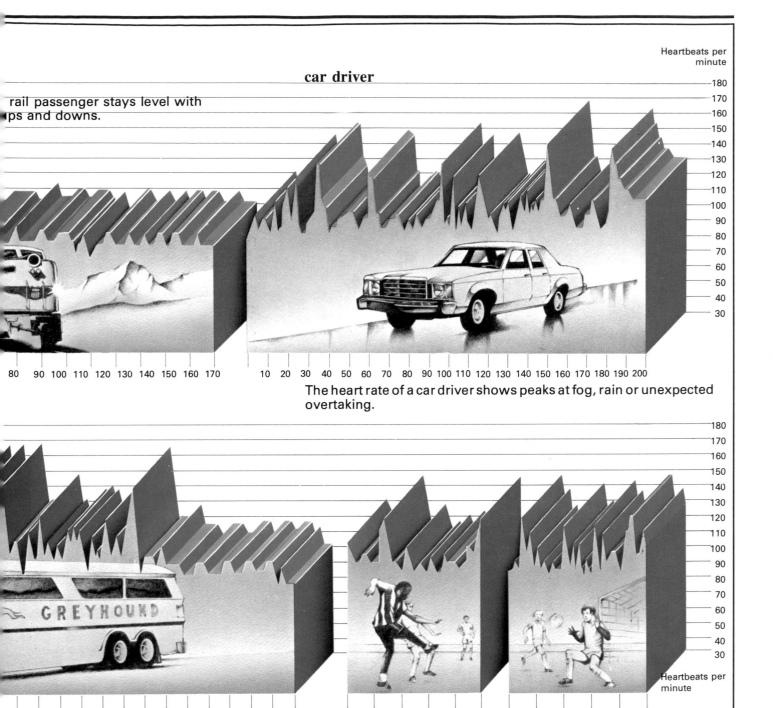

car driver

rail passenger stays level with
ups and downs.

The heart rate of a car driver shows peaks at fog, rain or unexpected overtaking.

on-stop traveling, showing the normal
t the journey's start, recording a high 150

Watching a live soccer match, the heart rate peaks at goals, near-misses and fouls—in both halves.

traits. Two American heart experts, Dr Meyer Friedman and Dr Ray Rosenman, have dubbed the typical heart disease personality the Type A. The Type A man suffers from hurry sickness. He does things rapidly, he is always conscious of time, impatient, doing two or three things at once, guilty about relaxing, obsessed with numbers and measurements, competitively ambitious, deadline-conscious, and an obsessive worker.

Sir William Osler, who was leading physician at Johns Hopkins Hospital at the turn of the century, gave a shrewd description of Type A: "It is not the delicate neurotic person who is prone to angina, but the robust, the vigorous in mind and body, the keen ambitious man, the indicator of whose engine is always at full speed ahead."

THE EFFECTS OF STRESS ON THE HEART

Stress is caused by a threat to which the body responds. The threat may be physical, the need to hurry to avoid missing a plane, or mental, the fear that something will go wrong and the plane will crash. The graphs above show the dramatic effects on the heart of traveling a few hundred miles by different means. The graphs also show that just being a spectator at a ballgame can be stressful, although there is no physical danger at all.

The graphs show the heart rate, measured in beats per minute, of the normal healthy subjects who were monitored while driving their own cars a distance of about 200 miles. The peaks of the heart rate relate to normal freeway hazards such as bunching of cars in the fast lane, overtaking, rain, hazardous moves by other drivers, and driving at high speeds. There was a sustained increase in heart rate while driving in the cities and on the freeway, with frequent peaks of 110–140. Stress is indicated by heart rates of over 100–120 beats per minutes, depending on the age of the subject. Normal resting heart rate is between 70 and 80. (The effects of the same test on those with heart disease were obviously more worrying, with up to 150 beats per minute.)

When the subjects were being driven in the front seat of a car doing the same journey, maximum heart rates ranged from 90–110 with situations of sudden or potential danger.

When they were traveling the same distance by plane their heart rates were recorded at between 100–150. The high rates were associated with events such as the closure of the aircraft's door before take-off, and landing procedures and sudden changes in altitude. Rail travel was by far the least disturbing with the heart rate rarely going above 80 beats per minute.

The subjects showed very little or no physical activity when the heart rate was at its highest, and one subject was unaware of what was happening to his heart, even though the heart rate was up to 150 beats per minute.

People were also monitored while watching live and televised soccer matches. The peaks here relate to goal-scoring, near misses, fouls on home team players and mis-interpreted decisions by the referee. Viewers of live transmissions of the matches show a lower heart rate than those who were actually seeing the match live.

Many experiments have also shown that people find it stressful to do arithmetic in their head. There is an increase in blood pressure and pulse, and an increase of blood flow in the limbs together with a decrease of blood flow in internal organs such as the kidney. And the same happens in real life: Drs Friedman and Rosenman have shown that cholesterol increases in the blood, and risk of heart attack goes up, when accountants are under stress preparing annual accounts.

Primitive man, faced with an experience that aroused emotion, would either attack or run away. Modern man has also got this flight or fight reaction. Strong emotion produces adrenaline and noradrenaline, hormones that pour into the system. The heart beats more strongly and the blood vessels narrow to make blood available for the muscles. Breathing becomes faster. The whole body is ready for action.

Unfortunately, physical action is not usually required. We cannot fight the boss or the income-tax demand – nor can we simply run away from a marital quarrel. So the body's emergency response turns inward on itself, taking a toll of the body, either immediately or sometimes later after the emotions have disappeared, resulting in nervous diarrhea, indigestion, or even a rise in blood pressure.

Doctors who believe that many of the changes in illness statistics, like the increasing amount of migraine and heart disease, are due to stress, blame modern life for producing this reaction too often. Caught in a traffic jam on the way to work, worried by a boss's demand for better performance, made anxious by the news that the firm is going to announce lay-offs, the modern executive is permanently on the alert. His or her body is going into this emergency response over and over again, and never being able to react in a physical way with a good fight or a fast getaway.

But it is not just stress that is the enemy: it is how the individual responds to stress. The theory is that the key may lie in the body's automatic response to emotions like fear, anxiety, anger or even joy.

However, the good news is that we *can* learn to cope with stress. For some people, particularly those who are in the grip of a serious illness like heart disease, this will mean avoiding stress – changing jobs, perhaps, stopping driving or traveling overseas. In the same way migraine sufferers, who know that family quarrels, say, produce the headache, can try to avoid the trigger moments that set off the pain.

RELAXATION

For stresses that cannot be avoided, a different strategy is needed. A regular relaxation period every day is what Dr Friedman and Dr Rosenman recommend for their Type A potential heart attack victims, and it does seem to work. Measurements on people practicing meditation, which involves mental and physical relaxation, have shown that their oxygen consumption drops, their breathing slows down, their heart beats more slowly and (if they are people with high blood pressure) their blood pressure drops. However, other researchers have found that the same amount of time spent sleeping seems to have a similar effect.

Even more interesting was a trial carried out by Dr Chandra Patel, a British doctor. She treated twenty patients suffering from high blood pressure by persuading them to carry out twenty minutes of meditation and relaxation twice a day. She compared their progress with a group of similar hypertension sufferers, who were getting the same regular attention from her but not doing any meditative relaxation. The blood pressure of the regular meditators dropped over a yearly period, and their need for drugs was reduced. The patients who were not doing the meditation did not improve, and they needed just as many drugs at the end as they had at the beginning.

Deep relaxation, like the sort experienced by meditators, is therefore the key. Of course, it may be a skill that you already possess. Hot baths, a quiet drink with the feet up, a real rest after sport or gardening – these are ways many people relax. Others find that these are not enough and find difficulty in relaxing body and mind into real quietness.

So how can we learn to relax? Here are some of the ways people have been helped to relax. Everybody has different preferences, so choose the one you think might appeal. Relaxation should be enjoyed, otherwise it will not work.
Massage. Try rubbing the back of your partner's neck and shoulders using the thumbs to roll up the muscles towards the head. Or massage the back and buttocks with the flat of the palm in a regular firm rhythm. Feats such as walking up

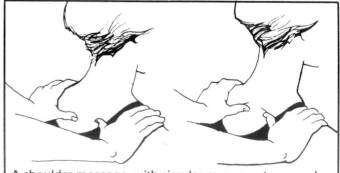

A shoulder massage, with circular movements, can relax you.

and down somebody's back are strictly for the professionals. If you do belong to a health or sports club where massage is available after exercise, indulge yourself.

Muscle control. Classes are sometimes available to teach muscle control. It is relatively easy to know when the muscles are tensed, but difficult to feel when they are relaxed. Relaxation classes can help teach this. In principle, if one can relax each major muscle group, one's mind will relax, too, and deep relaxation will follow. Classes can sometimes teach the trick of relaxing, which can be turned on at will during stressful experiences. It is worth checking to see if any classes are held in your area.

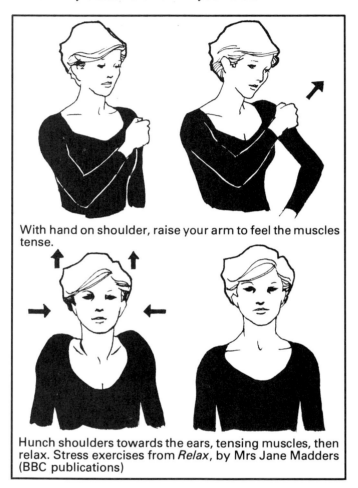

With hand on shoulder, raise your arm to feel the muscles tense.

Hunch shoulders towards the ears, tensing muscles, then relax. Stress exercises from *Relax*, by Mrs Jane Madders (BBC publications)

The most common method of learning to identify a relaxed muscle is the tense-and-let-go method. For instance, when shoulders are tensed, they tend to rise up towards the ears. By deliberately hunching them into a tense position then letting them go, it is possible to feel what a relaxed muscle should be like. Try sitting down hands on lap, and legs slightly apart. Then clench the jaw, and relax it; frown and screw up the face, and relax it; squeeze your thighs together, then let them relax outwards; clasp your hands and then relax them. There are several helpful books describing different methods of relaxation – see Appendix 2.

Some people find deep breathing useful. If you are emotionally upset, your breath comes in short sharp pants from the top of the rib-cage; so deep breathing from the diaphragm is the opposite. Place your hands at the bottom of the rib cage so that the fingers lightly touch. Take a deep breath inwards, pulling the air into the diaphragm so that your fingers are drawn apart as the diaphragm swells. Do this three or four times.

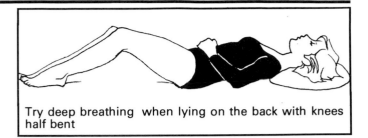

Try deep breathing when lying on the back with knees half bent

Some people find three or four deep breaths useful before a potentially stressful experience. A variant of this kind of relaxation trick is recommended for Type A potential heart victims by Friedman and Rosenman. If faced with a particularly long-drawn-out stressful experience – like writing a long report or having to do a series of complicated manual maneuvers – take the occasional break from it, to stop the nervous tension building up. Stop doing it altogether, and read a newspaper for a while. Stroll out of the office or workroom for a chat with a friend. Take a proper tea or coffee break – *not* with the work still before you.

Biofeedback machines are available which can actually measure relaxation. They consist usually of a small electronic box which gives out a continuous tone. The simplest method uses two electrodes strapped on to the skin to measure the skin's electrical resistance, which in turn is affected by the relative dryness or moisture on its surface. In the same way that panic makes one break out into a cold sweat, so the minute changes of less obvious tension produce skin moisture. The electrodes measure this, and their measurements are translated into sound. As the tension rises, and the skin sweats, the tone from the machine rises.

You can use the machine, therefore, to measure whether you are relaxing properly. Some people who are very tense cannot relax because they are not able to recognize what it feels like to be relaxed: the machine is most useful for such people. However, the noise it makes may interfere with relaxation in some people; it is perhaps most useful as an occasional check. Machines are not cheap, so it is probably only worth buying one if you enjoy gadgets. You can always play party games with biofeedback machines.

Meditation. Relaxation by meditation is common in yoga, Zen, and, of course, transcendental meditation. The principle is to use a mental device – a mantra, a single word, or a visual symbol – to relax the mind, from which bodily relaxation will flow. In its simplest form it means giving the mind something fairly unexciting to think about to blot out distracting thoughts, just in the same way that counting sheep is used to produce sleep. When a distracting thought comes into the mind, it is replaced by either a word, a mantra or a symbol. Again, it is probably easiest to learn this practise from a class, so check if local educational services have any yoga lessons or whether there is a meditation center in your area.

But if you want to try meditating by yourself, why not? You need to start in a quiet and warm environment, free from noisy distractions. You will also need to put yourself in a comfortable position, but not so comfortable that you fall asleep. Sitting should do. Choose a word or a symbol and think about it. If distracting thoughts occur, don't try to stop thinking of them: keep a passive mental attitude but let them pass out of the mind, replacing them with the repetitive word or visual symbol. If you find you can do it for yourself, it will save the fairly high fees of classes.

STRESS QUIZ

Are *you* under stress? You can measure the amount of stress in your life, using Dr Richard Rahe's stress scale. He has calculated the amount of stress that is caused by major life-events, and given each a numerical value. Have any of these events happened in your life in the last six months? If so, score for each that occurred, then check your total to see if your life is overstressful.

1. Death of spouse	100	23. Son or daughter leaving home	29
2. Divorce	73	24. Trouble with in-laws	29
3. Marital separation	65	25. Outstanding personal achievement	28
4. Jail term	63	26. Spouse begins or stops work	26
5. Death of close family member	63	27. Begin or end school or college	26
6. Personal injury or illness	53	28. Change in living conditions	25
7. Marriage	50	29. A change in personal habits	24
8. Fired at work	47	30. Trouble with the boss	23
9. Marital reconciliation	45	31. Change in work hours or conditions	20
10. Retirement	45	32. Change in residence	20
11. Change in health of family member	44	33. Change in school or college	20
12. Pregnancy	40	34. Change in recreation	19
13. Sex difficulties	39	35. Change in church activities	19
14. Gain of new family member	39	36. Change in social activities	18
15. Business readjustment	39	37. A moderate mortgage or loan	17
16. Change in financial state	38	38. Change in sleeping habits	16
17. Death of close friend	37	39. Change in number of family get-togethers	15
18. Change to different line of work	36	40. Change in eating habits	15
19. Change in number of arguments with spouse	35	41. Holiday	13
20. A large mortgage or loan	31	42. Christmas	12
21. Foreclosure of mortgage or loan	30	43. Minor violations of the law	11
22. Change in responsibilities at work	29		

How to Score

Below 60: your life has been unusually free from stress lately.

60 to 80: you have had a normal amount of stress recently. This score is average for the ordinary wear and tear of life.

80 to 100: the stress in your life is a little high, probably because of one recent event.

100 upwards: pressures are piling up, either at home or work, or both. You are under serious stress, and the higher you score above 100 the worse the strain.

Sleep

Few things are more important than a good night's sleep. After a good sleep you are much more alert and capable of working or enjoying yourself to your full capacity. When you are short of sleep you are slower, duller and less fun to be with. However, different people need different amounts of sleep: most adults average just under eight hours' sleep per night but old people need less and young people need more.

During sleep, the body is busy repairing itself. Growth hormone pours into the blood and stimulates the various tissues and organs of the body to repair themselves and grow. This is one reason why growing children need more sleep than adults. Even the brain is growing and repairing itself during sleep, and while it is doing this the blood supply to the brain increases and a person goes through a more wakeful period of dreaming sleep. Good sleep is essential for this process of bodily renewal, and if a person is deprived of sleep for a number of nights, then they* will oversleep later in order to catch up. If a person does not catch up on lost sleep, then they lose their ability to concentrate and to deal with anything but the simplest problems.

When we are awake, the hemispheres of the brain are very active, enabling us to respond to what we feel, hear and see. The activity in the brain hemispheres is dependent upon stimulation coming from the brain stem, which lies at the point where the brain is attached to the spinal cord. Thinking and consciousness occur in the hemispheres, but without the constant stimulation of the brain stem activity in the hemispheres declines and we fall asleep.

The brain stem itself works as if it were a clock with a 24-hour cycle of activity. However, some people seem to have a 25-hour cycle and tend always to stay up late, and others have a 23-hour cycle and tend to go to bed early and wake early. The hemispheres also stimulate the brain stem and may override it. This happens when we are worried or excited – the hemispheres then stimulate the brain stem to keep up its activity so that it is very difficult for them to switch off. On the other hand, a monotonous, warm environment makes us sleepy because the hemispheres cease to stimulate the brain stem, which in turn ceases to stimulate the hemispheres.

There are two kinds of sleep. We start the night with deep sleep, but after one and a half to two hours we experience lighter dreaming-sleep, when our eyes make rapid movements and our electric brain waves are faster than in ordinary sleep. Psychologists call the period of dreaming-sleep paradoxical or "rapid eye movement" sleep. When people are woken up during this period they say they have been dreaming; these periods of dreaming-sleep recur about every one and a half hours during the night. Both types of sleep are needed, and if someone is deprived of dreaming by being constantly woken up whenever they dream, then the following night they will have more dreaming-sleep.

Inability to sleep properly may be a sign that a person is worried, depressed, drinking too much or taking insufficient exercise. The majority of people who complain about their inability to sleep properly are worriers. They are people who feel they carry a great burden of responsibility, have great ambitions or perhaps carry a burden of guilt. Relaxation may help people with these problems.

A little alcohol may help a person to sleep at night. It is effective as an occasional remedy for difficulty in getting to sleep. However, regular or heavy drinking in the evenings can cause sleeping problems. A person who has had plenty of drink is liable to wake up early in the morning, when the effects of the alcohol are wearing off, and then find it very difficult to get to sleep again.

One of the best ways of getting a good night's sleep is to get some exercise in the evening before going to bed: take a walk, go jogging or if you cannot get out of the house try running up and down stairs.

People who suffer from depression often find it extremely difficult to sleep. Depression sometimes follows a personal crisis such as a death or a feeling of failure, or continues after a physical illness such as flu or jaundice. A person who is depressed, often feels at their worst in the morning and wakes up at 2 am and again at 4 am with their mind racing. During the daytime a person who is depressed does not have normal energy and is not able to do the normal tasks of life. When this has lasted for weeks and cannot obviously be put right by a change in circumstances, then your doctor may be able to help. Several drugs (anti-depressants) are available which are effective in treating depression.

Other drugs can be prescribed to help a person to sleep but none of them provide such good sleep as natural sleep. Barbiturate sleeping tablets used to be the type most commonly used. However, barbiturates carry some risk of addiction when they are used for prolonged periods. Also, a relatively small overdose can prove fatal when combined with alcohol. Sleeping tablets should never be the first choice – try the practical suggestions listed at the bottom of this page. An alternative to barbiturates is to take one of the minor tranquilizers, Librium or Valium, at night because they usually cause drowsiness. Moreover, there is very little danger of overdosage with these drugs. However, like other sleeping-drugs they reduce the amount of time spent dreaming and reduce the intensity of dreams. When coming off sleeping tablets, dreams become more vivid and it may take up to two months before sleep returns fully to normal.

Sleeping tablets taken before going to bed continue to have an effect the next day. They may cause a person to feel dreamy and to lack concentration; they may cause simple errors to be made in driving or any kind of brain work or mechanical work. This effect may last until lunch time the next day. Old people particularly (see Chapter 10) may become confused if given sleeping tablets or tranquilizers.

Sleeping tablets should always be considered to be a short-term solution. There are many alternative ways of promoting sleep. For example:

1. get more exercise. Take a walk or jog before sleeping.
2. have a milky drink or a snack before turning in. Avoid tea, coffee, rich or spicy food late at night.
3. wear ear plugs or install double glazing to cut out noise.
4. read a book until you drop off. If you wake in the middle of the night and worry, try reading a thriller to take your mind off your problems.
5. do not smoke in the bedroom. Stuffy air may stop you from sleeping.
6. if the bed is uncomfortable, buy a new one or put the mattress on the floor. If you are cold try bedsocks or a hot water bag.

* Please excuse the grammar, but "they" means both men and women. To say "he or she" each time is as pedantic and boring as it would be inexcusable to exclude either sex on grounds of brevity. Better for both sexes to feel involved, even at the price of our grammatical purity.

Yoga

Yoga is a pleasant and absorbing way for people of all ages to improve fitness and ease stress. The United States is one of the world's largest centers for yoga study outside India, but the subject is still widely misunderstood as suitable only for mystics or contortionists.

What is yoga? The word "yoga" means union or communion, and is a pragmatic science evolved over thousands of years which deals with the physical, moral, mental and spiritual well-being of man. The traditional path to a mastery of yoga is the Eight Limbs of Yoga first described by Patanjali in about 200 BC.

The first two "limbs", Yama (moral commandments) and Niyama (purification through discipline), control passions and emotions. There are at least 200 Asanas (postures) which keep the body healthy and strong. The next two stages, Pranayama (rhythmic control of the breath) and Pratyahara (freeing the mind from the senses), are known as the inner quests. Dharana (concentration), Dhyana (meditation) and Samadhi (a state of super-consciousness brought about by deep meditation) finally allows the yogi to realize his self. Yoga has several branches or divisions,

OUR LESSON EXPLAINED

The nineteen positions demonstrated by Maxine Tobias, a full-time yoga teacher, can be performed by nearly every novice yoga student within three months of starting weekly classes. Beginners can expect to find postures like these taught in one-hour classes all over America, and to feel increasingly relaxed and revitalized after each session. Yoga is not a competitive activity. By working intelligently, a person hampered by stiff joints and weak muscles can derive as much benefit as someone who finds the postures easier to perform. The movements and final positions are precise and require instruction. The diagram below indicates the three major categories of pose and the time devoted to each in a one-hour session. The numbers refer to the postures demonstrated by Ms Tobias. These individual postures bear their original Sanskrit names and a brief description of their effects.

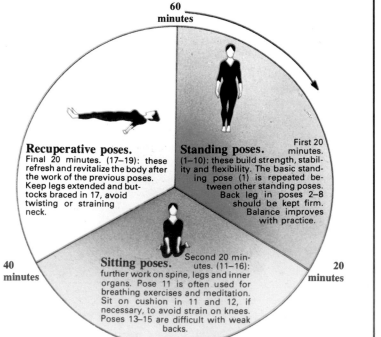

60 minutes

Recuperative poses. Final 20 minutes. (17–19): these refresh and revitalize the body after the work of the previous poses. Keep legs extended and buttocks braced in 17, avoid twisting or straining neck.

Standing poses. First 20 minutes. (1–10): these build strength, stability and flexibility. The basic standing pose (1) is repeated between other standing poses. Back leg in poses 2–8 should be kept firm. Balance improves with practice.

Sitting poses. Second 20 minutes. (11–16): further work on spine, legs and inner organs. Pose 11 is often used for breathing exercises and meditation. Sit on cushion in 11 and 12, if necessary, to avoid strain on knees. Poses 13–15 are difficult with weak backs.

40 minutes

20 minutes

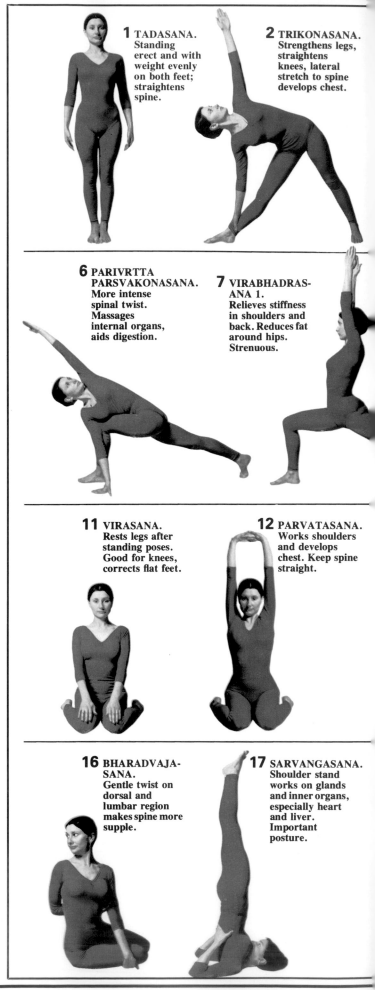

1 TADASANA. Standing erect and with weight evenly on both feet; straightens spine.

2 TRIKONASANA. Strengthens legs, straightens knees, lateral stretch to spine develops chest.

6 PARIVRTTA PARSVAKONASANA. More intense spinal twist. Massages internal organs, aids digestion.

7 VIRABHADRASANA 1. Relieves stiffness in shoulders and back. Reduces fat around hips. Strenuous.

11 VIRASANA. Rests legs after standing poses. Good for knees, corrects flat feet.

12 PARVATASANA. Works shoulders and develops chest. Keep spine straight.

16 BHARADVAJASANA. Gentle twist on dorsal and lumbar region makes spine more supple.

17 SARVANGASANA. Shoulder stand works on glands and inner organs, especially heart and liver. Important posture.

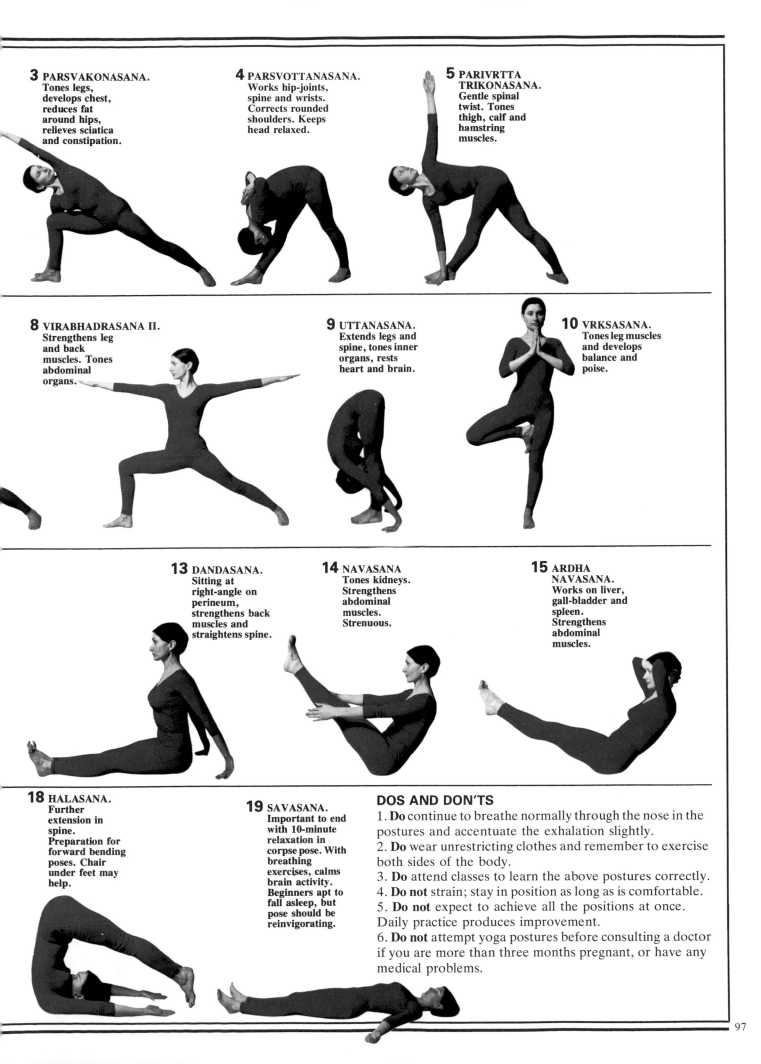

3 PARSVAKONASANA. Tones legs, develops chest, reduces fat around hips, relieves sciatica and constipation.

4 PARSVOTTANASANA. Works hip-joints, spine and wrists. Corrects rounded shoulders. Keeps head relaxed.

5 PARIVRTTA TRIKONASANA. Gentle spinal twist. Tones thigh, calf and hamstring muscles.

8 VIRABHADRASANA II. Strengthens leg and back muscles. Tones abdominal organs.

9 UTTANASANA. Extends legs and spine, tones inner organs, rests heart and brain.

10 VRKSASANA. Tones leg muscles and develops balance and poise.

13 DANDASANA. Sitting at right-angle on perineum, strengthens back muscles and straightens spine.

14 NAVASANA Tones kidneys. Strengthens abdominal muscles. Strenuous.

15 ARDHA NAVASANA. Works on liver, gall-bladder and spleen. Strengthens abdominal muscles.

18 HALASANA. Further extension in spine. Preparation for forward bending poses. Chair under feet may help.

19 SAVASANA. Important to end with 10-minute relaxation in corpse pose. With breathing exercises, calms brain activity. Beginners apt to fall asleep, but pose should be reinvigorating.

DOS AND DON'TS

1. **Do** continue to breathe normally through the nose in the postures and accentuate the exhalation slightly.

2. **Do** wear unrestricting clothes and remember to exercise both sides of the body.

3. **Do** attend classes to learn the above postures correctly.

4. **Do not** strain; stay in position as long as is comfortable.

5. **Do not** expect to achieve all the positions at once. Daily practice produces improvement.

6. **Do not** attempt yoga postures before consulting a doctor if you are more than three months pregnant, or have any medical problems.

but in the West students largely concentrate on Hatha Yoga, an approach concerned primarily with bodily posture – the Asanas. The relaxation and physical benefits achieved from practicing even just once a week are a sufficient reward for many beginners, and quickly become apparent.

How does yoga affect diet? The only special dietary rule to observe when taking up Hatha Yoga is always to practice on an empty stomach. It is not advisable or comfortable to perform postures within about four hours of having eaten, but you need not change your diet in any way. Those who become serious yoga followers do usually lose the taste for meat, and often stop or cut down on tobacco and alcohol. These measures are also good for health as described elsewhere in this book. One of the classic yoga texts, the Hatha Yoga Pradipika of Svatmarama, says: "The yogi should take a nourishing and sweet food mixed with milk. It should be pleasing to the senses and nutritive."

Will yoga affect my health? Considerable claims are made for the medical benefits of correctly practiced postures. The medical profession remains divided over some of the wilder claims, which range from alleviating appendicitis to ulcers, but supports the general notion that the physical postures, like other exercises, can be useful preventive medicine and that particular postures may help to relieve certain medical complaints such as backache, constipation, insomnia and flat feet.

The calm, relaxing effects of yoga are accepted as a valuable antidote to urban stress and strain. Serious ailments should not, however, be treated with yoga unless medical advice has been given and a qualified teacher consulted. It is also all too easy to damage muscles, joints and the spine without proper supervision.

If you suffer from heart trouble, dizziness or back disorders, you should never take up yoga, or any other strenuous activity, without consulting a doctor. Women should not perform all the postures during menstruation, for the last six months of pregnancy or for three months after giving birth.

Charles T. Kuntzleman and the editors of *Consumer Guide* in their book *Rating the Exercises* produced an eight-point summary of yoga's most frequently claimed benefits for general health and fitness. It is:
1. Yoga can improve flexibility and grace.
2. Yoga does not improve endurance or stamina.
3. Yoga is probably a good way to release tension and stress.
4. Yoga does not maintain proper circulation (although it may be helpful in reducing high blood pressure).
5. Yoga does not improve the strength of the vital organs and glands.
6. Yoga may improve the firmness and strength of selected muscles and muscle groups.
7. Yoga does not produce a taut, smooth skin.
8. Yoga makes only a meager contribution to weight control.

Yoga alone is therefore an inadequate program for diet control or physical fitness. This is firstly because it expends too few calories to have a significant effect on overall weight. Secondly, it does not have the beneficial effects on the heart and lung – the so-called cardiovascular exercise – that stem from such activities as running, swimming, cycling or walking. Use these activities therefore to build up your endurance (and the consequent heart-lung training effect) and use yoga for its beneficial effects on flexibility and general lessening of stress and tension.

Where can I learn? No longer a freak clique, yoga teachers can now be found in virtually every community, from YMCAs to American Legion halls. There are hundreds of yoga books in the shops and regular programs on TV. Simply looking in the telephone directory will reveal the names of many yoga practitioners, both individual and corporate, but there are also many adult education courses in yoga. Check local newspapers or ask at your nearest YMCA for details. Always ask about a teacher's qualifications, and check costs.

What will I need to practice? Yoga demands extensive stretching of the body and it is therefore most comfortable to wear loose clothing. T-shirts and footless tights, cotton trousers or shorts, are ideal. Avoid clothing that has buttons, belts or buckles. Try to find a clear patch of floorspace in a quiet, clean, airy room where you can practice regularly without interruption. The only equipment necessary is a folded blanket used for the sitting and recuperative postures. It can be instructive to observe yourself in a mirror, but it must be perpendicular to the floor and full-length to be of benefit.

The Iyengar method

Many yoga students in the West follow a method developed by the Indian yogi and guru, B.K.S. Iyengar. He began teaching in India in 1936 and has subjected the practice of yoga to detailed examination, which he continues at his Institute. One of his first pupils in the West was Yehudi Menuhin, who describes the Iyengar method as "a technique ideally suited to prevent physical and mental illness and to protect the body generally, developing an inevitable sense of self-reliance and assurance." The beginner first learns the Asanas (postures) before being led on to Pranayama (control of breath). Iyengar is an advocate of an integrated approach to yoga, known as Astanga or Raja yoga. Although the goal remains the same, there are other paths of yoga, each with a different emphasis, such as Bhakti, Jnana and Kundalini yoga.

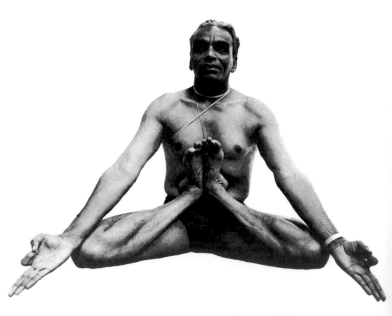

The doyen of yoga students, B. K. S. Iyengar, demonstrates an advanced posture at his Institute.

Signs of Suicide

Suicide is one of the most common causes of death for 15–34-year-olds, and one of the top ten causes of death at all ages. Yet tragedies can often be averted if the problems that cause them are recognized early enough – if not by the sufferer, by his family and friends. Suicide is increasing. A decade ago there were 20,000 suicides a year in the United States – now there are 36,000.

Loneliness is perhaps the commonest cause of suicide. People who have moved from one country to another or from one area to another are the most vulnerable. Immigrants, young housewives within two years of moving house, elderly people who retire to the shore, young people living in rented rooms and old people without children, are all at more than average risk. Bankruptcy, lay-offs and unemployment, the death of a loved one or even the anniversary of a death may trigger a suicide attempt. Divorce, disorganized home life, abortion, and medical verdicts are other common causes.

The most common disorder is depression, which affects perhaps two-thirds of all suicides; about 13 per cent suffer from excessive drinking and about 3 per cent from fears and anxiety. All these conditions can be treated with a fair degree of success if the seriousness of the person's state is recognized by a doctor. Often the depression is caused by physical illness and once the crisis is over, the suicidal feelings pass; a doctor may be able to correct the physical illness which is the basic cause.

But doctors often fail to recognize or help the potential suicide. Many people who commit suicide have consulted their family doctor *in the previous week*. In many of these cases, the family doctor obviously fails to recognize the danger, often prescribing tranquilizers or sleeping tablets instead of anti-depressants. Anti-depressants can be very effective; whereas barbiturate sleeping tablets can be used to commit suicide.

Voluntary agencies such as the National Save-a-Life League (see Appendix 2) can also be highly effective. They will offer friendship and help. They will listen to your problems and they will phone wherever you are two or three times a day for as long as you need them.

Practical advice. Most people who kill themselves give a warning. They may talk in detail about how they intend to do it or may simply hint at it. If you suspect a serious problem, ask about it; but do not raise the subject of suicide first because it may suggest the idea. When someone *does* talk of suicide, let them do the talking and listen. Do not tell them to snap out of it and do not offer too much advice. If they are too depressed to talk, just sit with them – all night if necessary. Try to persuade the person to call a doctor or the National Save-a-Life League. Accept the person who is threatening suicide as human and their feelings as real. Try to get them to professional help, and do not leave them alone.

Eric Zvi Hadar, a counselor for the National Save-a-Life League, says that the symptoms of depression, which can be recognized by anyone, should be seen as a call for help. This is his advice:

How to recognize depression:
1. Hiding from the problem, often a great reluctance to get up in the morning and face the world.
2. Sitting in the dark.
3. Acknowledging a fear of failure.
4. Saying things like: "One of these days I'm going to pack it all in" or "I can no longer cope with the situation."
5. Putting affairs in order and canceling plans for the future.

How a friend can help:
1. Listen carefully, be friendly and appreciative of what is being told you.
2. Don't be in a hurry to give advice. Don't generalize.
3. Don't sympathize, but be compassionate.
4. Try to understand what is being said, but do not make moral judgement. Do not be shocked or attempt to avoid the subject.
5. Ask specifically about the plan for suicide and the reason for the decision. The more detailed the plan for suicide the more pressing the problem.

What a friend can do:
1. Try not to let the person who has threatened suicide be alone for any length of time.
2. Try to shift the attitude and attention completely away from the problem as it appears.
3. Readjust the point of attention to a solution if possible. If no solution seems apparent, then recommend professional help.
4. Make a sincere effort to reinforce the self-worth of the individual. Try to assure them that you are a friend who cares whether they live or die.
5. Try to establish a new goal for the sufferer. A goal that they feel can be accomplished.

MAINTAINING THE BODYWORK

The Back

The twenty-four separate vertebrae of the spine are probably the most troublesome bones in the world. In America some 28 million people are estimated to suffer from back pain. Almost certainly, more working days are lost through back trouble than industrial disputes. Yet much back pain is avoidable.

It used to be believed that back pain was a consequence of our upright posture. Apart from being unhelpful – we cannot really spend our lives on all-fours – this belief is probably also untrue. We and our ancestors have been shuffling around on two feet for some millions of years, which should be long enough to have got used to the position.

The truth is that nobody knows for certain why backache is increasingly common. It could, like some headaches, be a sign of a more stressful world. It could be that, as part of the harder lives our parents and grandparents lived, backaches were accepted almost unnoticed.

But if we do not know why complaints about back pain are more common, we do know a lot about the causes of back pain, and this can help us to avoid much of it.

Back strains
These are the most common source of back pain. Fortunately, they are also the least serious, because if reasonable care is taken they usually cure themselves.

We frequently risk these temporary injuries, since whenever we lift a heavy weight or move awkwardly – let alone when we do both together – we subject the muscles of our back to enormous stresses. Some of the bundles of fibres that make up muscles may become fatigued: ligaments and tendons may become torn. (Ligaments join bones or cartilages; tendons join muscles to bones or other muscles.)

Disabling muscle pain can be caused by lifting weights awkwardly or by twisting or bending the joints of the spine beyond their normal range. In general, the pain is felt immediately and is sufficient to stop the activity that is causing the damage. Usually, too, the damage will repair itself, given time. But complete rest is not the answer. Muscles benefit by movement, and they need a circulation of blood. The process of self-repair will therefore be helped by gentle exercise such as walking or swimming, and by mild bending and stretching. The pain itself can be relieved by keeping the muscles warm. This is why infra-red lamps are recommended for muscle strains, although hot baths and hot-water bags are cheaper alternatives.

If the pain does not start to get better after a few days, it is usually sensible to see your doctor, in case the cause is something other than a simple strain.

Slipped discs
Disc trouble is much rarer than muscular pains, and it is slower to mend. The discs are the shock absorbers of the spinal system. The back itself, including the neck, is basically twenty-four moveable vertebrae that together form the spine. They link to form an S-shaped curve, as seen in the illustration on page 103.

The diagram on page 102 shows in detail how the spine can be moved. Each vertebra is linked to its neighbors by bony projections above and below. The rounded part of each vertebra is separated from its neighbor by a tough shock absorber known as a disc, and more properly called an intervertebral disc.

The disc is a fairly rigid ring surrounding a pulpy center. These discs operate healthily if the vertebrae they cushion remain in the proper alignment. If they are continually misaligned, and especially if they are heavily loaded while misaligned, the disc may slide, slip, or even burst. If the disc slips or bursts backwards it may cause pain, because it can then press on one of the nerves leading to the spinal cord. The spinal cord is the column of nerves that is an extension of the lower part of the brain, and it runs in a protective sheath down the spinal canal, passing through an approximately circular hole in the vertebrae and behind the discs. The roots of the nerves of the spinal column pass in and out of it, and carry nerve messages. As they pass between the bones of the spine, they are at risk of pressure from a displaced or burst disc, and the pressure may be sufficient to produce pain. Usually, the pain is felt in the part of the back where the disc has been disturbed; very occasionally, our idiosyncratic nervous system reports the pain as coming from an area of the skin to which the nerves of the spinal cord go.

Posture
The human body is self-repairing and to a certain extent muscles become stronger if they are frequently loaded. In the case of an arm or a leg, repeated movements against a resistance develops strength – and also the muscles sought by the body-builder. But the muscles of the back show this strengthening less markedly. Repeated abuse, or the

cumulative effect of relatively small stresses may cause painful muscle strain.

Posture is generally important, as explained on page 104, but it is particularly important for the back. If we habitually sit in motor cars so as to put our back into a stressed position, or ride where there is a series of unpredictable shocks – over rough ground, for example – the stressed part of the spine may yield to the repeated onslaught, and the disc may move.

An activity as simple as washing up or typing can produce incapacitating back pain if it involves prolonged stooping: it need not involve heavy work. Even walking, especially when carrying an awkwardly balanced load such as a suitcase, can strain the back. And because carrying an internal load can be as harmful as carrying an external one, over-weight people are much more vulnerable to back problems than those of normal weight.

Back pain and age
As we get older, our joints are increasingly likely to become inflamed and painful. About half the people over sixty suffer from this problem, known as *osteo-arthrosis* or *osteo-arthritis*, from time to time. It hits the joints of the neck and the small of the back as well as such joints as the hip and knee, which are discussed in more detail elsewhere.

Arthritis is not the only medical term associated with back pain in the later years. The word *rheumatism* is some-times used by doctors as a label for virtually any kind of pain that involves muscles, ligaments, bones or joints. *Rheumatism* is not the name of the disease, only shorthand for a number of afflictions that can often be more precisely described. *Lumbago*, again, is not the name of a disease: it means simply pain in the lower part of the back – the lumbar region.

As rheumatism and lumbago are not the precise names of diseases – the terms are clinically vague, in fact – there are no cures for rheumatism or lumbago as such; the remedies depend on the precise nature of the problem. It is worth while consulting your doctor before spending money on drugs, lotions or equipment advertised as rheumatism or lumbago treatments.

Sciatica is the name given to pain felt in areas of the buttock, back of the thigh, and in the leg, ankle and toes, all of which are supplied by the sciatic nerve, which runs down the back of the leg. Like *lumbago* and *rheumatism*, *sciatica* is the name of a symptom. The pain may be caused by disc trouble in the lower back – the sciatic nerve is formed by the joining of a number of nerves from the spine – or by joint disease affecting the lower spine.

Back pain in women
The muscle strain that produces backaches makes no dis-tinction between the sexes: men and women are equally vulnerable. However, there are a few causes of backache that are peculiar to women. The slackening of the joints of the pelvis that is associated with pregnancy can lead to pain in the back. Furthermore, the nerves from the lower end of the spinal cord feed into the womb, so period pain often includes backache. Some specifically female disorders, such as a prolapse of the womb or an infection in the tubes, may also produce pain in the back. But as a general rule, if it is back *movement* that elicits the pain in that region, then it is specifically the muscles or joints of the back that are the cause, rather than problems affecting other internal organs.

HOW TO AVOID BACK PAIN
Back pain is debilitating, it can keep you from work and spoil your pleasure, but it is not normally serious, in the sense that people do not, in general, die from it. Usually it goes away on its own; sometimes, recovery can be helped by medical treatment. But it is always unpleasant: that is the natural function of pain, as otherwise you would ignore it. And there is always the risk that the damage may not cure itself completely, and that there will be a weakness in the back that is vulnerable to a repetition of the damage.

There is, too, always a risk of injuring the back by sub-jecting it to unexpected stresses. A sudden awkward and energetic movement can present a hazard. Swinging a suit-case on to a luggage rack, or pulling one from the trunk of a car, for instance, can strain muscles or suddenly load par-ticular vertebrae so that the disc between them is damaged. Unfortunately, we cannot always avoid the risks. There are, though, ways of reducing the general vulnerability of the back.

Two ways have already been mentioned: the need for a good posture (which is explained more fully on page 104); and the need to avoid being overweight, since this is a steady abuse of the spine which can lead to serious back pain. A third general way of minimizing the chances of suffering back pain is to take regular physical exercise. Dr Hans Kraus, a New York physician and back specialist, estimates that up to 80 per cent of back pain is due to a general physical deterioration which can be reversed through exercise.

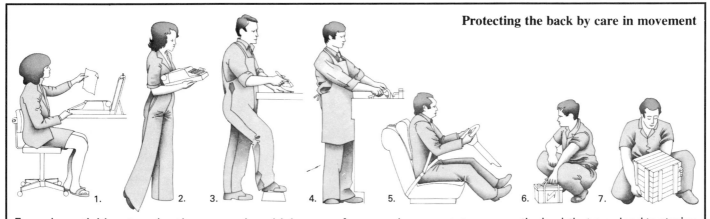

Protecting the back by care in movement

1.   2.   3.   4.   5.   6.   7.

Everyday activities at work, at home, or when driving a car, for example, can put stresses on the back that may lead to strains. Moving properly keeps the risk to a minimum: see overleaf for detailed descriptions – and advice.

Thus physical exercise is as good for back problems as it is for many other afflictions. A supple, mobile back is less likely to give trouble than one that is stiff and unused to movement, and if you exercise your back, there is a good chance that you won't damage it by the way you type or do the dishes or drive. Walking, swimming and yoga are all good exercises. If you are taking up exercises as prevention, you should start gently, of course, otherwise your attempts at prevention could themselves cause trouble. Take your exercise daily rather than in bursts at weekends.

You should also learn techniques for everyday activities that will reduce the risk of back damage. Some backs are weaker than others, and therefore more vulnerable. But everyone can lessen the likelihood of back pain by following the few simple rules illustrated by the drawings on page 101. From left to right:

1. Many workers sit down at their work. They, or their employers, should choose chairs so as to reduce the risk of back pain. The chair shown here supports the lumbar – lower – spine well. This is important, because this is where pain is most common. Ideally, the back of the chair should be adjustable for people of different height. The seat of the chair illustrated is less satisfactory. It should be deep enough, front to back, to support the thighs, and the front should not dig into the thighs. The seat should, as shown, have a slight slope backwards, and the height should be such that the feet can rest comfortably on the ground, with the user's knees bent to no more than ninety degrees. The height of the seat, therefore, must be adjustable. Furthermore, the design of the seat must suit the line of vision and the actual activities of the person who uses it.

The chair shown is fairly typical of those provided for typists. Office workers who have to use uncomfortable chairs should try to improve them – with a cushion, for instance – to support the lumbar spine. Another worthwhile, though less easy, modification is for shorthand- or copy-typists to clip their notebooks or copy directly in front of them. The traditional method, which involves continuously looking at copy fixed to the side, keeps the spine twisted. If you can avoid this, even if only by changing the work from one side to the other, the stress on the back and neck is reduced.

2. *Lifting weights.* If you think of the spine as a curved, flexible rod that must be kept in shape by its muscles, you can understand the rule for weight-handling. When carrying even a rather commonplace weight, such as a typewriter, keep the weight in front of you, so that you do not bend the spine sideways. Moreover, you should keep the weight as near to you as possible. In this particular example, it is worth remembering that the keyboard is the lighter part of the machine: carry a typewriter keyboard-forwards.

3 and 4. When working at benches or sinks, as in these two drawings, the danger is one of frequent small abuses. You should not stoop over a sink; if you can, make sure that the sink is high enough and that you can get your feet underneath it. Most of us, unfortunately, cannot rebuild either our sinks or our work benches. We must therefore compensate for bad design by extra care. There are a few simple modifications that can help. We can, of course, reduce the stress on our backs simply by leaning on the sink with thighs or stomach, wearing some protection against the wet. Quite often, the working height of a sink can be raised by standing a plastic bowl on a block of wood inside the sink. Equally, a block of wood (figure 3) at the side of a work-bench will

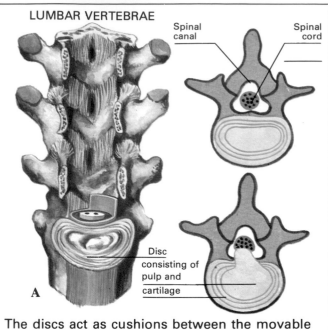

LUMBAR VERTEBRAE

Spinal canal

Spinal cord

Disc consisting of pulp and cartilage

A

The discs act as cushions between the movable vertebrae of the back. A disc that slips may press on a nerve and cause pain and disability.

help to reduce back pain. It enables you to take the weight off one foot at a time and so vary your posture, rather than having to bend over your work.

5. Many people get backache while driving a car. This is not surprising; we are ill-designed for the positions that car-driving puts us into. There are a few people whose back is so sensitive to stress that they shouldn't really drive a car at all. Most people cannot avoid driving at some time or another, but they *can* minimize the risks to their back. The aim is to keep the back upright and supported, and the legs extended with support along the thighs. Ideally, the seat should be as high as it can be without getting riskily near to the roof; low seats mean that the hips and the lumbar spine must be unduly bent. The seat can often be raised on wooden blocks; an easy modification – a firm cushion on the seat – can give the same effect. You cannot usually do much about changing the amount of leg support your car seat gives, but carefully arranged cushions can improve the backs of most car seats. The seat back should come up to the top of your head, but many car seats still do not. Head support can be added, but add one that reaches only to the base of your head, and which therefore supports the spine but not the head itself.

6 and 7. When heavier weights have to be moved, use your head to save your spine. Older people, and those who are unfit, should try to avoid lifting heavy weights if at all possible. If you are unused to the task, it is quite easy to damage the back by awkwardly lifting a weight of as little as twenty pounds. People who are traveling, for example, should think about the weight of their baggage when they are packing, rather than traveling in the hope that there will always be some strong-backed assistant at every stopping-place.

When moving furniture such as wardrobes or cupboards, try to avoid lifting. See if they can be rocked and turned and inched around. If you do have to lift, keep the load on the spine in the direction it is built for: vertical, or as near to as possible. Don't stoop, but bend the knees, keep the spine straight. Lift, if you can, between the bent knees, so that the

The machinery of the back.

The movable vertebrae of the spine (below) end in the forward curve of the very flexible lumbar region. Below these are the fused bones of the sacral region and the coccyx— the remnants of our tail. The powerful muscles that are attached to the spine (right) contract as the body moves, sometimes loading the spine heavily. Usually backaches represent strain in these muscles and can disappear quickly. But sometimes repeated stressing affects the spine itself.

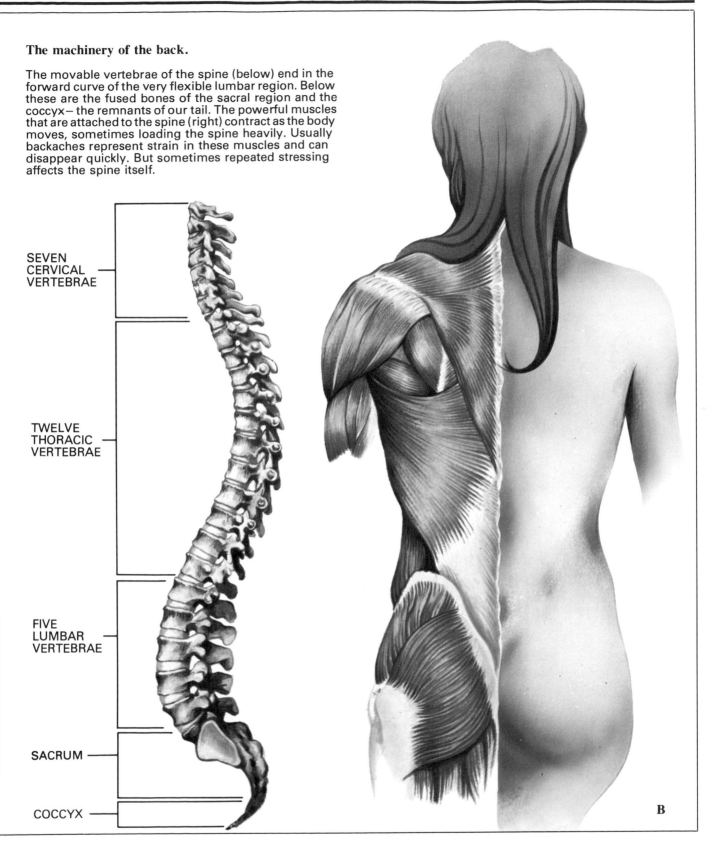

SEVEN
CERVICAL
VERTEBRAE

TWELVE
THORACIC
VERTEBRAE

FIVE
LUMBAR
VERTEBRAE

SACRUM

COCCYX

B

load is as near the body as possible, and lift by straightening the legs, where you have powerful and resilient muscles. In lifting, as with other tasks, the damage can come from one heavy load or a succession of small ones. You should lift a baby from a crib as you would lift a heavy weight: with bent knees and the weight near the body. In lifting a case from the trunk of a car, you can use one hand to lift and the other to press against the car's body to relieve the strain on the back.

Pushing a car puts a heavy stress on the back, but medical research at a British university suggests that pulling involves very much less. The stress on the back can be derived from a measurement of the pressure inside the stomach, because it turns out that the stomach muscles, in men at least, play an important part in straightening the back. They compress the fluid contents of the stomach and thus assist the back muscles. You can measure the effort of the stomach muscles by using a radio pill that is swallowed, and the results make it quite clear how preferable pulling is. It is, of course, difficult to arrange to pull a car, but the muscles of the back are, fortunately, concerned only with the direction of the effort, not in the actual way the effort is exerted. Leaning with your back against a car and pushing it counts as pulling to the muscles, and minimizes the risk to the back.

Back pain and beds

We spend a third of our lives in bed, generally asleep, so it is important to make sure that the bed is beneficial to the back. So-called orthopedic beds are available, but these are not essential. All you need is a bed that supports the body. The base must be firm, since a sagging bed allows the spine to curve to an undesirable extent, but it should not be hard. *Any* bed can be prevented from sagging by placing two or three nine-inch planks across it under that part of the mattress which supports the trunk. The boards should be about a foot shorter than the width of the bed. Other ways to achieve the same desirable effect are to use a thick foam rubber mattress on a hard base or a thinner one on a stiff-spring base. Any bed, in fact, which has a firm base and a mattress resilient enough to follow the contours of the body without letting it sag, will help avoid back pain. In emergencies you can always put your mattress on the floor and sleep there: this gives all the firm unsagging support you need. Pillows are less important than the bed itself, but they are worth some thought. If there are too many pillows they tend to get into odd places under the shoulders. They should also be soft rather than hard for comfort, while small pillows can be used to support the knees and the lower back when you lie down.

When back pain strikes

Despite precautions, you may still be laid low with back pain. Always see your doctor before contemplating any of the many cures which, considering the affliction is so widespread, have not surprisingly been proposed for back troubles. And as the human system varies as widely as it does, most of them have worked on someone. Acupuncture, which involves the use of needles on "sensitive" points of the body, has worked; plaster supports have worked; osteopaths, who manipulate joints, have succeeded; and some sufferers have been helped by changes in diet. If we accept that back pain can also result from psychological tension, then some people will cure their pain by learning to cope more successfully with stress.

But none of these should be the first remedy you try. Sufferers should always first see their doctor. He or she should know you and the kind of life you lead, and can at least tell you how to avoid making the problem worse. In fact, if the pain is severe, get your doctor to come to see you. Keep warm, stay in bed on a firm mattress – get someone to slide some boards underneath if it is soft – and wait for the visit. The doctor may recommend drugs: analgesics or pain killers help some people to sleep or exercise when they have a strained back; or the doctor's advice may be massage, manipulation, some form of physical support or a mixture of all these different approaches.

Muscle or ligament strain is the most common diagnosis, usually because nothing else can be found wrong. There are then several possible approaches to treatment, all of which are worth trying although there is no agreed order of priority. The general rule is that rest is the first treatment to be tried. Young people are generally advised to strengthen muscles and restore the full range of movement, though some preliminary treatment including rest will almost certainly be needed. Physiotherapy, heat treatment and massage may also help. If the pain still persists after several weeks, perhaps a surgical corset may be recommended – especially for older people. If there is local tenderness, then injections of hydrocortisone and local anesthetic may be advised. In other cases manipulation by an osteopath may bring relief, but always ask your doctor about this first. Time cures most backaches but sometimes nothing seems to work and the sufferer has to live with it. An operation is not advisable unless a doctor has found something positive in their investigations. Once you are cured, always remember that you are probably more vulnerable than before. You are also likely to know at least one activity which is risky – the one that set off the attack – and therefore to be avoided if at all possible.

POSTURE FOR HEALTH

Good posture is an important part of good health. It is something that we can all improve for ourselves without any special equipment or drugs. Improving your posture is more than a step to improving your health; it will also improve your personal appearance. Some people think of posture as simply the body's position when standing to attention. Posture is not just this. It is the attitude of the body, whether it is lying down, walking, sitting or moving in any way. A good posture is one that gives the highest efficiency for each individual with the lowest amount of muscular effort. As individuals vary, so will posture vary. One can therefore describe a good posture only in general terms.

A good posture is one which gives the body easy balance and poise; is aesthetically pleasing; enables the muscles to work to the best advantage and in harmony with each other; and provides the internal organs with room in which to work.

A bad posture is one where the balance of the body is maintained by muscles ill-prepared for the task. The result not only looks unpleasant; the muscles have to work more than necessary; and the internal organs are cramped.

You can feel the difference between a good and a bad posture by trying to stand in the right way. The body's weight should be distributed so that the line of gravity falls just behind the ear, through the cervical vertebrae, through the shoulder and in front of the thoracic vertebrae, through the lumbar vertebrae and the hip-joint, and just in front of the knee to about 1½ inches (4 cm) in front of the ankle-joint. To get this ideal posture, every part of the body has to be placed gently in the right position. The head should be centrally placed, neither leaning on one side nor jutting forward. The shoulders must be relaxed and low but neither hunched nor pressed back. The pelvis should be tilted so that the stomach is gently (but not fiercely) held in. The feet should face forward. Try standing like this in front of a mirror.

In order not only to see but also to *feel* what a good posture is like, try some bad attitudes. It is often assumed that standing to attention is a good posture. Thrust the chin up, the shoulders back and the chest out. You will feel that the shoulder muscles are rigid rather than relaxed – an unnecessary muscle effort. They will probably also have crept upwards. Though the thrust-out chest gives plenty of

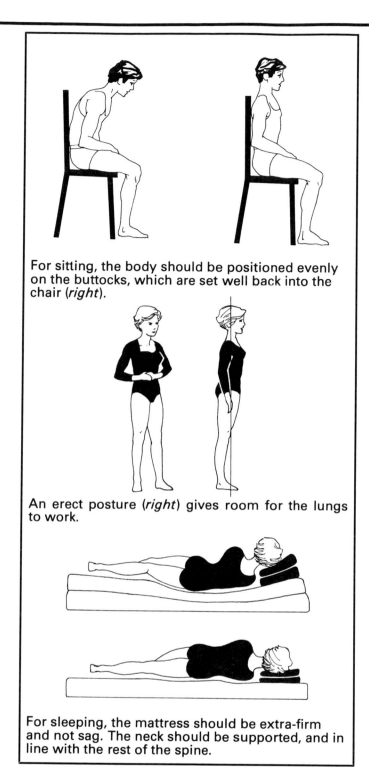

For sitting, the body should be positioned evenly on the buttocks, which are set well back into the chair (*right*).

An erect posture (*right*) gives room for the lungs to work.

For sleeping, the mattress should be extra-firm and not sag. The neck should be supported, and in line with the rest of the spine.

and proper weight distribution.

Sitting. Sit with legs firmly planted on the floor, slightly apart, the body positioned evenly on the buttocks, which are set well back into the chair. Try to make sure this is the way you watch television or read, although you will obviously change position from time to time. Rest the head on the back of the chair if possible.

Walking. An erect posture gives room for the lungs to work. Keep a rhythmical stride, stepping out freely and letting the arms swing naturally. If you have to carry anything heavy, try to split a load into two bags or suitcases, so that you can balance one on either side rather than have to walk with the weight all on one side.

Sleeping. Invest in an extra firm mattress. Do not assume it will last a lifetime. Buy a new one if it begins to sag or go lumpy. The base of the mattress should be hard: put in enough planks to support the whole mattress, not just one under where you think your back will be. Make sure the neck is supported, if you sleep on your side. The shoulder should be on the mattress with enough pillow or pillows to hold up the neck in line with the rest of the spine. Some people find special neck pillows helpful. You can make one by taking a loosely filled pillow and tying it in the middle into a butterfly shape.

Some people re-learn body attitudes by special teaching in various so-called "techniques". But these can be expensive. Most people can improve their posture by following these simple rules:

1. Practice a good posture, when standing, sitting or kneeling, whenever you remember.
2. Check any habitually bad body-movements and attitudes, and try to convert them into properly balanced ones.
3. Give the muscles a fair chance of rest by having adequate sleep (see also page 95).
4. Dress sensibly. Working clothes should permit free movement and be such that if necessary you can hold "dirty" weights closely.
5. Take up some sport, exercise or dancing. Anything which teaches bodily co-ordination and rhythm helps towards good posture.
6. Cultivate a healthy and optimistic mental attitude. This will have a positive effect on your posture.

Pregnancy, by adding an extra weight load, can give temporary posture problems (see Chapter 1). Walking is perhaps the best exercise. Don't worry unnecessarily. But make sure that when the baby is born, you go back to your old upright posture without too much hollow in the back.

room for the lungs, it also hollows the back unnecessarily, putting a strain on the spine. It is significant that armies, recognizing that standing to attention is a strain, make use of the "At ease" position.

At the other extreme is the slouching attitude. Round and hunch your shoulders forward, sinking the chest downwards and backwards. Usually your head will automatically jut forward, and your pelvis tilt too. If you try to take a deep breath, you will find there is not enough room to inflate the lungs fully. The weight of the head is a strain on the upper spine, and the pelvic tilt means that the lowest spine is under unnecessary strain.

Obviously a good posture applies to moving or sitting as well as standing. In all activities the same principles apply: balance, minimal muscle work, room for internal organs

The Feet

A healthy body owes a great debt to the feet. Your feet propel you through the day, down streets, up stairs, over sportsfields – but all too often the only care they receive is a fortnightly assault on stubbornly tough toenails.

Feet, then, are a down-trodden part of the body. They are squeezed into badly fitting shoes, constricted by sweaty, tight stockings or socks, and made to function for days at a time in fashionable footwear that would make an infantry regiment mutiny. No wonder they wreak their revenge in old age with bunions and – the most common complaint – corns.

Foot lib should begin with babies. Give a child badly fitting shoes and too-tight socks, and you have doomed them to foot deformity for life. Add fashionable shoes for the next twenty years and you have probably doubled the size of the developing bunions. Yet all feet need is a little bit of freedom.

1. *Choose shoes with care.* Shoes that hurt don't fit properly. Wear your normal sort of socks or stockings when you try on new shoes. Try on both shoes. Walk, stand on tiptoe, and wiggle your toes inside the shoe. If there is any discomfort, don't buy them. There should be at least half an inch from the end of your longest toe to the end of the shoe. Children's shoes should be fitted with particular care.

2. *Change shoes at least once daily.* If you wear sensible shoes in the day time, then it is fine to wear fashionable ones at night. Different shoes for dancing, walking, and daytime wear should ensure that at least the feet are not repressed in the same places.

3. *Wash feet daily with warm water, and dry between the toes.* Dust with talcum powder. It is very relaxing, apart from being good for the feet. If you get blisters, don't break them. Stop wearing the shoes that caused them. If the blisters break, cover them with a dressing.

4. *Change stockings and socks daily.* Men are particularly bad about this. Not only do socks that are worn too long make your feet smell, they go stiff and rub against the skin.

5. *Go barefoot as much as possible, within reason.* Trampling around the woodlands and fields will simply leave you with scratches, thorns and possibly worse. But a good way to give your feet a rest is to go barefoot in the house, or on the lawn whenever it is warm enough. Babies, indeed, should never wear shoes till they start to walk: check then that their bootees or socks are not tight.

6. *Consult experts for serious foot-trouble.* Minor conditions such as athlete's foot can, of course, be treated with lotions or powders bought in a drugstore. Hard skin on the sole can be gently pumiced off. But use common sense. Don't use too many lotions, and if soreness develops, or if athlete's foot won't go away, see a chiropodist.

Verrucae (or warts), *corns*, *bunions* and *ingrowing toenails* will also benefit from being dealt with by somebody who knows how. Slashing away with corn-cutters or files can do more harm than good. Consult your local pharmacist, if not a chiropodist.

This is particularly important for elderly people and for diabetics. The problem is that for these people foot problems sometimes occur without pain, and the subsequent delay in getting treatment makes matters worse.

The Hair

Hair matters to us all more than we probably realize. Too much of it or too little, or hair in the wrong places, can cause considerable emotional distress. What can we do to keep our hair and our feelings about it healthy?

Hair itself cannot be hurt or diseased, though it can show signs of disease elsewhere in the body. Many problems about hair are really problems about our attitude to it. Left to itself, hair manages quite well. It is shed regularly, and new hair starts forming in the base of the hair follicle and eventually pushes out the old. Its color, waviness, length and texture are part of a general body program which makes hair on the arms, for instance, shorter than hair on the head.

Hair can be washed twice a week without upsetting the natural balance of body oils. It can be waved, permed and generally cut without much trouble. The worst that might happen is that it might break off a few inches from the scalp, if it is permanently waved too often. Even so, it will grow again. Any sudden loss of hair should be reported to the doctor. There are a variety of possible causes, including pregnancy, drug side effects, illnesses or glandular abnormalities. Usually when the cause has been removed, the hair just grows again. But it is important to go to a doctor, not to a so-called hair clinic or trichologist. They are not qualified to diagnose illnesses.

Baldness is part of the body's genetic program that is fixed at birth. Many men suffer from what is known as "male pattern baldness" as they grow older, and some women also go thin on top. Although baldness can be alarming, it

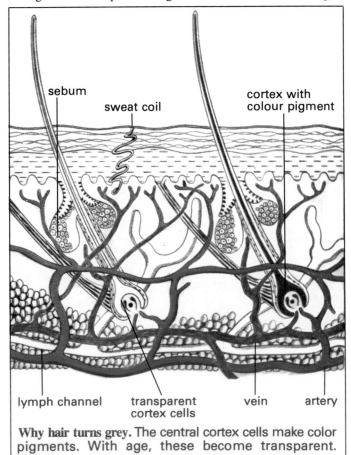

sebum — sweat coil — cortex with colour pigment

lymph channel — transparent cortex cells — vein — artery

Why hair turns grey. The central cortex cells make color pigments. With age, these become transparent.

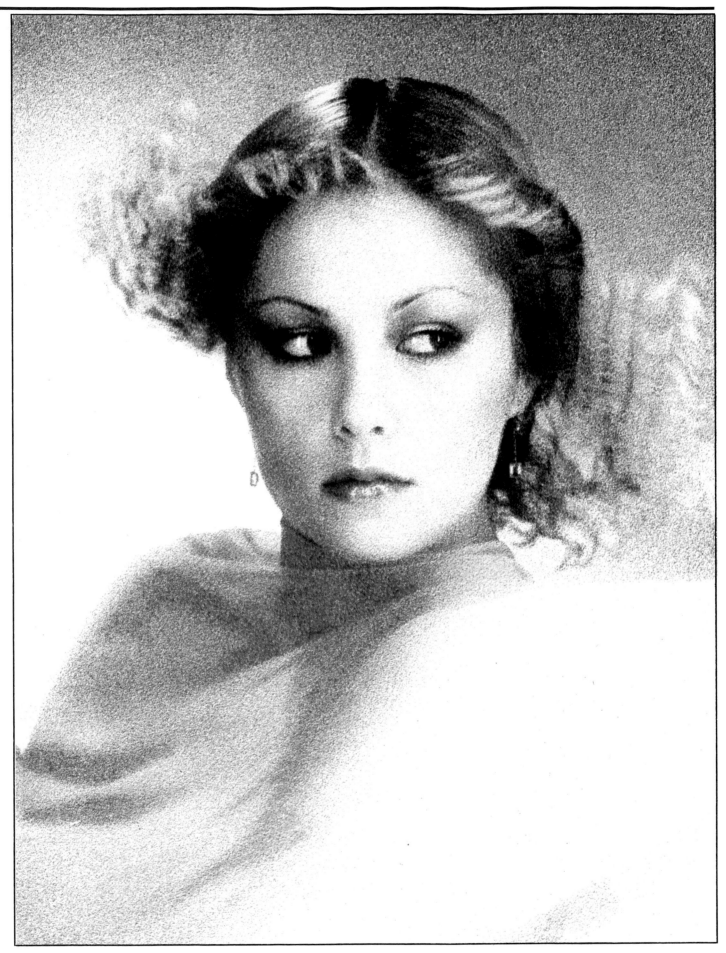

You can have your hair streaked or dipped in natural vegetable colors to avoid health risks of dyes. A rinse in gold and green (or even pink and purple) can be reversed with a shampoo. Or buy a switch of colored hair to pin in an exotic streak.

quite often stops at a certain point. So if the hair at your temples is receding, it does not mean you will end up as bald as an egg. There is no cure for baldness short of castration, and even castration would not bring back hair which is already lost. Yet a variety of hair clinics, treatment centers and hair specialists still offer expensive cures such as shampoos, creams, massage, motions, electro therapy, ultra violet and infra red radiation.

Sometimes it may seem as if clinics *do* work. This is because some people suffer a "transient moult". Their hair is shed then grows back again. If in the meantime they have been to a clinic, they think it is the result of the treatment, not knowing that the hair would have re-grown anyway.

If you must cover up your baldness, a hairpiece is probably the easiest answer. Hair transplants also work, but they are expensive and do not always look much better. Besides, you have got to use the hair from the side and back of your head, and when this is transplanted it might fall out too. Experienced plastic surgeons can estimate the chances of a transplant being successful for a particular person, depending on the type of hair and degree of baldness. If you are seriously considering a transplant, go to a reputable surgeon who values his reputation and ask him what your chances are of a good result.

Unsightly hair in the wrong places is the main female worry. Very occasionally this is caused by a glandular abnormality, so if hair suddenly sprouts it is worth checking with your doctor. Normally, like male baldness, it is just part of the genetic make-up of the individual. The only permanent way to remove hair is by electrolysis. Make sure that the electrolysist is a member of a reputable trade organization. Do not try to do it yourself with a home kit. Bad electrolysis can leave scars.

Electrolysis works by inserting a needle into the root of the hair, then killing the root with an electrical impulse. It is a slow process and can be expensive, so make sure you get a realistic estimate of the time and cost of treatment before committing yourself. There are commercial sharks that prey on women's worry about superfluous hair, just as some do on men's fears of baldness.

There are many old wives' tales about removing hair. Shaving it off does not make it grow strong: it makes it feel stronger or more bristly because of the blunt ends of hair. Likewise if you take out a hair with a tweezer, you will not find two growing in its place. Tweezing, however, does distort the follicle and may make subsequent electrolysis more difficult.

Hair dyes have become controversial ever since some research biologists suggested certain dye chemicals might cause cancer after being absorbed through the skin. So far there is no firm evidence that they do, and no firm evidence that they do not. Indeed, the problem of proving that anything causes cancer in human beings is particularly difficult, since it may take several decades before the disease emerges. The main scare centers round a series of chemicals that have been found to cause mutation in bacteria. Substances that cause cancer in humans also cause mutation in bacteria: but there are also some substances that do *not* cause cancer in humans which nevertheless have this effect on bacteria. So the bacteria test only works as a rough initial screen.

Seven of these hair dye chemicals have now been found to cause cancer in animals. The names of these as they usually appear on hair dye packages are: 4-methoxy- m-

phenylenediamine (4MMPD), 4-methody-m-phenylene-diamine sulfate, 2-nitro-p-phenylenediamine, 2-nitro-p-phenylene-diamine sulfate, 4-amino-2-nitrophenol. Direct Black 38 and, finally, Direct Blue 6. Many shades of both permanent and semipermanent hair dyes and some temporary dyes contain these chemicals. Some hair care products designed to cover up grey hair contain lead acetate, which has also been linked to cancer in animals. These chemical names will probably not appear on packages of dyes used in salons, as labeling of these packages is not required by law. To be certain that you are not getting one of these given to you at your salon, you will have to write to the manufacturer.

Dyes put on the scalp are absorbed through the skin of the scalp, enter the blood and are then carried to all parts of the body before they are excreted in the urine. Certain hair dyes have had to be removed from products sold to men because some men noticed that their urine had become a brown or black color. Women are not so likely to notice the color of their urine, and so these dyes have remained in the products for women.

The dyes used for hair are banned from use in food and other cosmetics because of the cancer risk. They are permitted for use in hair dyes under a Congressional Statute passed in 1938 as a result of industry lobbying. So the Federal Drug Administration has no authority to control the formulation or use of hair dyes.

It takes an average of twenty or more years of constant use of a chemical to cause cancer in human beings, and hair dyes have only been in widespread use for this length of time. It is impossible at present to assess the degree of risk that is taken by the 33 million US women and unknown number of men who use hair dyes, but it is certainly much less than the risks of smoking or of a high fat diet. However, these might be a major risk to the fetus, so at least avoid hair dyes in pregnancy, especially the first months.

The simplest way to play safe is just not to dye your hair. Vegetable dyes such as that old stand-by henna are probably all right, because henna does not enter the hair and scalp but coats it. Plain bleaching peroxide is all right too, but be careful because it often comes packaged with a dye. Streaking, highlighting, sunlighting, tipping, frosting, tortoise-shelling are also safe, because they involve selecting just a few hairs and changing their color. The dyes usually do not touch the scalp.

If you feel you must dye your hair, do so as little and as infrequently as possible. Have it done with a streaking technique which means the dye does not get on the skin of the scalp: as long as the dye does not touch the skin, it cannot enter the body, and can therefore do no harm. Use rubber gloves to put the dye on. And avoid if you can dyes which have been shown to cause cancer in animals. Light shades usually contain less potentially carcinogenic chemicals than dark shades.

The Environmental Defense Fund has compiled a list of brands which contain these chemicals. It can be obtained for a small handling charge of 50¢ from the fund at 1525, 18th Street NW, Washington DC.

Quite apart from any possible cancer risk, some dyes can set up an allergy. So before you use any hair dye, make sure you have a patch test on your skin. Even so, an allergy may develop as a result of use.

Dandruff is not a disease. The white flakes are simply dead skin scales off the scalp. It is more likely to be noticeable when the hair is greasy, so wash your hair more often. If you have severe dandruff look for a shampoo that contains either zinc pyrithione or selenium sulphide. These seem to be the only ingredients that really make any difference. However, medicated shampoos can cause scalp irritation, and frequent washing with a mild shampoo may be more effective.

Lice. Most of us think of lice or nits as something that cannot happen to our children. Yet the head louse is on the increase and no respecter of persons. Perfectly clean, nice and well-brought up children can, and do, catch lice. Indeed the head louse is having a population boom in almost every developed country. The head louse, or nit – *Pediculus humanus capitis* – is an ingenious and determined insect. A full-grown louse is about the size of a matchstick head with six legs. Each leg has a claw with which it clings on to the hair near the scalp. On the louse's head is a needle-like apparatus, with which it probes into the skin till it finds a blood vessel. It sucks up the blood, meanwhile pumping an anti-coagulant into the wound to make sure the blood keeps flowing. By the time the small bite begins to itch, the louse has moved on to another drinking hole.

The eggs are laid on hairs close to the scalp and fixed there with an insoluble glue. After eight to ten days they hatch out into larvae of a lighter color. Nine days later these mate, the males mating several times, since there are more females in the population. Each female then lays about five to eight eggs daily and can produce a total of up to 300. These are light-colored balls the size of pinheads, known as nits. The louse has evolved different strains, suitable for different hair. European lice have claws adapted for clinging to European round hair, while African lice have claws that are better for oval African hair. These two strains can mate and produce hybrids.

The spread of the new super louse, resistant to DDT, has been enormously helped by people's reluctance to admit to lice. The main reason why people are so ashamed of them is because they believe lice are only found on dirty people. In fact the reverse is true: the head louse actually prefers clean, non-scurfy hair, so that it can get at the scalp more easily. Nor can lice be caught from seats in public transport, theaters or other public places. Since the insect moves by clinging on to hairs, it cannot travel far. Lice are spread by head-to-head contact. Even long hair, sometimes blamed for lice, is not the cause. Short hair spreads lice just as well, if not better, since the louse always lives close to the skin rather than at the end of the hair.

Symptoms: The first sign is itching. If you look carefully you will see the dead lice which fall out of the hair after scratching, and may see the live insects which move quickly amongst the hair. White nits, the eggs of the lice, can also be seen. These first appear at the hair roots, but in severe cases may occur in clusters along the length of the hair.

Leave malathion lotion on for at least twenty minutes and preferably for twenty-four hours. The longer you leave it, the less likely is re-infestation. The malathion kills not only the adult lice and the larvae, but also the eggs. To comb out these, after you have treated them with malathion, you need a metal-tooth comb. Comb out the hair while it is still wet, pulling the comb through the hair after starting right at the scalp. Merely combing, without using malathion, will not do the trick. Malathion is a potent insecticide which may be absorbed through the scalp, so do not use it as a preventive in the absence of infestation.

The Skin

The body's first line of defense against disease is the skin. Its protective layer has to fend off germs, withstand temperature changes, cope with injuries, yet at the same time report back to the brain, via the nerves, what goes on in the tactile world outside.

The skin is made up of a barrier of cells, with a support system of nerves, glands and blood vessels below it. The top layer is called the epidermis and is made up of living cells that, in turn, rise to the surface and die. So the surface layer of the epidermis is continually being shed. This layer is kept soft, flexible and to a certain extent free from infection by a kind of natural cosmetic emulsion. The sweat glands feed liquid into the hair follicles, secreting more or less according to the body's mental and physical activity. The sebacious glands secrete a kind of grease called sebum into the same follicles and out onto the surface. This mixture of grease and liquid lubricates the skin.

Some people, especially adolescents, suffer from too much sebum and have greasy skins. Others, especially the elderly, suffer from too little of it and have dry skin. Greasy areas look greasy and may produce acne: dry skins look flaky and may be sore. Most of the time the body, if left to itself, will get the mixture of grease and moisture right. But we do not leave the body to itself. We have been brainwashed into washing too often. Most dermatologists reckon they see far more skin problems from clean people who wash too much, than from dirty people. So how often should we wash?

Face-washing once a day with soap and water is enough. If your face is greasy, wash more often: teenagers often need to wash three or four times a day. If your face is dry, use a cleansing lotion. Simple mineral oil obtainable from drugstores is the cheapest. A moisturizing cream may help too, but a cheap one is just as good as an expensive one. All that a moisturizing cream does is to put back water and grease on to the skin.

Daily baths are all right, but older people may need to take them less often. As their body oil decreases, a daily bath can produce dry skin which itches and cracks. If this happens to you, cut down on baths. Use a bath oil (any oil, even cooking oil, will do, though the smell may not be pleasant). Do not use bath salts or powders since these increase the dehydrating effect on the skin.

Diet probably does not make a great deal of difference to the skin in Western countries, although old people quite often suffer from mild scurvy, causing irritation of the skin and gums. This is easily treated by eating more fruit and vegetables, or drinking orange juice or vitamin C drinks.

Sunshine is another thing that many people think is good for skin. It is not. A sun tan is merely the skin's way of protecting itself against harmful rays. Be sensible about tanning. Anything which makes the skin blister and burn is too much. If you are going to be out in brilliant sunshine, look for a sunscreen lotion or cream with PABA (p-aminobenzoic acid) to protect you against harmful rays; or wear a hat, light shirt with long sleeves and trousers.

In the northern states most people usually need not worry about more than the occasional burn, but in hotter areas, cancer of the skin may be a danger for people whose skins are continuously exposed by working out-of-doors. The remedy is simple: do not let your bare skin be exposed continually for long periods.

The magical claims for cosmetics are mostly illusory. What you pay for is the perfume, the packaging and the *je ne sais quoi*. So some rules are worth remembering.

1. Skin cannot be fed from the outside, only lubricated.
2. Soaps with added fat are not likely to do anything. The fat is in small quantities, and anyway we rinse ourselves after washing, thus rinsing off the fat.
3. "Natural" ingredients such as avocado, strawberries and peaches will not do any harm. But neither are they likely to do much good. On the whole, vegetable matter will not act as a moisturizer and may make the skin dry.

Skins can suffer from diseases and in these cases go to the doctor just as you would with any other disease. People have the false impression that skin diseases do not matter. Children with an unexplained rash should be taken to the doctor: any rash on an adult's skin that lasts more than a week should also be seen by a doctor. Here are some of the most common problems:

Acne is usually suffered by teenagers, who are told that age will clear it up. Age does, but it can leave scars behind. So if your acne is severe, go to a doctor for help. He can prescribe antibiotics, lotions and in severe cases may suggest hormone treatment. If acne is not that severe, do not spend a lot of money on specially medicated soaps and lotions. Ordinary soap will dry up the greasy skin that produces acne, and special soaps (if over-used) can simply do harm. Cut out fatty foods and chocolate. There is no proof that this will help, but it is worth trying.

Contact dermatitis or contact eczema is a rash, with patches of red, itching and sometimes sores. The cause may be an allergy, which you can develop even to substances you have been safely and happily using for years. A dermatologist will help you track down the offending substance. The skin will never forget the allergy, so you will have to avoid touching that substance in the future (see Chapter 7).

Eczema, known as atopic eczema, is the term given to a similar rash when its cause is constitutional. Some people seem to have an inherited tendency to eczema, and it is often associated with asthma and hay fever. Babies are particularly prone to it, but the condition often clears up in later life. Eczema is not infectious or contagious. Go to a doctor for help and keep in regular contact with him. The steroid creams that are often prescribed can be strong, so use them sparingly and according to his instructions. Never lend or borrow such creams.

Psoriasis is the other major skin disease. Again it is neither infectious nor contagious. Red patches covered with silvery scales appear on the skin, often on the knees, elbows and scalp. Psoriasis comes and goes for no apparent reason and a doctor's prescription for ointments will be necessary. Careful sun tanning helps some people.

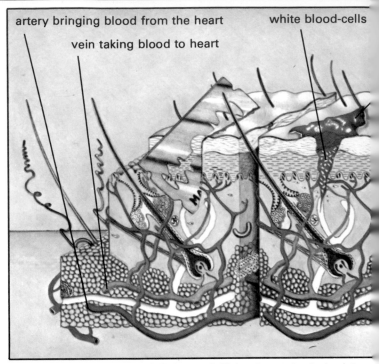

How skin heals: fine threads of fibrin start bridging the cut, hardening into a

The Joints

There are no fewer than 187 joints in the body – all of them working to make the rigid skeleton flexible. Keeping your joints working efficiently is something that the body does automatically. But you *can* help its maintenance work.

The name usually given to any disease or trouble with the joints is arthritis. It is a loose term that covers many different types of trouble, but it can roughly be divided into two main groups of diseases: **rheumatoid arthritis** and **osteo-arthritis** (properly known as osteo-arthrosis).

Rheumatoid arthritis is a generalized disease, which usually leads to ill health and affects many joints at the same time. Osteo-arthritis, on the other hand, just affects the joints without any general ill-health. It can be a "wear and tear" disease, affecting just one joint at a time, or affect many joints – perhaps on a hereditary basis. The cause of neither is fully understood, but both diseases become increasingly common as people grow older. Arthritis is estimated to cost the national economy $13 billion a year in lost wages and medical care bills.

Treatment can control the disease and prevent crippling, but since arthritis is not fully understood there are no certain "cures" and no certain ways to avoid getting it.

Arthritis can also be part of many other diseases. There is, for instance, a transient form of arthritis that occasionally accompanies German measles.

Some general rules, however, are of interest. Diet does not usually make much difference, though you will find a host of old wives' tales about raw onions, orange juice, and the like. A balanced diet with plenty of vegetables and not too many fattening foods is all that is needed. Don't get overweight. It makes arthritis more severe in weight-bearing joints such as the hips and knees.

Gout is an exception to the general rule. People who

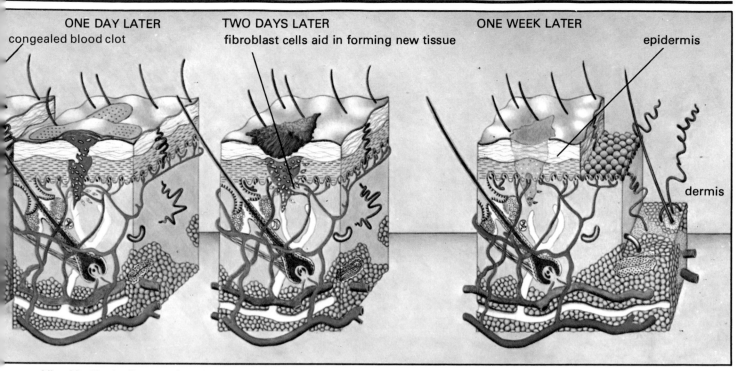

ONE DAY LATER
congealed blood clot

TWO DAYS LATER
fibroblast cells aid in forming new tissue

ONE WEEK LATER
epidermis

dermis

scar, while white blood cells swarm into the wound to attack foreign matter.

have an inherited tendency to gout will probably find that it may worsen, if they eat and drink too much. Even so, some unlucky teetotal vegetarians still get gout.

For many years it was thought that exercise was likely to produce arthritis. Since some forms of osteo-arthritis were wear and tear diseases, doctors concluded that exercise would just add to the wear. Yet a recent study in Finland showed the opposite. Seventy-four former athletes were X-rayed for signs of osteo-arthritis. The athletes were, on average, about fifty-five years old and had competed for twenty-one years. They were compared with non-athletes of a similar age – in fact, hospital patients but excluding those who had complained of problems with their hips.

Only three athletes – or 4 per cent of the total – had true osteo-arthritis, compared with 8.7 per cent of the hospital patients. Among the three unlucky athletes was one who had competed for only eight years, retiring from the sport

after he had collected an Olympic gold medal.

The sample was admittedly small and only applied to osteo-arthritis, not rheumatoid arthritis. However, a study of soccer players seemed to bear out some of its conclusions. Some 50 professional footballers, 15 ex-pros and 1,490 amateurs were involved in the study, which found that only 3.2 per cent had arthritis.

Even more interesting was the fact that it was the standing leg, not the kicking leg, which was more likely to suffer. This implied that it was *being* kicked rather than kicking that did the damage. As it was already known that injury to a joint can result in subsequent arthritis, athletes' arthritis may be due to injuries, not sport itself.

Indeed, the Finnish survey suggests that exercise can be positively good for joints – perhaps because the joint cartilage is nourished by a joint fluid. This nourishment is facilitated by movement. Regular but not violent exercise, therefore, will do the joints good. If you do get injured, make sure you give the injury time to heal. One English soccer club claims to have cut down on arthritis by making sure injured players do not go back to the game too quickly.

Stiffness in the joints can in many cases be eased by simple remedies such as flexing the muscles before getting up in the morning, sleeping in a warm bedroom, hot baths and regular exercise. Walking is often sufficient to loosen stiff joints in the legs, while other joints can be kept mobile by generally flexing appropriate parts of the body. But if you do get serious problems apparently arising from the joints – pain, perhaps accompanied by swelling, heat or redness – go and see your doctor. Much can be done, if arthritis is treated early, to limit the problem. If you are merely being treated with pain killers, do not be afraid to ask your physician for a second specialist opinion.

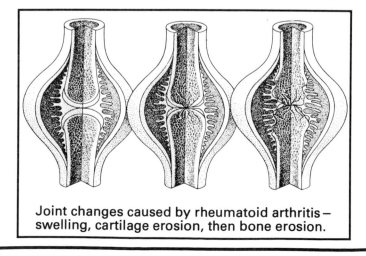

Joint changes caused by rheumatoid arthritis – swelling, cartilage erosion, then bone erosion.

The Eyes

The eye works like an automatic camera. Light reflected from an object in front of the eye enters the eye through the lens. The lens is flexible and can be moved by a tiny muscle so that an image of the object is accurately focused on the back of the eye. The iris just in front of the lens acts like the diaphragm in a camera, and prevents too much light from entering. The back of the eye, the retina, contains light-sensitive nerve endings which pass messages back to the brain, informing the brain of the quantity and color of the light falling upon them. So the retina is comparable with the film in a camera. The most sensitive part of the retina, the fovea, is near its center. When a person looks directly at an object, the image of the object is focused on the fovea, where it can be seen most clearly.

Just like a camera, the eye must be "made" to precise proportions. If the retina is a fraction of a millimeter out of position, then the image will not be precisely focused upon it. This incredible accuracy has to be maintained from birth, when the eye is 14mm long, until adulthood when the eye has grown to 24mm long.

If the eyeball is too long, so that the image cannot be properly focused upon it, then a person is short-sighted. *Short sight* may develop at any time but particularly while a person is growing. It is readily corrected with glasses, which give clear distance vision that is essential for driving. If the eyeball is too short, so that the image again cannot easily be focused upon it, then the person has *long sight*. A small degree of long sight can frequently be compensated for by the eye itself while a person is still young and the lens of their eye flexible. But when such a person gets older, they find it increasingly difficult to see things near-to, and may require glasses for reading or close work.

Poor eyesight can also be caused by a third condition called *astigmatism*. When someone suffers from astigmatism, they see an object as blurred and distorted, although they do not realize this until their eyesight is corrected with glasses.

There is no way of preventing the development of long sight, short sight or astigmatism. To some extent these conditions may run in families, but more often they are probably simply the result of chance effects on growth and development of the eyes. It is important that any defect in vision is corrected as early as possible so that children do not have any unnecessary difficulties in learning to understand their surroundings or to read. Children should have their eyes checked at any age if a defect is suspected.

Ideally, all children should have their eyes checked before starting school. A rough test is often done at the school itself, but this is sometimes left until most children can recognize letters at six or seven; by that time a short-sighted child may already have suffered difficulty in learning because of poor sight. If parents, brothers or sisters have poor sight, then a child should have a full check-up before going to school. If a child has any difficulty in learning to read, a full eye check-up is advisable.

The lens in the eye starts out in children with the consistency of a liquid such as molasses, but as a person gets older the lens becomes less flexible and ends up in old people almost as dense as the nails of the fingers. This means that as a person gets older they find it increasingly difficult to see close objects. Most people who have normal eyesight up to the age of forty begin to need glasses by their middle forties, especially for reading in artificial light. Check-ups every two years are advisable after the middle forties.

People are not usually aware of poor eyesight until it is corrected, and so some simple tests are useful. Anyone who cannot read a telephone directory at nineteen inches using *each eye separately*, has difficulty reading newspaper print with *each eye separately*, or cannot read a car license plate at twenty-five yards with *each eye separately*, may need glasses and should get their eyes checked.

Good lighting from behind is essential for easy reading. Eye exercises may help a person to interpret blurred images better and so may improve eyesight in that sense, but the most important way of correcting blurred vision will always be with glasses. Contrary to popular belief, it is not possible for an adult to damage his eyes, either by using them excessively or by using them in poorly lit conditions, although such "eye strain" may cause headaches (see page 148) which should be relieved by the correct spectacles or by relaxation (see page 90).

Infection

A bloodshot eye is often caused by a small blood vessel bursting; this should not be a cause of worry and will heal without treatment. When the eye is red, or sticky, or watery, and also painful you should consult a doctor. The irritation may be caused by a foreign body in the eye or by an infection, often a virus. Any mild inflammation of the eye or soreness which does not clear up in two days should also lead you to consult your doctor. Most eye infections are contagious, and so it is important that a person with infected eyes uses separate towels and wash cloths.

Accidents

In many jobs it is important to wear protective glasses to prevent damage to the eyes. Strong infra red light, such as

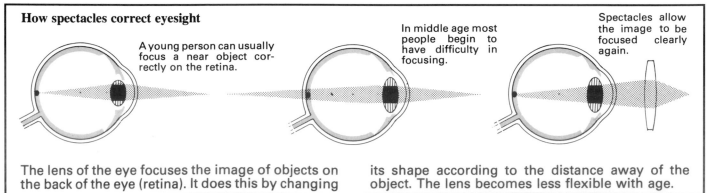

How spectacles correct eyesight

A young person can usually focus a near object correctly on the retina.

In middle age most people begin to have difficulty in focusing.

Spectacles allow the image to be focused clearly again.

The lens of the eye focuses the image of objects on the back of the eye (retina). It does this by changing its shape according to the distance away of the object. The lens becomes less flexible with age.

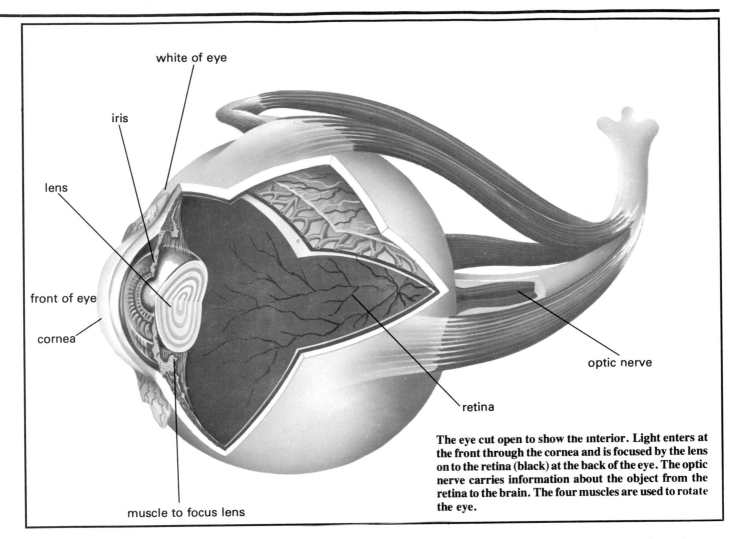

white of eye

iris

lens

front of eye

cornea

optic nerve

retina

muscle to focus lens

The eye cut open to show the interior. Light enters at the front through the cornea and is focused by the lens on to the retina (black) at the back of the eye. The optic nerve carries information about the object from the retina to the brain. The four muscles are used to rotate the eye.

that given off by molten metal, can burn the lens or the retina, causing cataract or other forms of blindness. Ultra violet light generated during welding may cause flash-burns to the cornea, which may cause temporary blindness: always use protective goggles or shields. Intense ultra violet light reflected from snow can cause the same condition, known as snow blindness. Intense light reflected from water or sand may also cause discomfort, but is unlikely to do harm. Polaroid or reflecting sunglasses or a broad-brimmed hat provide the best protection.

Protection of the eyes against injury from foreign bodies is particularly important for people employed in workshops and factories. Goggles or special spectacles with cup-type side shields may be sufficient, but more elaborate protection in the form of face- and head-shields are available. (See Chapter 7 for information on how to obtain advice about industrial safety.) Do-it-yourself enthusiasts should take special care and invest in protective glasses. The greatest danger comes when hitting metal with metal, because small chips may fly into the eye at high speed.

A person who wears glasses and is also exposed to the possible hazard of flying objects hitting the eye should invest in plastic or toughened glasses with special side cups for extra protection. It is vital that whatever eye protection is used it is comfortable to wear, otherwise it will tend not to be used. If a chemical enters the eye, wash the eye out immediately with water by immersing the head in a basin and opening the eyelids with the fingers so that all the chemical is removed. Alternatively, the person may sit down with their head back, and while they hold the eye open a helper may gently pour about two pints of water over the eye; a teapot is ideal for this. Seek hospital attention at once unless the chemical is known to be mild.

Prevention of blindness

Two of the most common causes of blindness in Western countries are glaucoma and the retinal changes associated with diabetes. These can usually be treated if discovered early. The common type of glaucoma usually gives no warning signs, and is only picked up during a routine eye examination. People who have a close relative with glaucoma should have their eyes examined regularly after the age of forty, as this disease tends to run in families. The less common acute glaucoma may be indicated by pain in the eye, headache, transient blurring of vision, especially in dim light, and the presence of colored haloes around lights. The occurrence of any of these symptoms should lead a person to consult a doctor. Diabetics should have regular eye examinations, and close relatives of diabetics should have regular checks for diabetes, because this disease also tends to run in families.

Even more common than glaucoma and diabetes as causes of blindness are macular degeneration and cataract. Patients with macular degeneration are usually elderly and notice a slow deterioration in their ability to read and to recognize people's faces. They can often be helped by glasses or by other aids for low vision. Cataract, a condition in which the lens of the eye becomes opaque, produces a gradually increasing mistiness of vision which, if necessary, can be treated by an operation.

The Ears

Deafness is a terrible handicap affecting one in every twenty adults, and anything that can be done to prevent it is worthwhile. Most communication is based on the spoken word, and inability to follow conversation means social isolation and often difficulty in finding work. Our ears are very delicate structures and are easily damaged in a number of ways – many of which can be avoided.

Types of deafness
Sound waves entering the ear are transmitted to the organ of hearing, the *cochlea*, which is situated in the inner ear. The cochlea is connected with the brain via a nerve called the auditory nerve. Damage to the cochlea produces a **nerve deafness** (also called perceptive or sensori-neural deafness). This is the commonest type of deafness. It cannot be cured by surgery but can often be helped by a hearing aid.

Conductive deafness occurs when sound is blocked in its passage to the cochlea. The cause may be something simple, like wax blocking the outer ear canal, or there may be disease of the eardrum or the cochlea. Many forms of conductive deafness may be corrected by surgery, and for this reason a specialist's opinion should always be sought. Simple hearing tests can in most cases quickly indicate which sort of hearing loss a person has.

CAUSES OF HEARING LOSS
Congenital deafness
Being born deaf is a special handicap. Although many children who are born deaf learn to lip-read and to use what residual hearing they have, without the ability to hear their own voice their speech is always very strange and often unintelligible to strangers. The deafness may be due to a genetic abnormality that is inherited. If early deafness occurs in a family, or a partner is deaf, it may be advisable to seek genetic counsel before planning a family. One form of inherited deafness called otosclerosis, which causes severe conductive deafness in adult life, can now be cured by surgery.

German measles caught by a mother in the first three months of pregnancy produces a high incidence of nerve deafness in the child – see Chapter 1.

During childbirth it is not uncommon for the baby to become temporarily deprived of oxygen. The ear is very sensitive to the lack of oxygen, and deafness may result. It is now possible to measure hearing very early in childhood, using special electrical tests linked to a computer. Eventually, these methods will be available as a screening test for all young babies. When there is any doubt about a child's hearing ability these tests should be used, and if necessary a program can be begun to make use of what hearing there is.

Childhood
Earache in childhood can be alarming, but infection rarely nowadays results in permanent hearing impairment. This is largely due to the use of antibiotics. Any earache in a child which is not relieved by a pain killer such as aspirin, or is associated with general illness or temperature, should be referred to the doctor.

If there is a profuse and smelly discharge from the ear, this too is serious and needs immediate attention to avoid damage to the middle ear.

Mumps and measles very occasionally result in profound deafness. Measles can be avoided by vaccination (see page 155).

Injury
Small children tend to push things into their ears and into those of their friends. More damage may be done in removing these than by pushing them in. Never make an attempt to remove them yourself but seek expert advice. The best way to remove foreign bodies from the ear is either by gentle syringeing or the use of a small suction apparatus. Poking and probing usually causes pain and bleeding, and pushes the object further down the ear.

A blow over the ear from a ball or from the flat of the hand may rupture the drum and occasionally disrupt the small bones of the middle ear. A conductive deafness results and there may also be pain and bleeding. For this reason never hit anyone over the ear. In fact, many perforations of the eardrum caused by a blow heal without treatment, but expert advice is always needed. More serious blows to the head which cause head injury may also result in deafness. Sometimes this is due to damage to the middle ear which may be correctable, but more commonly there is concussion of the inner ear, and the cochlea receives permanent damage. If there is a skull fracture this may involve the inner ear, and bleeding from the fracture may damage it permanently. Always wear proper head protection when working in heavy industry, when riding a motor cycle or in any other potentially dangerous situation.

Wax
Wax can also cause conductive deafness but usually only if it is pushed down the ear canal. It is a popular misconception that the outer ear should be cleaned out with cotton buds, corners of towels and fingers. This pushes the wax, which is normally produced in the outer ear canal, further down against the eardrum. In this position it causes uncomfortable blockage of the ear and mild deafness. If this happens, medical advice should be sought and the wax removed by expert syringeing.

Irritation in the ear is also common and this may provoke more finger- and towel-poking. In addition to causing blockage of wax, infection may be introduced into the outer part of the ear. The majority of these cases can be avoided by leaving the ear canal entirely alone. If you do develop an irritation in the outer ear, seek medical advice.

Noise exposure
It has been known since the last century that loud noise can damage the ear, but still many people exposed to this risk fail to wear simple ear protection. The louder the noise, the shorter the length of exposure that is necessary to produce hearing loss. To begin with, this loss is temporary but eventually it becomes permanent. The most damaging sort of sound is that produced by a gunshot, especially rifles and sporting guns. The sudden negative shock wave following the explosive noise is particularly damaging to the cochlea. Damage may easily be prevented by the use of a special

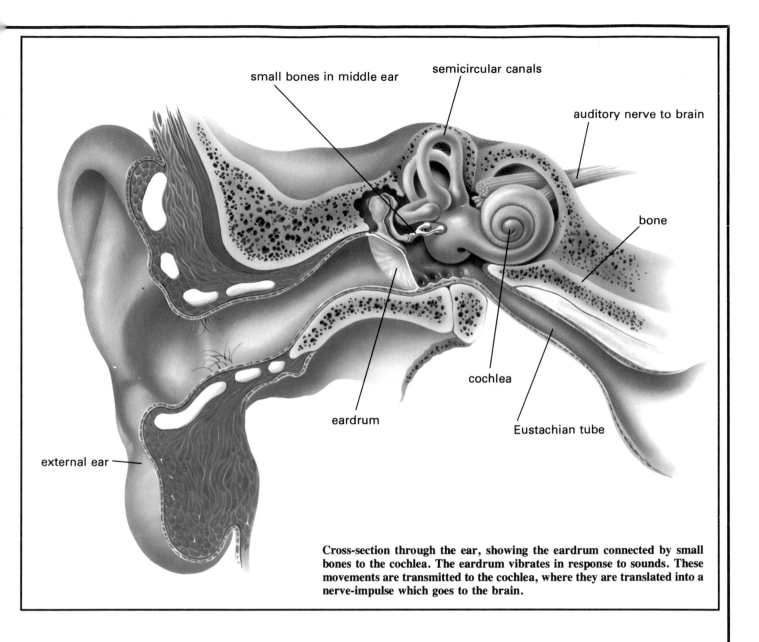

small bones in middle ear

semicircular canals

auditory nerve to brain

bone

cochlea

Eustachian tube

eardrum

external ear

Cross-section through the ear, showing the eardrum connected by small bones to the cochlea. The eardrum vibrates in response to sounds. These movements are transmitted to the cochlea, where they are translated into a nerve-impulse which goes to the brain.

diaphragm ear protector, which does not reduce the sound level of conversation.

Continuous noise in heavy industry can also produce permanent deafness, although the full effects may not be felt for many years. Where noise levels in a factory exceed ninety decibels – equivalent to the sound of a road drill at five yards – ear protection should be provided and worn at all times. A rough guide is that no one should be exposed to noise for any length of time which is so loud that normal conversation is impossible – although workers in such conditions often learn to lip-read and cease to be aware of the intensity of noise. A great deal can frequently be done to reduce noise in factories by surrounding noisy machines with baffles, or introducing noise-absorbing materials – but this is a job for experts. A wide variety of earplugs and earmuffs are available which, while they do not exclude all sounds, do reduce it to safe levels. In addition to deafness, excessive noise exposure may produce severe tinnitus. This takes the form of ringing, buzzing or machinery-like noises generated in the damaged ear. It continues incessantly and can be extremely disturbing.

Sudden deafness

Sometimes, profound deafness occurs quite suddenly. It usually affects only one ear, and it is often difficult to find an exact cause. Sometimes the blood supply to the cochlea is interrupted, owing to a spasm or a small clot in a blood vessel. Prompt treatment aimed at increasing the blood supply to the sensitive cochlea can sometimes restore hearing. It is always very important to seek specialist advice following sudden deafness.

HOW TO MANAGE A HEARING LOSS

The first thing is to get expert advice. If the hearing loss is conductive it may be amenable to treatment or surgery; a hearing aid may help and should always be tried. Everyone makes use of visual clues during conversation, especially if there is a lot of background noise. People with a hearing loss need to make an effort to watch the face of the person speaking to them.

The speaker should make every effort to speak clearly and not to shout. Make sure you are in a good light and that your face is not covered by a hand or pipe. All these things make lip-reading much more difficult. Above all, it is important to be patient. Deaf people find their difficulty in communicating extremely frustrating. Try not to treat them as if they were weak-minded.

The Teeth

Cleaning your teeth is a bore. That is partly why so many people have such rotten teeth. But we also make our teeth worse every day by eating the wrong things and, if we clean our teeth at all, often looking after them in the wrong way. The result: 25 million Americans have no teeth of their own and the rest have an average of four cavities each. And many of those who still have their own teeth regularly suffer from pain, bad breath and infected gums. Yet neither pain nor a toothless middle age are inevitable.

Diet: the positive way to protect your teeth

You may never flash a film star's smile, but you will be saved a lot of pain and embarrassment if you think about what you eat. The basic rule is this: cut down on sugar. And cut out sweet things between meals. There is ample evidence to prove the link between sugar and tooth decay. Tooth decay became worse as the sugary content of our diet increased over the last hundred years. Eskimos, for instance, rarely suffered from tooth decay until they adopted the sweeter Western-style diet. And there was less tooth decay in Europe during the Second World War when sugar was scarce and candy rarer still.

If you must eat sugary things, do so at mealtimes. In 1954 the unfortunate inmates of a Swedish institution were subjected to an experiment which showed that sweet things taken at meal times caused less decay that sweet things taken between meals. Continually drenching the teeth in sugar liquid makes the plaque produce more acid, which continuously dissolves the protective enamel of the teeth. Many people believe that the unhealthy effects of a sweet diet can be avoided by eating honey instead. No such luck or, at least, no such evidence.

A sweet tooth is a habit which can be gradually altered by cutting down on sugar in cooking; the amount of sugar in cakes, for instance, can usually be halved without making much difference. But it is better never to allow children to develop a sweet tooth. Cut out all sweet snacks between meals and avoid sweetened drinks, such as sodas, colas and also the syrupy fruit extracts, advertised as being so full of vitamins. Children will learn to enjoy water as their regular drink if they are encouraged. Never put sugar in babies' bottles. Offer people fruit or nuts as snacks. An apple a day will not by itself keep the dentist at bay but it is better for teeth than candy.

If cutting out sugar is the most negative way toward better teeth, adding fluoride to our diet is the most positive way to reduce decay. The latest figures from the Netherlands, for example, show that fluoridation of the water supply has reduced the amount of dental decay by some 50 per cent and the number of extractions by 85 per cent. Fluoride is a chemical compound which, in essence, hardens teeth to increase their resistance to decay. It can do this in two ways:

1. *Added to the diet*. This is especially effective for children since their teeth are still growing. The fluoride is absorbed into the bloodstream and incorporated in the tooth enamel.

2. *Brushed on to the teeth*. This hardens the exposed surface enamel of the teeth and thus enables them to resist decay.

About half the population of the US now drink fluoridated water, and fluoridation has the support of the American Medical Association, the American Dental Association, the American Academy of Paediatrics and the US Public Health Service. Fluoridation is the simplest way of adding fluoride to the diet, but it is also controversial. An alternative open to individuals is to buy it in tablet form from chemists. These can be swallowed one a day or, what might be a better idea for children, crushed and added to food. Or drink lots of tea – unsweetened, of course – since this contains extra fluoride. And use fluoride toothpaste.

Plaque

Plaque is your enemy. It is a sticky white substance, consisting of millions of bacteria, which grows on the surface of everyone's teeth, feeding on the debris and food in the mouth. Plaque commonly accumulates between the teeth and at the edge of the gums where the attack begins. It attacks on two fronts. Firstly, bacteria in the plaque produce an acid which attacks the enamel surface of the teeth causing them to decay. Secondly, it produces poisons which cause the gums to recede leading to pyorrhea (see below).

Acid from plaque bacteria gradually dissolves a hole in the enamel where other bacteria take over, causing *caries*, the familiar tooth decay. This is the major dental problem for people under thirty. If the the caries is not removed by the dentist, then the decay will continue until it reaches the living pulp deep within the base of the tooth. Up to this point, the tooth will be painful only if it is stimulated by hot, cold or sweet food. But when the softer dentine beneath the enamel becomes infected, real toothache begins. When the pulp at the center becomes infected, the tooth will become extremely painful. But this pain will suddenly cease as pressure builds up, cutting off the blood supply and killing the nerves in the pulp. The relief is only short-lived. The infection passes through the minute nerve channel to create an abscess which causes more swelling of the gum and jaw.

Save your gums

"I had to have all my teeth out although the dentist said they were perfect." This unlikely tale is only too often true. Gum disease is the major dental problem for over thirties, and again plaque is the cause. It collects at the base of the teeth, continually attacking the gums, and forms tartar, a hard white deposit which irritates the gums, causing further soreness and swelling. The first symptoms of this attack are bleeding gums and a pink toothbrush; the gums themselves may be painless. These warning signs should be taken seriously and an urgent visit made to the dentist.

You can treat mild gum infection between just a few teeth yourself by removing offending plaque with a toothpick or floss and by thorough cleaning. Gum disease that is allowed to become really advanced through neglect is called pyorrhea, and it may have to be treated surgically by scraping and cutting away the unhealthy tissue. If gum disease is not treated it spreads to the root of the tooth which loosens in its socket and finally falls out. Regular careful toothbrushing is the only way to save your gums, although dentists can help through scaling and polishing.

Cleaning your teeth

Most of us skimp the tooth cleaning chore and many do it

What a mouth

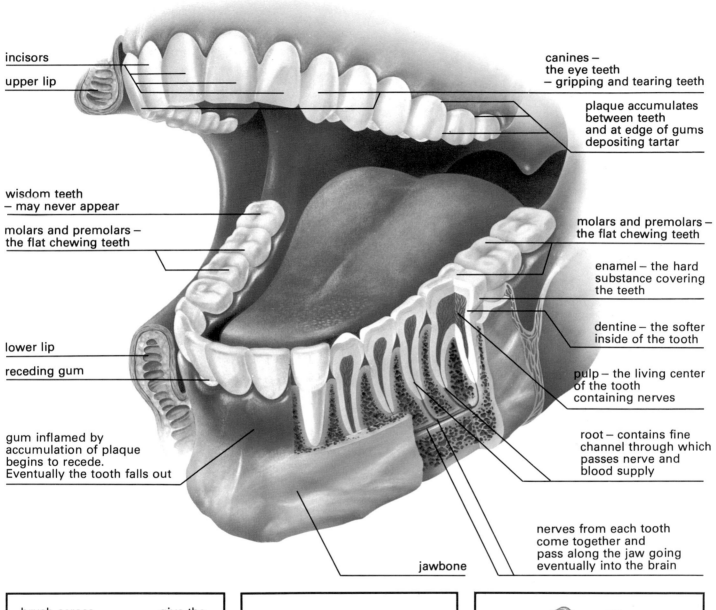

incisors

upper lip

canines –
the eye teeth
– gripping and tearing teeth

plaque accumulates
between teeth
and at edge of gums
depositing tartar

wisdom teeth
– may never appear

molars and premolars –
the flat chewing teeth

molars and premolars –
the flat chewing teeth

enamel – the hard
substance covering
the teeth

dentine – the softer
inside of the tooth

lower lip

receding gum

pulp – the living center
of the tooth
containing nerves

gum inflamed by
accumulation of plaque
begins to recede.
Eventually the tooth falls out

root – contains fine
channel through which
passes nerve and
blood supply

nerves from each tooth
come together and
pass along the jaw going
eventually into the brain

jawbone

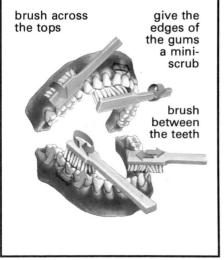

brush across
the tops

give the
edges of
the gums
a mini-
scrub

brush
between
the teeth

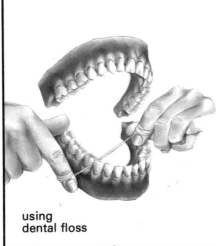

using
dental floss

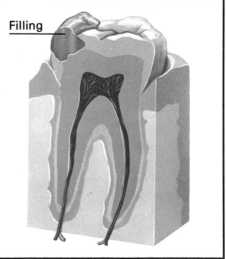

Filling

Brush with small circular movements first, then up and down, but
not backwards and forwards.

Dental floss is useful for removing
stubborn pieces of food from *between* the teeth.

Cross section of a molar tooth
showing a filling – the most common of all dental repairs.

incorrectly, often doing more harm than good. To clean teeth effectively you must remove plaque from the crevices, gaps between the teeth and from around the edge of the gums. Plaque takes a long time to build up so it is probably sufficient to clean once a day, *if* you do a thorough job. Too many people push the brush in and out of the mouth backwards and forwards. This wears a trough in the teeth and can damage the gums. To brush correctly, manipulate the bristles between the teeth into the areas where the plaque accumulates. Give the crevices and the edges of the gums a mini-scrub in a small circular motion, and then brush up and down to remove plaque between teeth.

There are sixteen surfaces of the teeth which should be cleaned: the insides, outsides and tops of the big chewing teeth in the upper and lower jaws, and the inside and outside of the cutting teeth at the front. It should take you at least three minutes to clean all these surfaces thoroughly.

Is an electric toothbrush a con? Yes and no. They don't do anything that an ordinary toothbrush cannot do. But there are three things to be said for the electric brush if you use it in the right place: (a) the motor provides the right scrubbing action; (b) the small head enables you to clean all the teeth; (c) you are more likely to do it long enough.

For manual cleaning use a soft or medium, nylon or bristle brush, not a hard one since this can damage your gums. Choose a brush with a small head (one inch or less), so that each tooth gets individual attention.

Are fluoride toothpastes best? Yes. Fluoride in toothpaste hardens the exposed surface enamel of the teeth and this enables them to resist decay. Choose one which carries the American Dental Association seal of approval.

Dare you pick your teeth? Once only Hollywood tycoons (*circa* 1933) picked their teeth. Now nearly everyone does it, either discreetly in public or privately. A toothpick does two things: it removes awkward debris, and massages the gums where they meet the tooth. If your gums have already receded some way, you may need a thick pick; if the gaps are small, a slimmer birchwood pick is better. But be careful you do not injure the gums. Aggressive use of a pick may make gum disease worse.

Is dental floss worth the fuss? Yes. Some stubborn pieces of food cannot be shifted with toothpicks and then you must use dental floss – a strong waxed thread which can be passed between the teeth. You must do it in front of a mirror and take care not to damage the gums. Removing the stubborn pieces of food helps to prevent bad breath.

What about the kids? Dentists would like parents to clean their children's teeth for them until they get to the age when they can do it themselves. Good luck, if you have the patience to try. Children should be taught to clean their own teeth from the earliest practicable age, which is not likely to be before they are four or five. Toothbrushing can be introduced earlier, at three or four, as a game but it should never be made a chore and it would be fruitless at this age to insist on technically correct brushing. But tooth brushing should become routine, if possible, by the age of six, when the first adult teeth appear at the back of the mouth before any of the milk teeth have been lost. The American Dental Association suggests a first visit to the dentist before age two, but this will seldom be necessary if the advice on diet given here is taken.

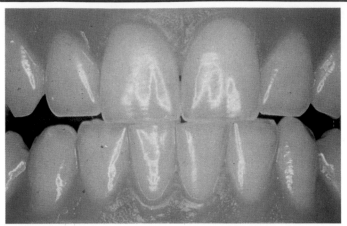

Perfect teeth: white and gleaming, all present (32 in all) with no gaps, and tight healthy gums.

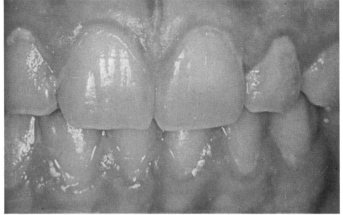

These teeth have not been cleaned for three days, and the result can be seen more clearly below.

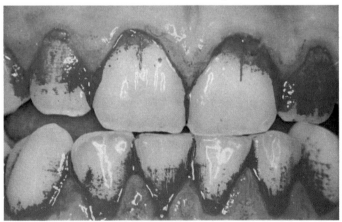

The same teeth washed with a pink 'disclosing' solution to reveal the full horror of plaque.

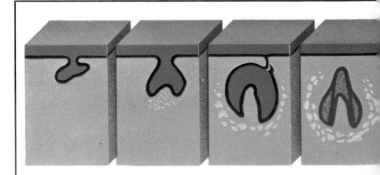

Stages in the growth of a tooth, originating (*left*) in the sk and above the skin.

TOOTHACHE

So you have eaten the right things, brushed away zealously night and morning, picked away assiduously after meals, devotedly used fluoride toothpaste, regularly seen your dentist and your teeth are hurting like hell. Don't despair and give up all your bad habits; you have probably had bad habits for longer. But do see a dentist urgently.

If you are really unlucky, of course, the toothache will strike at the weekend. You may be able to get emergency treatment at a large hospital with a dental department. Most people will not be so lucky and will have to bear it until Monday. This is what you can do to relieve the pain:

1. Take aspirin, acetaminophen or any proprietary pain killer. *Swallow* it – never hold it in the cheek against the aching tooth since this will cause a painful ulcer or aspirin burn on the gums.
2. Try not to lie down, since this increases the blood pressure in the head, and the pain.
3. Hot mouthwashes of salt and water may relieve the pain a little if gums are the problem, but not if the tooth is sensitive to heat.
4. Finally, if things look really bleak, you could try a little whisky or other spirits. But if you have already taken some aspirin, spit out the whisky and use it simply as a mouthwash. Otherwise the combination of alcohol and aspirin may cause serious stomach irritation, which since the toothache will also still be there may not make drowning your sorrows seem quite such a good idea.

AT THE DENTIST'S

Not even the prettiest nurse, the softest music, the most comfortable bed-type chair or the most riveting television program is ever going to make the dental surgery particularly popular. Dentists are trying all these ideas to woo their patients, but none have had remotely the impact of the high-speed drills developed over the last ten years. These mean the nastiest part of the dentist's work is over more quickly and less painfully. Anesthetics are better, too, but be wary of the total anesthetics favored by some dentists. The American Society of Oral Surgeons recommended in 1971 that there should be at least three trained people in the surgical team when a total anesthetic is given so that help can be given if problems arise. Local injections in the gum are certainly safer and normally just as effective. The three most common running repairs undertaken by dentists are:

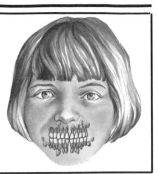

'Adult' teeth are present beneath the skin long before they begin to push out the baby teeth when a child is around six years old.

1. *Scale and polish.* This removes the tartar and thus gives the gums a new lease of life and prevents decay. If you are lucky, scaling and polishing will be all the dentist prescribes on your six-month visit.
2. *Fillings.* The dentist begins by removing the decayed matter from the cavity with the drill. He then dries the cavity before filling it. The filling sets hard within about three minutes and continues to harden for several hours afterwards. The cavity must be shaped so that the filling cannot fall out after it sets, and so that the teeth can actually bite; the filling must be shaped so that food doesn't collect between the teeth.
3. *Crowns.* When a tooth is badly damaged, the only way to repair it may be to make an entirely new crown. The existing tooth is ground down to a peg and then an artificial crown is glued on to the peg. Even when the entire tooth has been lost, it is sometimes possible to insert a screw or peg into the jawbone and build a peg on that.

Remember that you should in any case see your dentist twice a year. Remember, too, that postponing a visit to the dentist doesn't make your teeth any better. The odds are that it will be still more painful next time.

If you notice any of the following symptoms, you should consult your dentist immediately:
1. Bleeding of your gums when brushing and flossing.
2. Persistent bad breath.
3. Soft, swollen, or tender gums.
4. Pus between the gums and the teeth.
5. Loose teeth.
6. Gums shrinking away from the teeth.
7. Any changes in the fit of your partial or complete dentures.
8. Any change in the spaces between your teeth or in the way your teeth come together.

Dos and don'ts

Do visit your dentist twice a year for a check-up.
Do eat fruit or nuts if you must eat between meals.
Do brush your teeth properly at least once a day.
Do cut down on sweet things to eat and drink.
Don't put sugar in babies' bottles or drinks.
Don't give sweets as presents to children (or adults).
Don't give a baby a sweetened pacifier to suck on for hours.
Don't be embarrassed about using toothpicks.
Don't take a sweet drink last thing at night.

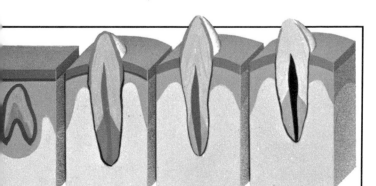

…ver itself before its later development beneath

Smoking

If you are a smoker trying to give it up, you are a member of a large club. One in three adults in the United States smokes, and nine out of ten would probably like to quit. Unfortunately, more than four-fifths of all smokers continue to their last breath, even though they know how painful that last breath is likely to be.

The high failure rate in attempts to give up smoking is because, for most smokers, it is more an addiction than a simple pleasure. Many smokers might deny this. But smoking is obviously not a pleasure in the sense that watching an exciting movie, listening to Mozart or riding on ferris wheels can be pleasures. People are not normally bad-tempered because they have not had their first Mozart record or ferris wheel ride of the day. And there cannot be many people so driven by a passion for movies that they regularly scour a deserted town at night looking for a late, late show.

Breaking an addiction is different from giving up a pleasure. The reasons for breaking this particular addiction are numerous. For whatever the disagreement about the extent of smoking's contribution to various illnesses, there is no medical expert who claims that it does you good.

Why give it up? Everyone knows about the link between smoking and lung cancer, but not everyone appreciates what this means. Young people, in particular, can be vague about this hazard. This is a pity since they will have smoked, if at all, for only a short time and will not be strongly addicted. Cancer is a disease in which the cells that make up some part of the body, in this particular case the lungs or larynx (voice box), multiply wildly, without any control. The sufferer, in the early stages, will be unaware of this, but in the case of cancer of the larynx will soon notice a persistent cough or a change in the quality of the voice. In the case of lung cancer, the sufferer may spit up blood when coughing, or develop a severe pain in the chest.

Operations for lung cancer are only possible in one in five cases, and less than one in twenty are cured. In the United States nearly 200 people die of lung cancer each day, over 60,000 a year. In all, smoking is responsible for some 250,000 premature deaths in the US each year and, in addition, heavy smoking causes $17 billion in unnecessary expenditure – $4 billion in medical care alone and $17 billion in accidents, absenteeism and lost output. More Americans die each year from smoking than died from battle injuries during the whole of the Second World War. This should be reason enough to give up smoking, especially as half the victims are under 65. But lung cancer is only one penalty of smoking.

Another is chronic bronchitis. It may sound more like a complaint than a disease but it, too, kills 44,000 people a

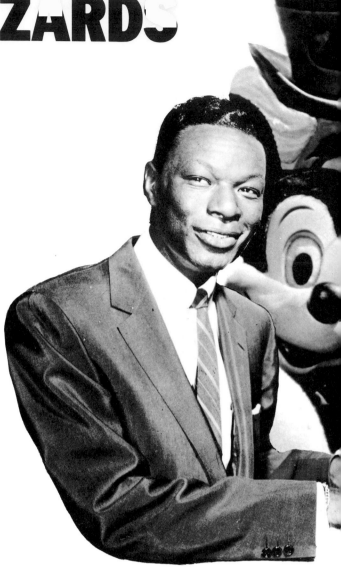

(Above) Nat "King" Cole, the husky-voiced singing star of the 1950s, died aged forty-five from lung cancer. He was a heavy cigarette smoker.

(Centre) Walt Disney, the pioneer of cartoon movies and leisure parks, died aged sixty-five from lung cancer without seeing Disneyworld completed.

(Left) Humphrey Bogart, the hard man of the cinema screen, died aged fifty-seven from cancer of the esophagus after two years of illness.

year. Bronchitis begins as a smoker's cough, clearing from the air-passages of the throat and lungs a slimy mucus produced by the irritating smoke that eventually starts to clog the lungs themselves. The smoke also damages the small air tubes and the air sacs, so that the victim cannot get enough air into the lungs and the blood cannot get the oxygen the body needs without desperate efforts to breathe. The shortness of breath may be so severe that the victim of chronic bronchitis cannot walk far without severe discomfort. In extreme cases, a victim may be confined to bed and only be able to move around the house on his hands and knees.

Other complaints caused by smoking are severe heart and blood vessel diseases which kill thousands of people every year. Smoking also causes cancer of the mouth and bladder, which together with cancer of the larynx account

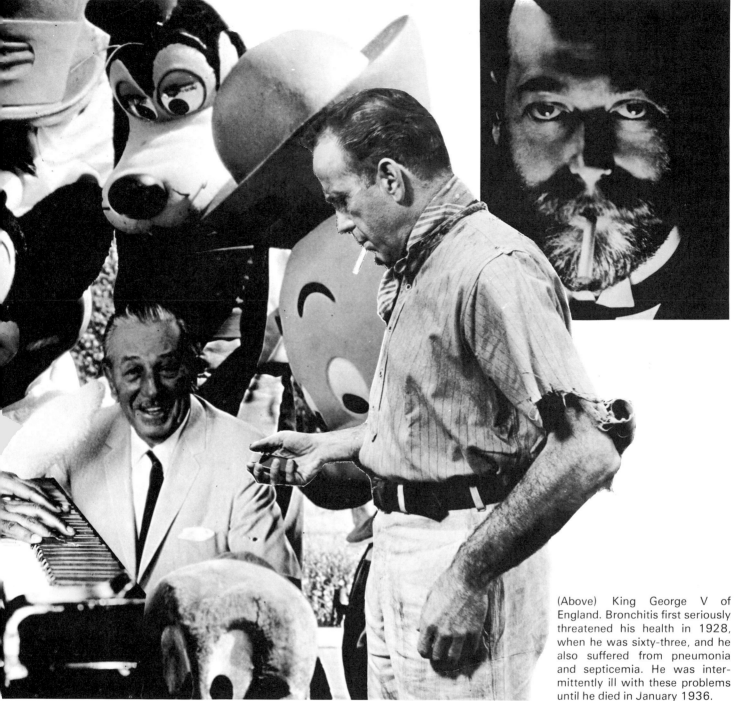

(Above) King George V of England. Bronchitis first seriously threatened his health in 1928, when he was sixty-three, and he also suffered from pneumonia and septicemia. He was intermittently ill with these problems until he died in January 1936.

for several thousand deaths a year. If these do not kill, they can cripple. Some people suffer from these illnesses without ever having smoked in their lives, of course. But *without exception* the risk increases dramatically if you do smoke. You are twice as likely to suffer from heart disease, for instance, and four or five times as likely in the 35–44 age group. Pregnant women have a particular incentive to give up smoking: it can harm the unborn child, as explained in Chapter 1.

The list of afflictions is so grim that many people need read no further, but avoiding diseases is not the only reason for not smoking. Very soon after you stop, you will discover that you feel better, suffer less of the clogged-up feeling common among smokers, and be better able to taste and enjoy food. And at whatever stage you stop smoking, it will lessen your chances of falling victim to the smoking-related diseases described above.

It really is never too late to give up. The first benefit you will notice is that cough and phlegm will gradually decrease and you become less liable to chest infections. If you suffer from breathlessness, that may also decrease on giving up. In some people permanent damage has been done and their breathlessness does not improve much; even for them, however, it stops getting worse, and a real benefit is still gained from being less liable to infection.

The long-term risks of premature death through lung cancer or bronchitis also begin to improve on giving up. A classic study of British doctors who gave up smoking shows that their health steadily improved. After five years the risk fell to about one half of the risk for men who continued to smoke, and after fifteen years the risk had nearly returned to normal. The heavy smoker has a two out of five chance of dying before retirement at sixty-five, while for the non-smoker the risk is one in five.

The 1976 follow-up study of the smoking habits of 34,000 British doctors, started over twenty years ago, confirms the risk of smoking cigarettes. Between a third and a half of those who continued to smoke died prematurely of it. The earlier they stopped, the less likely was a premature death. Giving up is always worthwhile.

The latest report of the American Cancer Society, *Task Force on Tobacco and Cancer*, says that 30 million Americans have stopped smoking since anti smoking campaigns began. In 1964, 42 per cent of the adult population of the United States was smoking. Now only 33–4 per cent smoke. Furthermore the average cigarette today has 60 per cent less tar and nicotine than it had twenty years ago. However, there has been a dramatic increase in the number of young teenage girls smoking compared to a few years ago, and the number of teenage girls and young women who smoke heavily has also increased dramatically. Since smoking is a form of drug dependence, the majority of young people who try it become dependent on it. So special efforts are needed to protect children against smoking. The latest report of the *US Surgeon General* (1979) says that research over the last fifteen years "overwhelmingly ratifies the original scientific indictment of smoking as a contributor to disease and premature death. . . . Today there can be no doubt that smoking is truly slow motion suicide." The report emphasizes that special risks for smokers attach to work in certain industries; in particular the asbestos, rubber, coal, textile, uranium and chemical industries.

If you smoke, anyone who shares space with you will effectively smoke the equivalent of perhaps one cigarette an hour by inhaling the smoke-laden air. The nearer and dearer people are to you, the more likely it is that they will share the afflictions your cigarettes produce. Husbands, wives, lovers and children may thus suffer the irritations and ill effects of smoke.

HOW TO GIVE UP

The simple answer is "Just stop". It is not that simple, of course, otherwise more people would succeed. You may be one of the lucky ones who can stop quite easily once they have really decided to. About one in three smokers are like this. You will have to *want* to stop smoking. Nobody can succeed against their will. Most anti-smoking experts say the only long-term guarantee of success is to stop altogether: compulsive gamblers and alcoholics face the same recommendation. But some half-measures are better than nothing. For instance, the most dangerous constituent of a cigarette is tar, which is known to contain the cancer-producing substances. And the most dangerous part of a cigarette is the final third, where the tar and nicotine tend to condense. These two facts alone suggest the following simple and sensible half-measures:

1. Leave long stubs
2. Smoke low tar filter cigarettes (see tables)
3. Avoid inhaling
4. Smoke fewer cigarettes
5. Take fewer puffs from each cigarette
6. Never leave the cigarette dangling in your mouth

Do not pin too much hope on the tobacco substitutes that are promised. Advertising and promotion of these cigarettes has left some people with the idea that cigarettes might one day be made safe. Cigarettes may be made less hazardous to health but they will never be made safe. The most likely prospect is a cigarette containing a mixture of tobacco and substitute, not necessarily lower in tars and nicotine than some all-tobacco cigarettes now available. An alternative approach, already in use in Germany, is very low-tar, low-nicotine tobacco with flavor components added so that it tastes, it is said, like a normal tobacco. It is important to remember that even the most technologically modified cigarette is not a safe cigarette. The only safe way is to give up smoking.

If you can cut down the volume of smoking to, say, five a day, then the effect of your action will obviously help. But few people in practice can keep themselves for very long to the "one or two a day after meals" that they claim. It is much better to aim for a complete break, and there are some ways of making the going a little easier. Begin by trying to recognize the kind of smoker you are.

WHAT KIND OF SMOKER ARE YOU?

Here are some statements made by people to describe what they get out of smoking cigarettes. How often do you feel this way when smoking? Answer every question, and score as follows: Always – 5; Frequently – 4; Occasionally – 3; Seldom – 2; Never – 1.

A. I smoke cigarettes in order to keep myself from slowing down.
B. Handling a cigarette is part of the enjoyment of smoking.
C. Smoking cigarettes is pleasant and relaxing.
D. I light up a cigarette when I feel angry about something.
E. When I have run out of cigarettes I find it almost unbearable until I can get them.
F. I smoke cigarettes automatically without even being aware of it.
G. I smoke cigarettes to stimulate me, to perk myself up.
H. Part of the enjoyment of smoking a cigarette comes from the steps I take to light up.
I. I find cigarettes pleasurable.
J. When I feel uncomfortable or upset about something, I light up a cigarette.
L. I light up a cigarette without realizing I still have one burning in the ashtray.
M. I smoke cigarettes to give me a lift.
N. When I smoke a cigarette, part of the enjoyment is watching the smoke as I exhale it.
O. I want a cigarette most when I am comfortable and relaxed.
P. When I feel blue or want to take my mind off cares and worries, I smoke cigarettes.
Q. I get a real gnawing hunger for a cigarette when I haven't smoked for a while.
R. I've found a cigarette in my mouth and didn't remember putting it there.

Scoring: Enter the points scored on each question below and then add up each of the six totals:

	+		+		=			+		+		=	
A		G		M		Stimulation		D		J		P		Support
B		H		N		Handling		E		K		Q		Craving
C		I		O		Pleasure		F		L		R		Habit

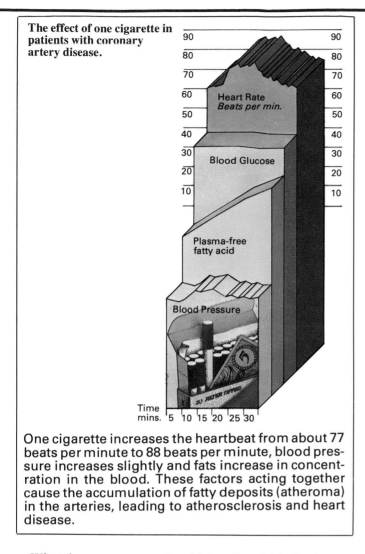

The effect of one cigarette in patients with coronary artery disease.

Heart Rate
Beats per min.

Blood Glucose

Plasma-free fatty acid

Blood Pressure

Time mins. 5 10 15 20 25 30

One cigarette increases the heartbeat from about 77 beats per minute to 88 beats per minute, blood pressure increases slightly and fats increase in concentration in the blood. These factors acting together cause the accumulation of fatty deposits (atheroma) in the arteries, leading to atherosclerosis and heart disease.

What the scores mean. Any higher than 11 indicates you smoke for that reason. Scores of 7 or less are low, scores in between are marginal. The higher your score (15 is the highest), the most important a particular factor is in your smoking.

Stimulation: If you score high or fairly high on this factor, it means that you are one of those smokers who is stimulated by the cigarette; you feel that it helps you wake up, organize your energies, and keep you going. If you try to give up smoking, you may want a safe substitute such as a brisk walk, moderate exercise or a cup of coffee whenever you feel the urge to smoke.

Handling: Handling things can be satisfying, but there are ways to keep your hands busy without lighting up or playing with a cigarette. Why not toy with a pen or pencil, or try doodling, or playing with a coin, a piece of jewelry or some other harmless object.

Pleasure: It is not always easy to find out whether you use the cigarette to feel good, to get real, honest pleasure out of smoking. About two-thirds of smokers score high or fairly high on the pleasure factor and about half of those also score as high or higher on the support factor. Those who do get real pleasure out of smoking often find that sufficient consideration of the harmful effects of their habit will help them to stop. They substitute eating, drinking and social activities – within reasonable bounds – and find they do not seriously miss their cigarettes.

Support: Many smokers use cigarettes as a kind of support in moments of stress or discomfort, and on occasions it may work; the cigarette is sometimes used as a tranquilizer. But heavy smokers, those who try to handle severe personal problems by smoking many times a day, are apt to discover that cigarettes do not help them deal with their problems effectively. When it comes to stopping, this kind of smoker may find it easy to give up when everything is going well, but may be tempted to start again in a time of crisis. Again, physical exertion, eating, drinking, or social activity – in moderation – may serve as useful substitutes for cigarettes, even in times of tension. The choice of a substitute depends on what will achieve the same effect without having the same appreciable risk.

Craving: Giving up smoking is difficult for people who score high on this factor, that of psychological addiction. For them, the craving for the next cigarette begins to build up the moment they put one out, so tapering off is not likely to work. They must stop dead. It may be helpful for them to smoke more than usual for a day or two so that the taste for cigarettes is spoiled, and then isolate themselves completely from cigarettes until the craving is gone; this may take several months. Giving up cigarettes may be so difficult and cause so much discomfort that once they do stop, they will find it easy to resist the temptation to go back to smoking.

Habit: This kind of smoker is no longer getting much satisfaction from cigarettes, but just lights them, frequently without even realizing he is doing so. He may find it easy to stop permanently if he can break the habit patterns he has built up. Cutting down gradually may be quite effective if there is a change in the way the cigarettes are smoked. The key to success is becoming aware of each cigarette you smoke.

Conclusion: If you do not score high on any of the six factors, the chances are that you do not smoke very much or have not been smoking for very many years. If so, giving up smoking – and staying off – should be relatively easy. If you score high on several categories you apparently get several kinds of satisfaction from smoking, and will have to find several solutions. Those who score high on both the Support and Craving factors may have a particularly hard time in giving up smoking and in staying off. They can try the half-measures suggested above, and after several months of this temporary solution they may find it easier to stop completely.

Many people smoke automatically. As they pick up a telephone, or finish a meal or settle in a car, or start to drink coffee, or even as they wake up, they suddenly find they have a cigarette in their hands. If you have noticed these habits you will not be surprised to find something missing when you stop. People who smoke out of habit should therefore try to change their routine. Don't smoke first thing in the morning. Try to delay your first cigarette by an extra fifteen minutes each day. Go for a short walk after dinner. Simply leaving a gap where once you smoked is a bit unnerving: a new routine will help break the addiction.

Changing to pipes and cigars, which can be less harmful, is not really the best way to avoid the risks. First, it is not available to everyone. Our society may be permissive, but it still looks at a pipe-smoking woman with a bit of surprise. What is more, most of the statistics about the relative safety of pipe and cigar smoking are based on people who have always smoked them and have never inhaled deeply.

There is no substitute for actually stopping smoking, and if you are to stop, there is no substitute for clearly wanting to. Some people go to smoking withdrawal clinics, for example, with a vague hope that somehow or other the clinic will stop smoking for them. But if you do sincerely want to become a non-smoker, there is a wide range of aids. There is no miracle cure, and the idea that there is one is harmful: people can try something, fail, and decide that their case is hopeless. Virtually every method of giving up has at best a low success rate: it works for roughly 30 per cent of those who try it. But the 70 per cent are not the same people for every method. Somewhere or other, there is a method for almost everyone, and if you have not succeeded with one, try another.

There is a range of what may be called pharmaceutical aids available from drugstores. They are much cheaper than the cigarettes you would smoke during the cure, let alone during the rest of your life. Aversion compounds form one group of chemical aids. These usually contain a silver salt that makes cigarette smoke taste foul: no one will continue smoking while using the tablets, mouthwash or gum, but of course a lot of people abandon the treatment. It is not necessary or advisable to use these silver salt products for more than about a week, because taken for long periods they cause poisoning. There are also tablets containing lobeline (Nicoban, Bantron), a chemical that the manufacturers claim gives the satisfaction of nicotine without the harmful or addictive effects. They may do so for some people, and while it is difficult to be sure what fraction of users this represents, it could turn out to be the method for you. However, many people find that their resolve weakens without support, and smoking withdrawal clinics may help them. (See Appendix 2.)

People, it is sad to report, will offer you cigarettes when they know you have given them up. Be firm, or abusive, or full of suspicious insight: why are they doing this? Or if they insist, accept the cigarette and tear it up. People who still smoke owe it to others not to offer cigarettes to anyone who is trying to stop. In fact, it is not a bad general rule never to offer cigarettes, as it leads to over-smoking in the same way as dutifully buying drinks for others leads to over-drinking. And as some people's smoking is limited by the cost, don't give cigarettes as presents, and don't bring people cheap cigarettes from foreign trips. Don't smoke when children are about: your example, as well as your smoke, is harmful. A Scandinavian survey of families found that if neither parent smoked, and both were vocally opposed to smoking, only 10 per cent of the children took up the habit; if both parents smoked and were permissive about smoking, 70 per cent of the children followed their parents. Anyone who smokes owes a lot of consideration to those who do not. And a smoker who thinks enough about this obligation may even decide to give the habit up.

Brand and Type[3]	Tar (mg/cig)	Nicotine (mg/cig)
Low Tar		
Carlton king, f	<0.5	<0.05
Carlton king, f, m	1	0.1
Now[2] king, f	1	0.1
Benson & Hedges reg, f	1	0.1
Now[2] king, f, m	1	0.1
Carlton king, f	1	0.1
Iceberg 100's 100mm, f, m	3	0.3
Luck 100's 100mm, f	3	0.3
Carlton 100mm, f	4	0.4
True king, f	5	0.4
True king, f, m	5	0.4
Decade king, f	5	0.4
Decade king, f, m	5	0.4
King Sano king, f	6	0.3
King Sano king, f, m	6	0.3
Pall Mall Extra Mild king, f	7	0.5
Tempo king, f	7	0.5
Tareyton Lights king, f	7	0.6
L & M Lights king, f	7	0.6
L & M Lights 100's 100mm, f	8	0.6
Kent Golden Lights king, f	8	0.7
Real king, f, m	8	0.6
Merit king, f, m	8	0.6
Merit king, f	8	0.8
American Lights 120mm, f	9	0.7
Lucky Ten king, f	9	0.7
Kent Golden Lights king, f, m	9	0.6
American Lights 120mm, f, m	9	0.7
Parliament king, f	9	0.6
Kent Golden Lights 100mm, f, m	9	0.8
Real king, f	9	0.7
Parliament king, f	9	0.6
Kent Golden Lights 100m, f	9	0.8
Newport Lights king, f, m	10	0.8
Hi-Lite 100mm, f	10	0.7
Salem Long Lights 100mm, f, m	10	0.8
Vantage 100m, f	10	0.8
Salem Lights king, f, m	10	0.8
Low to Middle Tar		
Merit 100's 100mm, f, m	11	0.7
Merit 100's 100mm, f	11	0.7
Multifilter king, f, m	11	0.7
Vantage king, f, m	11	0.8
Vantage king, f	11	0.8
Viceroy Extra Mild king, f	11	0.8
Doral king, f, m	12	0.8
Marlboro Lights king, f	12	0.8
Parliament 100's 100mm, f	12	0.8
Doral king, f	12	0.9
Fact king, f	12	0.8
Kent Micronite II king, f	12	0.9
Fact king, f, m	13	0.9
Multifilter king, f	13	0.8
Winston Lights king, f	13	0.9
Raleigh Lights king, f	13	0.9
True 100's 100mm, f	13	0.8
True 100's 100mm, f, m	13	0.8
Winston Lights 100's 100mm, f	13	1.0
Marlboro king, f, m	14	0.8
Kent Micronite II 100mm, f	14	1.0
Eve 120's 120mm, f	14	1.0
Kool Milds king size, f, m	14	0.9
Alpine king, f, m	14	0.8
Marlboro king, f, m	14	0.8
Belair king, f, m	15	0.9
Saratoga 120mm, f	15	1.0
Eve 120's 120mm, f, m	15	1.1
Kent king, f	15	1.0
Saratoga 120mm, f, m	16	1.0
Pall Mall 100mm, f, m	16	1.2
Sano reg, non-f	16	0.5

Tar[1] and Nicotine Content of Cigarettes from Federal Trade Commission Report, May 1978
(Shown in increasing order of tar values)

Low to Middle Tar

Eve 100mm, f, m	16	1.0
Galaxy king, f	16	1.0
DuMaurier king, f	16	1.1
Silva Thins 100mm, f, m	16	1.1
Raleigh king, f	16	1.0
Virginia Slims 100mm, f, m	16	0.9
Virginia Slims 100mm, f	16	0.9
Tall 120mm, f, m	16	1.3
Eve 100mm, f	16	1.0
Long Johns 120mm, f, m	16	1.3
Silva Thins 100mm, f	16	1.2
Philip Morris International 100mm, f, m	16	1.0
Viceroy king, f	16	1.1
Salem king, f, m	16	1.1
Kent king, f	16	1.1
Old Gold Filters king, f	16	1.1
Belair 100mm, f, m	16	1.1
Tareyton 100mm, f	16	1.2
St Moritz 100mm, f	16	1.1

Middle Tar

Twist 100mm, f, lemon/methanol	17	1.3
L & M king, f	17	1.0
Tareyton king, f	17	1.2
L & M king, f	17	1.0
L & M 100mm, f	17	1.1
St Moritz 100mm, f, m	17	1.1
Long Johns 120mm, f	17	1.3
Philip Morris International 100mm, f	17	1.1
Kent 100mm, f, m	17	1.1
Max 120mm, f	17	1.3
Marlboro king, f	17	1.0
Benson & Hedges king, f	17	1.2
Marlboro 100mm, f	17	1.1
Benson & Hedges 100's 100mm, т, m	17	1.1
Kool king, f, m	17	1.4
Raleigh 100mm, f	17	1.2
Newport king, f, m	17	1.2
Lark king, f	17	1.1
Chesterfield king, f	17	1.1
Chesterfield 101mm, f	17	1.1
Pall Mall king, f	17	1.2
Benson & Hedges 100's 100mm, f, m	17	1.0
Benson & Hedges 100's 100mm, f	17	1.1
Marlboro king, f	17	1.0
Max 120mm, f, m	17	1.3
Benson & Hedges 100's 100mm, f	17	1.1
Montclair king, f, m	17	1.3
Tall 120mm, f	17	1.4
Salem king, f, m	18	1.2
Kool king, f, m	18	1.4
Marlboro 100mm, f	18	1.1
Viceroy 100mm, f	18	1.2
Newport king, f, m	18	1.3
Kool 100mm, f, m	18	1.3
L & M 100mm, f, m	18	1.1
Old Gold Filters king, f	18	1.2
Oasis king, f, m	18	1.1
Kent 100mm, f	18	1.3
Pall Mall 100mm, f	19	1.4
Salem 100mm, f, m	19	1.3
Winston 100mm, f	19	1.3
Camel king, f	19	1.3
Lark 100mm, f	19	1.2
L. T. Brown 120mm, f, m	19	1.4
Winston king, f	19	1.3
Newport 100mm, f, m	19	1.4
Winston 100mm, f	19	1.3
Spring 100's 100mm, f, m	20	1.1
Winston king, f	20	1.3
Old Gold Straights reg, non-f	20	1.2
Philip Morris reg, non-f	20	1.1

Middle Tar

L. T. Brown 120mm, f	20	1.5
Kool reg, non-f	20	1.3
Home Run reg, non-f	21	1.5
Old Gold 100's 100mm, f	21	1.4

Middle to High Tar

Chesterfield reg, non-f	23	1.3
Picayune reg, non-f	23	1.6
English Ovals reg, non-f	23	1.6
More 120mm, f	23	1.7
More 120mm, f	23	1.7
Lucky Strike reg, non-f	24	1.4
Mapleton king, f	24	1.4
Piedmont reg, non-f	24	1.4
Raleigh king, non-f	24	1.4
Half & Half king, f	24	1.5
Stratford king, f	25	1.4
Old Gold Straights king, non-f	25	1.5
Philip Morris Commander king, non-f	25	1.4
Camel reg, non-f	25	1.6
Pall Mall king, non-f	26	1.6
Mapleton reg, non-f	27	1.2

High Tar

Stratford king, non-f	28	1.1
Fatima king, non-f	28	1.7
Chesterfield king, non-f	28	1.7
Herbert Tareyton king, non-f	29	1.8
Bull Durham king, f	30	2.0
English Ovals king, non-f	30	2.1
Players reg, non-f	35	2.5

[1] TPM dry (tar) – milligrams total particulate matter less nicotine and water
[2] Now cigarettes have been reformulated to produce 2mg "tar" and 0.1mg nicotine in the FTC test method, according to the manufacturer
[3] Abbreviations: king=king size, f=filter, m=menthol, mm=millimeters length, reg=regular size, non-f=non-filter

How to use the tar table: Check out the brand you normally smoke and see if you can find another brand which gives less tar but the same nicotine. Remember it is the nicotine which is most addictive and the tar which is worst for health. For example. Marlboro kings give 0.8mg nicotine and 14mg tar. You should get as much nicotine satisfaction from Kent Golden lights. which also deliver 0.8mg nicotine and at the same time get only 9mg tar. They are lighter tasting because they give a worthwhile reduction in your intake of damaging smoke. Gradually work your way down the tar table until you have reached the lowest nicotine and tar intake you can tolerate – next you have to make the big break and give up altogether.

As "tar" is regarded as a greater danger to health than nicotine. the brands are listed in order of tar yield. Differences between brands of up to 2mg of tar can generally be ignored. The Federal Trade Laboratory has measured "tar" (dry particulate matter) and "nicotine" (measured as total alkaloid) by smoking cigarettes to a 23-mm butt length or to the length of the filter and overwrap plus 3mm if in excess of 23mm. The samples of cigarettes were purchased where possible in each of 50 geographic locations throughout the United States. Tests were based on 100 cigarettes randomly selected from the samples of each brand.

Heart Disease

WHAT IS HEART DISEASE?

One half of all deaths in most Western countries are caused by atherosclerosis, the underlying condition responsible for coronary heart disease, strokes and other blood vessel diseases. Atherosclerosis is also the cause of much crippling illness and senile decay; it may also cause chest pain and leg pain on walking. But now the means of preventing, delaying or perhaps even reversing the disease are beginning to be understood.

Atherosclerosis is caused by the accumulation of a sludgy deposit called atheroma in the lining of arteries all over the body, including those arteries which supply blood to the heart – the coronary arteries. The build-up of atheroma (which contains a lot of cholesterol) causes the walls of the arteries to thicken and narrow. This accretion of fatty material may begin in childhood but the ill-effects are not usually found until the forties when men, apparently in the prime of life, begin to be struck down by coronary thromboses.

The reason for atheroma clogging up arteries is usually a diet that has been too rich in saturated animal or saturated vegetable fats. The condition is accelerated and aggravated by smoking, high blood pressure and stress. (The precautions that everyone can take to reduce the chances of heart disease in middle age are outlined below, along with the details of medical measures designed to produce marked improvements in health for angina sufferers and those coronary victims who get a second chance.)

Atheroma restricts the supply of blood flowing through the coronary blood vessels to the heart muscle, so that any physical or emotional stress which puts an additional burden on the heart may precipitate a crisis. This occurs when a rapidly beating heart needs more blood than is available to provide the heart muscle with sufficient oxygen. The narrowed vessels cannot supply it and so the heart is deprived of oxygen, causing patches of tissue to die which are replaced by inelastic scar tissue. One in every four people dies suddenly of heart trouble without any previous warning. Even when a person is aware of possible heart trouble, two out of three of those who die do so too quickly for medical help to reach them.

The immediate cause of a heart attack may be a blood clot – otherwise known as a thrombosis. This cuts off the blood supply to the heart muscle. Blood clots form easily in people who have a lot of atheroma because the normal duck's back lining of the blood vessels, which prevents clotting, is lost. However, many people survive a warning attack, because the area of heart muscle which dies following the interruption of the blood supply is small.

ANGINA

Some people learn that their heart is not working properly when they first suffer an attack of angina. This is a pain in the center of the chest which may spread to the neck, midriff and arms. It is brought on by exertion, emotion or cold weather and goes away with rest, and can generally be distinguished from heartburn, which is caused by indigestion.

In angina the supply of blood to the heart is unable to keep up with demand. When a person who suffers from angina takes exercise, the heart muscle works harder and requires more oxygen. If blood vessels, narrowed by atheroma, restrict the blood supply, then the heart muscle will be deprived of oxygen and will begin to burn up fats and sugars inefficiently, so that waste products accumulate. These stimulate nerves in the heart, causing a violent pain.

Angina may be caused by anything which makes the heart beat faster: sport, sexual intercourse or any other kind of excitement. A heavy meal, particularly if it is fatty, may bring on an attack. Smoking and exhaust fumes may cause angina, since carbon monoxide from the smoke replaces some of the oxygen in the blood. Smoking also increases heart rate and blood pressure, in the same way as emotional or physical stress, so that the heart may require more oxygen than can be supplied.

Angina can be relieved by medical treatment with drugs such as nitro-glycerine which expand the blood vessels of the heart. Other drugs, the beta blockers, prevent the heart responding to adrenalin and impose a type of speed limit on the heart so it cannot respond in the normal way to exercise or emotion. Operations have also been devised to relieve angina. It is sometimes possible to take a piece of vein from the leg and graft it on to the heart, by-passing a local blockage in one of the coronary arteries. However, if the harmful lifestyle is not changed, the graft itself may silt up and the problem return. So it is important for angina sufferers to keep strictly to a diet, to abandon smoking, to avoid stress, to reduce weight and to take as much exercise as they can without pain in order to improve circulation.

STROKES

Atheroma may cause trouble elsewhere in the body. A blood clot cuts off the blood supply to part of the brain, causing a stroke. Only half of the people who have a stroke are alive a month later. The survivors may be partially paralyzed, and their speech or other functions controlled by the brain may be badly affected. The factors which lead to a high risk of stroke are the same as those for heart disease: particularly smoking and high-fat diet.

Other symptoms of heart disease

Arteries narrowed by atheroma can reduce the blood supply to leg muscles and cause cramping pains during mild exercise – a condition known medically as intermittent claudication (limping).

Arteries generally become narrower and harder as atheroma accumulates. They are unable to respond flexibly to the demands of the heart during exercise, and so a person with narrowed arteries tires very quickly. Eventually, arteries become so narrow that the blood supply is inadequate even without exercise. When this happens to blood vessels in the brain, a person gradually loses normal mental functions and control of the body. This is the tragic waste of life we see as senile decay.

ARE YOU AT RISK?

Your chance of suffering from heart disease can be calculated fairly accurately from the chart overleaf which was devised by the Michigan Heart Association.* As no single predominant cause of heart disease has yet been identified, the degree of risk depends on the combined total of several separate factors. So study the eight columns, mark the appropriate box in each and then add up your score.

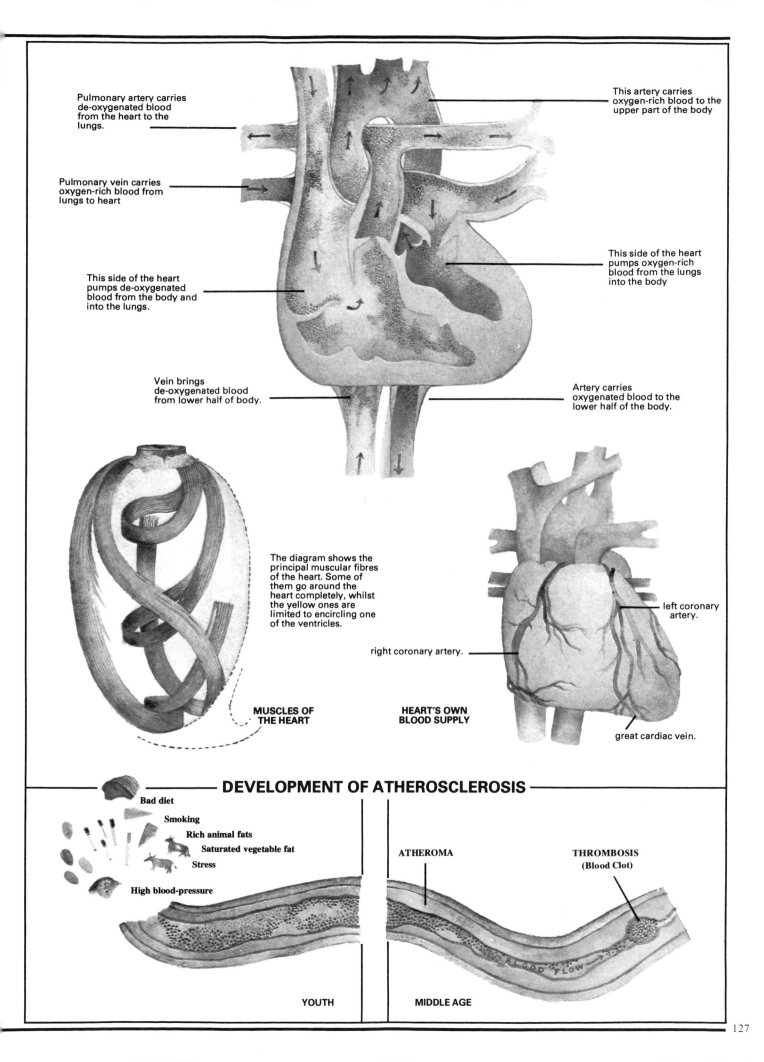

Pulmonary artery carries de-oxygenated blood from the heart to the lungs.

This artery carries oxygen-rich blood to the upper part of the body

Pulmonary vein carries oxygen-rich blood from lungs to heart

This side of the heart pumps oxygen-rich blood from the lungs into the body

This side of the heart pumps de-oxygenated blood from the body and into the lungs.

Vein brings de-oxygenated blood from lower half of body.

Artery carries oxygenated blood to the lower half of the body.

The diagram shows the principal muscular fibres of the heart. Some of them go around the heart completely, whilst the yellow ones are limited to encircling one of the ventricles.

left coronary artery.

right coronary artery.

great cardiac vein.

MUSCLES OF THE HEART

HEART'S OWN BLOOD SUPPLY

DEVELOPMENT OF ATHEROSCLEROSIS

Bad diet

Smoking

Rich animal fats

Saturated vegetable fat

Stress

High blood-pressure

ATHEROMA

THROMBOSIS (Blood Clot)

BLOOD FLOW

YOUTH

MIDDLE AGE

SEX	BLOOD PRESSURE	FAT % IN DIET	EXERCISE	TOBACCO SMOKING	WEIGHT	HEREDITY	AGE
Female under 40 **1**	100 (upper reading) **1**	Diet contains no animal or solid fats **1**	Intensive work and recreational exertion **2**	Non-user **0**	More than 5lb. below standard weight **0**	No known history of heart disease **1**	10 to 20 **1**
Female 40–50 **2**	120 (upper reading) **2**	Diet contains 10% animal or solid fats **2**	Moderate work and recreational exertion **2**	Cigar and/ or pipe **1**	−5 to +5lb. standard weight **1**	1 relative over 60 with cardiovascular disease **2**	21 to 30 **2**
Female over 50 **3**	140 (upper reading) **3**	Diet contains 20 animal or solid fats **3**	Sedentary work and intense recreational exertion **3**	10 cigarettes or less a day **2**	6–20lb. over weight **2**	2 relatives over 60 with cardiovascular disease **3**	31 to 40 **3**
Male **5**	160 (upper reading) **4**	Diet contains 30% animal or solid fats **4**	Sedentary work and moderate recreational exertion **5**	20 cigarettes a day **4**	21–35lb. over weight **3**	1 relative under 60 with cardiovascular disease **4**	41 to 50 **4**
Stocky male **6**	180 (upper reading) **6**	Diet contains 40% animal or solid fats **5**	Sedentary work and light recreational exertion **6**	30 cigarettes a day **6**	36–50lb. over weight **5**	2 relatives under 60 with cardiovascular disease **6**	51 to 60 **5**
Bald stocky male **7**	200 or over (upper reading) **8**	Diet contains 50% animal or solid fats **7**	Complete lack of all exercise **8**	40 cigarettes a day or more **10**	51–65lb. over weight **7**	3 relatives under 60 with cardiovascular disease **7**	61 to 70 and over **8**

1. If you are a smoker who inhales deeply and smokes to a short butt, add one to your total.
2. If you have passed an insurance company medical recently, your blood pressure will probably be below 140.
3. Don't forget that cream, butter and eggs are high in animal fat.
4. To calculate the hereditary factor, only count parents, grandparents, brothers and sisters as relatives.

If you are an aggressive person, live under a lot of stress or suffer from gout or diabetes, then these factors will increase the risk of heart disease. But they are too complicated to calculate on a points system.

Scores:
6 to 11 – well below average risk
12 to 17 – below average risk
18 to 24 – average risk
25 to 31 – moderate risk
32 to 40 – dangerous risk
41 to 63 – imminent danger: see your doctor

HOW TO PREVENT HEART DISEASE

All forms of heart and blood vessel disease are difficult to treat medically. The best hopes of preventing or alleviating them derive from a change of lifestyle. Apart from controlling diet and giving up smoking, it is particularly important to reduce the stress of daily living. Apart from causing a build-up of atheroma, stress can cause sudden death by interfering with the heart rhythm. Some people are addicted to a stressful life. They are ambitious, aggressive or uptight; they are not satisfied until they have drained themselves of all energy. Some doctors call this the coronary personality and this type of person faces a growing risk unless they learn to alter their lifestyle (see section on relaxation, Chapter 4).

What this means, according to authorities such as Britain's Royal College of Physicians and the American Heart Association, is summarized below; fuller details of each category will be found elsewhere in this book. People who scored highly in the coronary risk quiz at the start of this chapter are strongly advised to take immediate steps to alter their way of life. But do not try to do it all at once; you are likely to find it too great a change, and give up. Try to change your lifestyle slowly, over a period of weeks, months or even years. Even a small change may make a large difference.

Diet: Whatever your age or state of health, reduce the saturated fat in your diet.

1. Eat less meat and then choose lean meat, although even that contains 30 per cent invisible fat. Remove visible fat. Broil rather than fry.
2. Eat fewer eggs – one per day maximum. Eat more poultry, fish.
3. Use butter sparingly, prefer soft margarine high in polyunsaturates. Cut down generally on dairy products such as top-of-the-milk and cream.
4. Use polyunsaturated oils for cooking, e.g., corn, soya bean, sunflower or safflower oils. Olive oil is also acceptable. Avoid hard margarines, lard. Oils simply labeled vegetable oil may contain a lot of saturated oil.
5. Eat more vegetables, fruit.

Weight: The reason overweight people run a greater risk of coronary heart disease is because they are less likely to take physical exercise and more likely to have a badly balanced diet. It is more important to balance your diet correctly by cutting down on fats than to worry about weight itself.

It makes sense to lose weight, but make sure you do not cut down mostly on starchy (carbohydrate) foods: cut down on saturated fats or by calorie counting. Fats are a highly concentrated source of calories so if you cut down on fatty foods you can still maintain the bulk of your normal diet and are less likely to feel hungry. Cut down, too, on sugar and alcohol.

Smoking: The risk of coronary heart disease among smokers is almost twice that of non-smokers, and several times higher in middle age (35–54). But if you cannot give up smoking:
1. Smoke filters with progressively less tar.
2. Smoke less than five cigarettes a day.
3. Do not inhale; this is particularly important if you switch to cigars or a pipe.

Stress: Acute emotion may precipitate angina or a heart attack. In extreme circumstances a person may lose the will to live; their heart beats irregularly, then stops.
1. Guard against stress. Try to manage your life differently to avoid unnecessary, unproductive stress.
2. Try to cultivate methods of relaxation. Yoga or meditation may help.
3. Make sure of a good night's sleep. Make time to relax before going to bed. Sleep in once a week and catch up on lost rest. If necessary use an occasional sedative.
4. Discipline yourself to avoid exhaustion and fatigue. Be strict in refusing to take on more than you can do.

Exercise: Everyone should exercise regularly. Middle-aged people, who may not have exercised for years, can begin gradually. A medical is not essential except for older people, those who are seriously overweight or heart sufferers. If you develop unexpected symptoms during exercise, however, consult your doctor.

1. Get breathless some time every day. Climbing stairs instead of using escalators is a good way.
2. A minimum of 15 to 20 minutes vigorous exercise three times weekly (not on consecutive days) is necessary for your health. A daily walk is also excellent exercise. Gradually increase the distance, pace and slope.
3. Simple keep-fit exercises once or twice a day will work the main muscle groups in turn.

Contraception: Women over forty, those who have relatives with coronary artery disease, and women who smoke more than 10 cigarettes a day should avoid the pill and use some other form of contraception if possible (see Chapter 8).

HOW TO RECOVER FROM HEART DISEASE
Some people are lucky. They survive a heart attack to win a second chance to live. The clinical possibilities of improvement have been demonstrated in research involving monkeys at two American universities – those at Iowa and Chicago. The monkeys were first given a diet high in saturated fat and cholesterol, and their arteries became narrower. When the monkeys were returned to what the researchers called a prudent low-fat diet, their arteries widened again and their health improved. It is more difficult to establish that the same reversal of heart disease occurs in people. But there is evidence that the arteries of patients with high blood fats can get wider again after many months of dietary treatment. As the coronary arteries get wider it is possible that the danger of heart disease gradually decreases.

During the Second World War, when there was a general shortage of meat, eggs and animal fats, there was a marked decrease in fatalities from heart disease in every European country involved except Denmark. The Danes had stopped exporting dairy produce and so maintained something like their usual diet.

Isolated agricultural communities tend to suffer little heart disease. The Tarahumara Indians of Mexico, for instance, eat a diet based on maize and beans with very little meat or eggs. Both men and women can run distances of 100 to 200 miles over mountainous countryside kicking a small wooden ball. They do this in regular kickball races which show what endurance and stamina can be achieved on a diet far lower in fats, calories or proteins than would be considered appropriate for athletes.

For people at high risk of having a heart attack, including those who have already had one attack, the American Heart Association recommends : "A nutritious diet low in saturated fat and cholesterol, consumed at a low calorie level to maintain optimal body weight." A person who has already had one heart attack may be advised to have an even stricter diet than is necessary for simple prevention. Stricter measures should include the following:

1. Restrict meat meals to eight a week.
2. Always use soft margarines high in polyunsaturates.
3. Use skimmed milk.
4. Eat no more than three eggs a week.
5. Keep down cheese intake; use cottage cheese.
6. Restrict cakes, pastries and cookies unless they are homemade with suitable fats.

A vegetarian diet seems to be particularly effective in reducing the chances of heart disease. The Seventh Day Adventists, who mostly eat a vegetarian diet with eggs and milk and occasionally meat, have a much reduced incidence of heart disease and many other diseases. They also tend not to smoke or drink, which explains much of their good health and lower cancer rates but not all. So if you like the idea, it is well worth trying a vegetarian diet for rehabilitation from heart disease (see Appendix 2).

Other more extreme diets are sometimes recommended and may be beneficial, although they have not yet been proven scientifically. A diet consisting almost entirely of unprocessed vegetables and grains is recommended by the Longevity Research Institute in California. Their star patient, 87-year-old Mrs Eula Weaver, was chronically ill until she went on the diet. Mrs Weaver could not walk more than 100 feet without getting severe pains in her chest, and her legs were swollen to twice their normal size. She was found to be suffering from high blood pressure and arthritis. After following the diet for several years, Mrs Weaver won six gold medals in the veterans' Olympics at Irvine, California. At eighty-seven years old she was running two miles a day, riding ten to fifteen miles on a stationary bicycle and working out twice a week in a gym. Mrs Weaver attributed her rejuvenation to the diet and exercise regime recommended by the Institute. It consists of peas, beans, other vegetables and unprocessed grains such as rice, wheat, oats, buckwheat and corn. The patients also eat some cottage cheese made from skimmed milk and eat up to three pieces of fruit a day. They eat one ounce of fish *or* fowl every five days but no meat, eggs, milk, full-cream cheese or any extra fats and oils. This limits the fats and cholesterol in the diet to a fraction of that eaten in conventional diets.

The amount of exercise taken is gradually increased in the Longevity regime. Patients go for short walks three times a day and later every hour, until finally they are able to jog gently. Mr Nathan Pritikin, director of the Institute, says that this regime has been remarkably successful in rehabilitating heart patients who were waiting for by-pass surgery and has also been successful for treating patients who have had by-pass surgery and have since relapsed. People who are suffering from claudication (limping caused by artery disease) have also made spectacular recoveries.

Doctors will be skeptical of these results until they are repeated in other research establishments. In the meantime anyone can try this extreme diet for themselves. Strict vegetarians have pioneered a diet which contains no meat or animal produce. If you follow it rigorously there is no danger to health, but a little meat – particularly liver – once or twice a week will help to give you the B vitamins which must otherwise be supplied in the form of yeast extract.

HIGH BLOOD PRESSURE

At least one person in a hundred has severe high blood pressure and many more – perhaps one in ten people over forty-five – suffer from mildly increased blood pressure which is a threat to health. However, a person with high blood pressure often complains of no symptoms until the high blood pressure causes a stroke or heart failure. High blood pressure is aggravated by a stress lifestyle, and an individual can do a great deal to avoid it by cultivating a relaxed approach to life (see page 92) and changes in diet.

The pressure of blood in the body depends upon the force of the heartbeat and upon the tension in the 30,000 miles of arteries which spread throughout the body. Blood pressure is measured by putting a cuff around the arm and inflating it to a pressure which stops the flow of blood. Two readings are taken: one for the blood pressure at its highest when the heart is actually contracting, and one at its lowest when the heart is resting between one contraction and the next.

Blood pressure varies a great deal according to physical and mental activity. If the person has been running, working hard, or worrying, then their blood pressure will be higher: this is quite normal. However, this variation makes it difficult to measure a person's resting blood pressure accurately; all the doctor can do is measure the blood pressure on several different occasions. If it is always raised, then this indicates that a person has high blood pressure which may be confirmed by other tests. Blood pressure is raised if it exceeds about 160 millimeters of mercury for the high reading and 95 for the low reading. This would usually be written by the doctor in the form 160/95.

The first signs of high blood pressure may be dizziness, headaches, or impairment of memory or concentration. However, many people with high blood pressure feel per-

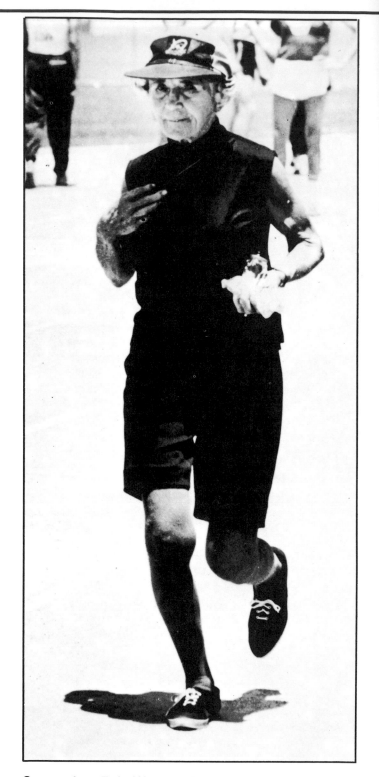

Star patient Eula Weaver, 87, was crippled. Now she wins medals in the senior Olympics. Exercise benefits the heart and circulation.

fectly well and only come to notice through routine examinations for insurance or eyesight, or other health checks. When high blood pressure builds up in the blood vessels in the brain, one may burst, causing a stroke. Alternatively, heart failure or damage to the eyes or kidneys may eventually result. These dangers are not immediate but steps must be taken to reduce them in the long term.

A full examination by a specialist is usually advisable when high blood pressure is found, in order to try and identify a cause. In the majority of people no cause can be found. In some cases kidney disease is found to be respon-

How to deal with a heart attack

During a heart attack a severe pain in the chest is experienced. This is often mistaken for indigestion but after the heart stops beating, a person collapses and turns pale or blue. Prompt action may save life.

Some doctors claim that it is possible for someone who is suffering a heart attack to restart their own heart and keep it going by coughing sharply and repeating as necessary. If there is no one else to help, cough sharply. If possible, phone for help.

If you are near someone who collapses with chest pains, put the patient on their back and lift the legs so that blood goes to the heart and thump the chest. Call an ambulance quickly. Loosen clothing around the person's neck, check the mouth for foreign bodies, remove false teeth. If breathing does not restart after thumping the chest, give mouth to mouth respiration: hold the nose and breathe into the mouth until the chest has risen; watch the chest fall, then repeat the operation.

If the victim does not begin to recover spontaneously, someone with experience of first-aid can look for signs that the heart has stopped: dilated pupils and no pulse in the neck. An experienced person may then attempt to restart the heart with cardiac massage. Cardiac massage squeezes the heart rhythmically to keep it going until expert help can be obtained. But inexperienced people are not advised to try this procedure. (For more information see Emergency!,

---

sible; more rarely, there may be disease of one of the endocrine glands which secrete hormones into the blood. Women at menopause sometimes suffer from high blood pressure which can only be detected by hospital investigation.

Salt in the diet is an important cause of high blood pressure. Investigations of several different kinds have now persuaded doctors after years of doubt that this is so. The Japanese have a diet high in salt. However, Japanese living in the North Island eat much more salt than those in the South and their blood pressure is on average higher. Solomon Islanders living beside the sea cook their food in sea water and eat about 11g of salt a day. They tend to have a much higher blood pressure than closely related people who live inland and cook their food in fresh water. And a trial in Belgium has shown that quite modest changes in salt intake from 11 to 5g a day is accompanied by an average reduction in blood pressure.

The average American consumes 12g of salt a day – much of it in consumer foods prepared already salted. However, doctors at Stanford University have shown in their Heart Disease Prevention Program that moderate salt restriction by people living in two northern California communities resulted in lower blood pressures. Our sense of taste adapts to different quantities of salt in the diet. But people who are accustomed to having large quantities of salt in the diet are unable to distinguish large additions of salt to the food. If salt in the diet is gradually reduced, people who were accustomed to very salty food will become sensitive again to small additions of salt to the diet and be able to detect once more when food is oversalted.

To reduce salt in your diet, first avoid all salted foods such as nuts, chips, salted popcorn, pretzels and cocktail snacks. Then stop using table salt and pickles. Finally, try to reduce the quantity of convenience foods such as canned vegetables, sauerkraut, canned soups, certain breakfast cereals, and salted meats such as ham, corned beef and sausages.

One of the commonest identifiable factors contributing to high blood pressure is the stress caused by emotional problems. Apprehension, fear, anger and prolonged resentment can all cause stress or raise blood pressure. The effect on blood pressure may be temporary and it may return to normal when the period of stress is over. However, the cause of stress often seems to be difficult or impossible to find. Sometimes people develop a style of life which is impossibly stressful, and then they must learn a new way of living.

It is important for a person who suffers from high blood pressure to learn to relax (see page 92), but it is also important for them to review their life and look for ways in which they can avoid stress. To begin with, it is important to aim at having nine hours in bed at night, and to wind down by reading something relaxing. Do not exercise immediately after a heavy meal. Delegate as much of your responsibilities as you can. Avoid working in the evenings or at week-ends. Take leisurely holidays which involve a minimum of traveling, and especially try to avoid driving, which can be particularly stressful. Compulsive drivers should try to minimize driving at weekends in order to have a thorough rest.

It is important for someone who suffers from high blood pressure and is also overweight to try to reach a normal weight. If a person has more or less normal weight it is still a good idea to adopt the low-fat diet and avoid overeating, by cutting down a little all round, and to avoid drinking excessive amounts of alcohol. It is best to give up smoking completely. Normal sexual activity can usually be continued, although it is best to discuss this with the doctor. It is best to avoid sex when unduly tired or suffering from any shortness of breath or pain, which may be signs of stress.

Regular walking is good for people with high blood pressure because it lowers blood pressure by dilating the blood vessels in the lower limbs. Swimming, running and cycling are also good exercises for people with high blood pressure, but care must be taken not to begin exercising suddenly after high blood pressure has been diagnosed. An exercise program should be introduced gradually (see page 74). Isometric exercises such as weight lifting, wrestling and water skiing clamp down on the muscles and so put up blood pressure – they should be avoided.

Many drugs are available for treating high blood pressure although a lot of them cause one side effect or another. Most effective drugs for treating moderate high blood pressure are diuretics, which increase urine flow and so remove more salt from the body. If side effects do occur it is usually possible to change the drugs so that they are avoided. Sometimes a person with high blood pressure may find that one day a week in bed resting, drinking fruit juice and taking very little solid food is a great help. Whatever treatment your doctor suggests, it is important to cultivate methods of relaxation.

Cancer

Cancer is not one disease but many, perhaps as many as a hundred or more, each affecting different parts of the body and each one caused in a different way. Now that infectious diseases have been largely conquered by better housing, vaccinations and modern drugs, cancer remains one of the major killers of our time. Over 385,000 Americans died of cancer in 1977, about 1,055 people a day. Yet most cancers can be cured successfully if caught in their early stages. Everyone knows their own body best and should pay close attention to any changes which could be a sign of cancer. This does not mean becoming a hypochondriac but simply taking your own health seriously and watching for things which do not go away. Most cancers give early signs that they are developing, although the smallest lump which can be felt already contains 1,000 million cells. These are too often missed because they are confused with the common symptoms of less serious complaints.

The warning signs: the International Union Against Cancer had identified eight warning signs of cancer. They may be caused by other less serious conditions but they may also be caused by cancer.
1. Chronic, persistent cough or hoarseness.
2. Any sore or ulcer which does not heal.
3. Unusual bleeding or discharge.
4. Any unexplained change in regular bowel or bladder habit.
5. Chronic indigestion or difficulty in swallowing.
6. A lump in the breast, neck, armpit or anywhere else in the body.
7. A change in a mole or wart.
8. Any unexplained loss of weight.

If you have any of these signs, do not panic. The explanation may be quite simple, but consult your doctor for advice without delay. Specific warning signs for different cancers and the chances of successful treatment are given below.

CANCER OF THE SKIN
Warning signs: Any change in the skin which grows larger; a sore which does not heal; moles or birthmarks which begin to grow, to bleed, to change color, or become painful.

There is no need to be alarmed if you have a small skin cancer, as most of them are easily dealt with and cause no trouble. Skin tumors occur most frequently on exposed areas of the body, particularly in fair-skinned people who are exposed to sunshine. These people should therefore take care to wear a hat or to keep in the shade where possible.

Rodent ulcer is the commonest type of skin tumor. It starts as a small raised lump which flattens out and grows at the edges while the center ulcerates. It is easily cured but should not be neglected. A similar type which has more irregular edges (*squamous cell carcinoma*) is more serious because it can spread to the lymph glands if ignored. But it can be dealt with easily if medical attention is sought promptly.

The most dangerous type of skin tumor is black in color

and called *melanoma*. If it is caught early and a lot of apparently normal tissue around it removed with it, then the prospects of cure are nevertheless good. There are many other completely harmless skin blemishes, particularly in old people, but if in doubt always consult your doctor.

CANCER OF THE BREAST
Warning signs: Any unusual lump or thickening in the breast, or any alteration in the shape of the breast; swelling in the armpit; retraction of the nipple; a bloodstained discharge from the nipple may have a variety of causes, but consult your doctor.

Many women delay seeking advice for breast lumps because they fear that treatment will make no difference. In fact early treatment of breast cancer can effect a complete cure, and a breast lump should always be treated as an emergency. However, the majority of lumps are not even malignant.

All women should examine their own breasts once a month (see below). Women who are particularly at risk should also try to get their breasts examined professionally in a screening clinic (see Appendix 2 for details). Those most at risk are women who have a relative who has had the disease; women with no children or with only one child; women who had their first child after thirty-five; those who have had benign breast lumps; women whose breasts have a knotty fibrous texture; and women with a late menopause whose periods continue after fifty-one years of age. New methods of treating breast cancer are being developed, and even late breast cancer can be given treatment which will extend life for years.

Self-examination of breasts
Every woman over twenty should examine her breasts at least once a month, and more frequently if possible, so that she will notice any change as soon as it is detectable. Some lumps can be detected in this way which do not show up on an X-ray. Lumps may be best detected by a woman who examines her own breasts regularly, because she will notice any change. The consistency of the breasts change during the menstrual cycle: some fluid-filled cysts get larger before a period and then go down or disappear altogether a week later. There is no need to worry about these. If a *persistent* lump appears, consult your doctor without delay; if you are unsure, wait for one cycle and go to the doctor if it does not go away. A few days after menstruation when the breasts are smallest is a good time to look for lumps.

How to examine yourself
Undress to the waist and stand or sit in front of a mirror. Look at your breasts first with your hands at your side, and then look again with your hands raised above your head, turning from side to side. Then put your hands on your hips and look again. Good lighting is important. Look for any differences between the breasts. Size is not important: breasts are frequently not exactly the same size. Look for a flattening or bulging in the surface or a puckering in the skin. Gently explore any part which looks different by feeling with the fingers. Any discharge from the nipple when it is gently squeezed, or any sore or scaly part, should lead you to consult your doctor. Lastly, lift each breast up in turn and examine the under-part in the mirror.

Now lie down on a bed – or you can do the next bit in the

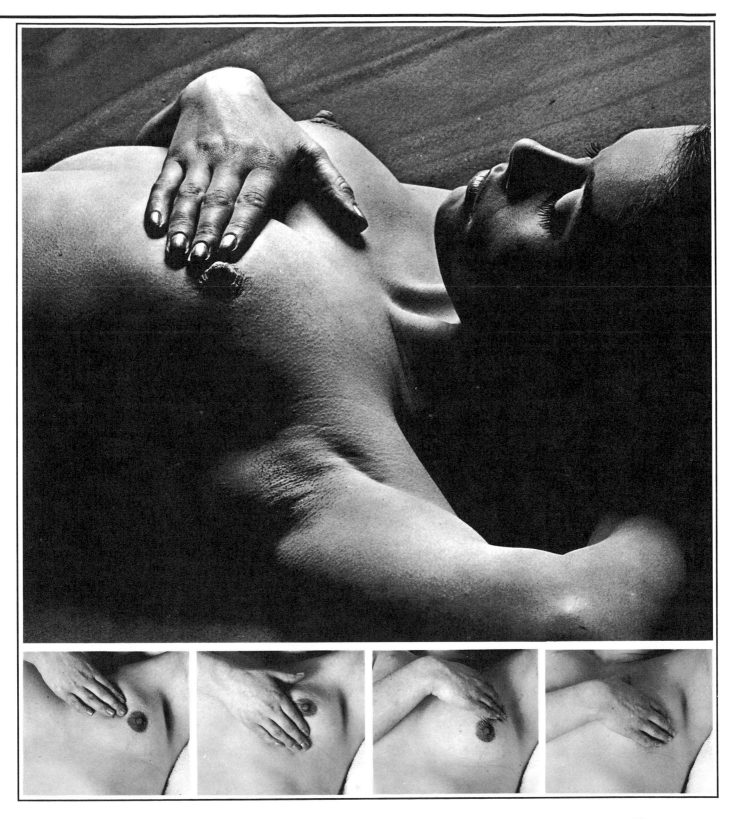

bath – and lift up one arm, putting your hand behind your head and keeping the elbow flat. Examine the breast on that side, gently feeling each quarter of the breast in turn. Repeat with the arm at the side. Then repeat the whole procedure for the other side, using the opposite hand. Tumors are most commonly found between the nipples and the armpit, so give that area special attention. Any slight thickening or lump which is different from normal and does not go away, however tiny, should be reported to your doctor for an expert opinion. If you do find a lump, your doctor will probably refer you to a specialist who may take an X-ray or ask you to have an operation for removal of the lump for tests. *Remember: the majority of lumps are not cancer.* If the lump *is* cancer it is probably best to have the breast removed, although it is sometimes possible to remove only the lump. Self-examination of breasts is most important, and most lumps are discovered by women themselves.

The removal of a breast is often profoundly disturbing for a woman, and support from the husband and family at this time is most important for a woman's mental well-being. A variety of attractive breast replacements are available which will return a woman's figure to an entirely natural line. Some can even be worn when swimming.

CANCER OF THE LUNG

Warning signs: Lasting cough; blood in spit; pain in chest; loss of weight. Rare in non-smokers.

There is as yet no good way of detecting lung cancer at an early stage and chances of recovery, except for a very few, are poor. Prevention is the only answer. It has been calculated that life expectancy may increase by a year for every three cigarettes fewer a person smokes per day. After a person gives up, their health slowly improves and the chances of getting lung cancer and other diseases caused by smoking slowly decline.

CANCER OF THE MOUTH, THROAT, NECK AND LARYNX

Warning signs: Any lump or swelling in the mouth or neck, a mouth ulcer or hard lump which refuses to go away; lasting hoarseness of the voice; persistent discharge of blood from the nose.

All these tumors can be treated successfully if caught early but if ignored may spread to the glands in the neck and become more difficult to treat. Pipe smoking, cigarette smoking, or even badly fitting dentures, may all cause irritation of the mouth, leading to cancer. Cancer of the larynx (voicebox) is commonest in people who both smoke and drink heavily. The larynx may have to be removed but it is possible to learn to speak again by a special method involving the swallowing of air, or with the help of an electronic gadget. Swellings in the neck are most commonly caused by infections. However, sometimes a swelling persists in the thyroid gland and it may occasionally be caused by a tumor. Surgical treatment is usually very effective.

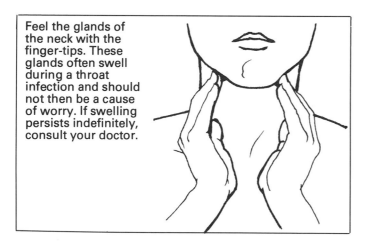

Feel the glands of the neck with the finger-tips. These glands often swell during a throat infection and should not then be a cause of worry. If swelling persists indefinitely, consult your doctor.

CANCER OF THE ESOPHAGUS AND STOMACH

Warning signs: Persistent indigestion; difficulty in swallowing, particularly of dry foods; loss of weight and anemia; poor appetite; vomiting and pain in the stomach; bleeding in the stomach may cause the stools to become black and tarry-looking.

These cancers are treated by surgery which can be successful if the warning signs lead to early treatment. People can live very well and eat almost normally even after large parts of their stomach have been removed. The cause of stomach cancer is not known but something in food or drink is suspected. Improvements in food preservation are thought to be responsible for a 50 per cent reduction in stomach cancer in the US over twenty-five years.

CANCER OF THE COLON AND RECTUM

Warning signs: Constipation or diarrhea or both, or other unexplained change in bowel habit; blood or pus in the stool; pain in the bowel; anemia; loss of weight and general ill-health.

Early diagnosis of cancers of the bowel and rectum is important because the chances of dealing with it effectively by surgery are good. Any bleeding from the rectum should be investigated by a rectal examination, even though in the vast majority of cases – at least 99 out of 100 – it is caused by piles. A good doctor will do this but unfortunately many still do not. If the cause of bleeding cannot be established by the family doctor, a specialist examination should be requested. The cause of cancers of the bowel is probably a diet too rich in fat and low in fibre.

CANCER OF THE WOMB OR CERVIX

Warning signs: Unexpected bleeding from the vagina; irregular bleeding between periods; prolonged bleeding during or after period; bleeding after intercourse.

Cancer may occur in the womb itself or in the neck of the womb (the cervix), the part where the womb is attached to the vagina. Women who have had children, and women who have had more than the average number of sex partners, are most at risk from cancer of the cervix.

Cancer of the cervix can now be diagnosed by the Pap smear test. Women are now automatically tested as part of their pre-natal examination, or during gynecological examinations or sometimes by their family doctors. When cervical cancer is found in its early stages it can be prevented from spreading by a simple operation. Cancer of the womb is also dealt with simply by surgery. Women most at risk of getting cervical cancer seem to be the most reluctant to come forward for screening.

The cause of cervical cancer is not known for certain, but all evidence suggests that it is connected with intercourse and with personal hygiene; the cause may be a virus or other infection spread by intercourse. Regular washing in the normal way may help prevent it, but measures such as douching are not recommended because they may cause other problems.

CANCER OF THE BLADDER OR KIDNEY

Warning signs: Blood in the urine but no pain; a small amount of blood in the urine may make it a pink or smoky color.

The chances of curing bladder cancer are good if it is caught in the early stages, because many bladder tumors are not malignant. Careful investigation is required to establish the type of tumor and to rule out other conditions such as bladder stones; the inside of the bladder can now be visually examined through a small tube. One cause of bladder tumors is chemicals which were once used in the rubber and dye industries. Smoking increases the vulnerability to bladder tumors. Blood in the urine accompanied by pain in the abdomen could be a sign of a kidney tumor. These are rare but with modern treatment the chances of cure are extremely good, especially in children.

PROSTATE ENLARGEMENT

Warning signs: Difficulty or discomfort in urination and increased frequency of urination; getting up in the night to pass only a small quantity of water.

The prostrate gland, found only in men, secretes part of

the seminal fluid. It is situated at the base of the bladder around the tube which brings the urine to the outside. It often becomes enlarged in old age and occasionally a tumor develops, but these are slow-growing and can usually be treated relatively easily, and much can be done to relieve the discomfort.

LEUKEMIA

Warning signs: Anemia, tendency to bleed, severe tiredness, fever and sore throat are the most common initial signs; these may be accompanied by ulcers in the mouth, pains in joints and muscles, and swollen glands.

There are several different types of leukemia but all are the result of an increase in the number of white cells in the blood. Some develop very quickly over a short period but others may develop slowly over the years. Treatment of leukemia has improved enormously in the last ten years, and there is now good prospect of a cure of certain types. The cause of leukemia is not known but it is thought that some type of virus infection or radiation may be responsible.

CANCER OF THE BONE OR SOFT TISSUES

Warning sign: Lasting swelling or pain in the bone.

Tumors in the bone are usually the result of the spread of cancer from another part, such as the breast. However, cancer does sometimes start in the bone, particularly in children. Cancers of the soft tissue are usually recognized as a painless lump which can generally be removed without difficulty.

CANCER OF THE BRAIN

Warning signs: Severe headaches over a long period, sometimes causing vomiting and disturbance of vision and personality; interference with speech or movement, or double vision.

Some tumors of the brain are benign but cause trouble as a result of pressure on the brain. Once they are removed, much of the trouble may disappear. Others can be more troublesome and the results achieved by surgery or irradiation depend on the type. The new X-ray brain scanners have made it much easier to locate difficult brain tumors.

HODGKIN'S DISEASE

Warning signs: Lasting enlargement of the glands, particularly in the neck, armpits or groin, which does not disappear as in a passing illness; tiredness, itching of the skin, loss of weight and fever may also be signs.

This disease used to be rapidly fatal but now the large majority of people are cured. Radiotherapy and drugs are the usual treatment. The cause is not known.

HOW TO AVOID CANCER

Scientists are still laboring to produce cures for cancers. It is difficult to identify all the possible causes because of the long delay that sometimes exists between cause and effect. Exposure to some noxious substance such as asbestos dust may cause cancer many years afterwards. This delay may be anything from five to fifty years. However, scientists estimate that 80 per cent of cancers are caused by something in our everyday pattern of life – the air we breathe, the food or water we drink, or chemicals or infections to which we are exposed – and these cancers are all in principle preventable.

Studies lasting many years have been necessary to establish the dangers of certain substances used in industry. And laborious studies of the changes in lifestyle and health of migrants from one country to another have established that diet can be an important cause of cancer. Nevertheless, the causes of many cancers remain completely unexplained. These are the latest clues to the causes as presently understood, and suggestions as to how you can endeavor to avoid some cancers.

Risks at home

Reduce the amount of fat you eat in your diet. The fatty diet of affluent countries appears to be linked with bowel and breast cancer. Bowel cancer is uncommon in Japan but common in the USA. When Japanese migrate to the USA they begin to suffer from bowel and breast cancer; one prime suspect is the change from a diet of rice and fish to a more fatty, meaty diet. To reduce fat in your diet, take the same measures as are taken to prevent heart disease (see page 128). Try not to eat more than one meat meal a day. Cut out butter and cream. Reduce cakes, pastries, ice-cream and chocolate. Limit cheese and eggs. Do not be afraid of eating the staple starchy foods such as bread, potatoes, spaghetti and rice.

Eat plenty of fresh fruit and vegetables. People who eat plenty of fresh vegetables seem to be less likely to get cancer. Lettuce, celery, cabbage, Brussels sprouts, turnips, cauliflower and broccoli are all good for stimulating the production of enzymes (biological catalysts) in the liver which help to destroy poisons and cancer-causing chemicals in food. Oranges and lemons are not only effective in stimulating these enzymes but also contain vitamin C, which may protect against chemical reactions in the stomach that produce cancer-causing chemicals.

Eat wholewheat bread and wholegrain breakfast cereal. Lack of cereal fibre (bran) in our diet is blamed as a contributory cause of bowel and rectum cancer. Although this theory is not proved, it is likely to benefit your health in other ways if you eat wholewheat bread. Eat wholegrain cereals or add All-Bran or natural bran to other cereals.

Avoid eating moldy food. Moldy food does not usually cause any immediate stomach upset, as would food spoiled by bacteria. However, one of the most potent cancer-causing chemicals known – aflatoxin – is found in moldy peanuts. Aflatoxin causes cancer in animals and is suspected of causing cancer in man although this has not yet been strictly proven. Many molds produce potent biologically active substances and so it seems wise either to throw away moldy food or to cut off the mold with a generous amount of the food. Improved preservation of foods by the food industry and increased use of refrigerators may be responsible for the decline in stomach cancer in the Western world. There is no evidence that cheeses ripened by introduction of molds – such as the blue cheeses – are bad for health and so there is no good reason to forgo them except that they are high in fat.

Beware of food additives, spices and seasonings. Only in recent years have food additives begun to be systematically screened for their cancer potential. Some 3,000 food additives are used in food in Western countries, many of them flavors which have never been tested for any cancer links. Tests are still in progress on the much smaller number of food *colors.* In other words, it is only sensible to restrict the amount of synthetic and processed food eaten at home.

Restrict the amount of ham, bacon, corned beef and frank-furters eaten: the nitrite preservatives which give these meats their pink color may cause the formation of nit-rosamines in the body. Nitrosamines cause cancer in animals but have not yet been shown to cause cancer in man. Be mean in your use of spices and seasonings such as black pepper and turmeric (the main ingredient of curry powder). They are powerful chemicals which can wreck living cells and have never been tested for their cancer-causing propensities.

Drink only in moderation, especially if you smoke. The risk of cancer from alcoholic drinks is greatest among heavy drinkers who also smoke. The risk that they will get cancer of some kind is up to fifteen times higher than for those who neither smoke nor drink. They are more vulnerable to cancer of the mouth, throat, esophagus, larynx and liver.

Do not smoke. One in fifteen men in the United States dies of lung cancer, and the proportion of women is increasing rapidly.

Risks at work (see also Hazards at Work, Chapter 7)

A relatively small proportion of all cancers, less than 3 per cent, are suspected of being caused by exposure to substances in the workplace, according to Dr John Higginson, director of the International Agency for Research in Cancer at Lyons, France. These are the cancers caused by substances such as asbestos, vinyl chloride and naphthylamine, which is used in the rubber industry. NIOSH, the National Institute for Occupational Safety and Health, is less precise and estimates that occupational hazards cause between 4 and 25 per cent of cancers. Even the lowest estimate, however, means nearly 20,000 new US cases a year.

The cancer-causing potential of some chemicals has only been noticed because they induce a cancer which is otherwise extremely rare. Vinyl chloride increases the risk of dying of a very rare type of liver cancer (*angiosarcoma*) some 400-fold but the average worker in a vinyl chloride factory is still ten times more likely to die of lung cancer and five times more likely to die of bowel cancer. There may be many other chemicals which cause cancer rarely that go unnoticed. Cancer of the scrotum was first observed in 1775 as a disease of chimney sweeps by the English doctor Percivall Pott. Today the same disease still causes the deaths of some sixty men a year. Mineral oils used in industry and the motor trade cause irritation of the skin and warts on the scrotum which may eventually turn into cancer. This cancer can be completely avoided by using clean overalls, not putting oily rags into the pocket, and regular bathing after work.

About 200 substances are suspected to cause cancer in man. Another 100 are known to cause cancer in animals and many more are under suspicion. The number of substances which have actually been *proved* to cause cancer in man is quite small (see table). Even everyday substances such as wood dust can cause cancer if people are exposed to it regularly over a period of years.

Each industry and each process in industry has to have its own special equipment and routines to prevent the escape of chemicals in hazardous quantities. Workers in America are protected by the Occupational Safety and Health Act of 1970, which obliges employers to take all reasonable precautions to ensure safe and healthy working conditions. Employers must inform workers of official safety standards and employees must take safety measures required. A major cause of skin cancer is ultra violet light from the sun. Most skin cancers are slow growing and present no threat to life provided they are caught early. However, others such as melanoma can be more difficult and worth taking simple measures to avoid. Farmers and other outdoor workers are more vulnerable to these cancers because of their continual exposure. A hat provides valuable protection.

Avoid unnecessary X-rays. Survivors of the atomic bombs exploded over Hiroshima and Nagasaki have to face increased chances of getting leukemia, breast cancer and cancers of bowel and brain. Each X-ray causes a tiny amount of damage to body cells and carries a minute risk of starting a cancer. Generally you can only rely on the doctor's judgement of whether an X-ray is necessary. Bear in mind that this may be a factor in the doctor's decision not to X-ray you.

Five-point safety program

1. Ask your employer for copies of official safety rules that relate to your own workplace – and follow them.
2. Treat chemicals, dusts, minerals, oils and smokes with suspicion. Avoid inhaling dusts and fumes. Always wear protective clothing and breathing apparatus when advised.
3. Do not eat food in the place of work. Remove dirty outer clothing and wash thoroughly before handling food, so as to avoid eating chemicals and dusts.
4. Protective clothing and overalls are best laundered by the employer and not taken home if dangerous materials and dusts are handled.
5. If you work outdoors all day, wear a hat.

Industrial substances known to cause cancer in man

Substance	Hazard	Cancer
p-biphenylamine	rubber industry	bladder
arsenic	vineyards, miners, copper smelters	lung and windpipe
asbestos	insulation, brake lining workers and handymen; also in air and water	lung
C.I. basic yellow 2	manufacturing industry	bladder
benzene	shoemaking	leukemia
benzidine	dye and rubber manufacture	bladder
sym-dichloro-methyl ether	industrial intermediate	lung
cadmium oxide	industry, food, cigarettes	prostate
chromate	production of chromate pigments	lung
hematite	mining	lung
napthylamine	rubber manufacture	bladder
nickel	refining	lung, nose
tars, oil, soot and smoke	industry metal working	skin, scrotum
vinyl chloride monomer	production of PVC	liver

Many other substances are suspected of causing cancer in man, and many more do cause cancer in animals.

Alcoholism

Alcoholism has long been portrayed by red-faced comedians as something of a joke. Or it has been associated with the stubbly-bearded casualties of society seen swigging cheap wine in TV documentaries about the slums. But the vast majority of alcoholics are also businessmen incapable of useful work in the afternoon, housewives not really up to preparing an evening meal, and people kept from work by a wide range of illnesses that have the common factor of striking the sufferer down on a Monday. Alcohol, unlike smoking, is not necessarily bad for you. A little can often be beneficial. But when a little becomes a lot, drinking can cease to be a pleasure and becomes an addiction. As many as 10 million people in the United States have been estimated to have a serious drinking problem. Some 40 million people in the United States are affected by a problem drinker in the family. The majority of problem drinkers are men, but almost 2 million in the US are women and the proportion is increasing.

Use of alcohol is also associated with an annual toll of 25,000 traffic fatalities, 15,000 homicides and suicides and almost half of all police arrests. The economic cost of alcohol abuse is conservatively estimated by the Institute of Medicine of the National Academy of Sciences to be \$25 billion per year in lost work, health and welfare services, accidents and medical expenses.

Nevertheless, the majority of people who experience problems with drinking are able to control or overcome them without any help. In one household survey seven out of ten American men aged 21 to 59 admitted having at one time experienced a problem with drinking, and half had such problems currently.

WHAT IS ALCOHOL?

If natural fruit juices are kept warm for a few days and exposed to the air, the sugars in them will usually ferment to form alcohol. Starches – grains, potatoes – can also, with no great difficulty, be persuaded to ferment. Alcohol, to the chemist, is a rather general name: the alcohol we drink is strictly speaking called ethyl alcohol. Beers contain between 2½ and 4 per cent of this alcohol by volume: strong beers and ciders may have as much as 8 per cent. Wines generally range between 8 and 12 per cent, and fortified wine (e.g., sherries and aperitifs) contain added spirits which bring the alcohol content up to 20 per cent. To make spirits, the fermented liquors must be distilled. Most distilled liquors – whiskies, brandies, gins, vodkas – have about 40 per cent of alcohol in them, but their strength is usually described in terms of proof spirit. This, in historic testing, was an alcohol that when mixed with gunpowder produced a mass that could still be ignited: it contains about 50 per cent alcohol by volume.

WHAT IS ALCOHOLISM?

Alcoholic drinks provide a source of energy for the body and may also contain nutrients and vitamins. Those who drink them moderately, in company, becoming drunk only rarely, are social drinkers. Some social drinkers become heavy drinkers, and may develop, without necessarily recognizing it, into excessive drinkers. These are people whose drinking leads to social, economic or medical problems, or a mixture of all three. An excessive drinker does not automatically become an alcoholic, and many people do not continue down this path. Once they recognize that alcohol is the source of their problems, they can cut down, or stop drinking. An alcoholic is someone who cannot stop drinking without help, and who drinks without control, although many seldom show visible signs of drunkenness. The World Health Organization defines alcoholics as, "Those excessive drinkers whose dependence on alcohol has attained such a degree that it shows a noticeable mental disturbance or an interference with their bodily or mental health, their personal relations and their smooth social and economic functioning or who show the prodromal (early) signs of such development."

The effects of alcoholism are not confined to the individual drinkers. It breaks up marriages, alienates children and loses people their jobs. Physically the effects can be disastrous. It is thought that around 70 per cent of chronic alcoholics suffer from fatty infiltration of the liver, about 10 per cent from cirrhosis of the liver – the death rate from this went up by a third between 1963 and 1973.

Many alcoholics have peptic ulcers, but whether this directly results from alcoholic abuse is not absolutely certain. Regular drinking causes chronic inflammation of the stomach which in turn causes most alcoholics to lose interest in food. As a result of eating a small amount of poor food, alcoholics are often short of vitamins. They may nevertheless maintain a normal weight or increase in weight because alcohol substitutes for carbohydrates in the diet.

Excessive alcohol may also weaken the heart muscle, causing the heart to enlarge and reducing the efficiency of the pumping action. Eating a balanced diet may protect a heavy drinker from some of these effects, but not all. Another effect is the nerve damage described as polyneuritis – a tingling in the hands and feet, and cramps in the legs, are among the symptoms – which can affect a fifth of all alcoholics.

Some of the mental complications, such as the shakes and delirium tremens (hallucinations), are withdrawal symptoms, and alcoholics who have reached this stage need treatment and special care. Others – severe memory loss, for example – may be permanent. Nobody who has ever drunk more than modestly needs to be told that heavy drinking reduces dexterity. Alcohol is very rapidly absorbed and begins to act on the brain in about ten minutes. Co-ordination of hand and eye begins to fail, as does the ability to judge distance – precisely the brain functions required to drive an automobile safely. But although these kinds of co-ordination fail – and sometimes brain damage can be permanent – verbal skill usually remains unaffected. So do not regard your ability to talk coherently as proof of your ability to drive safely. Drinking is also an important cause of accidents (and violence) at work and home.

However, these physical and mental effects are complications of the disease of alcoholism itself, and generally arise only years after the sufferer's personal, social and professional life has been destroyed. Alcoholism itself is the basic disease that must be treated.

The peculiar nature of alcoholism is that it starts as a pleasure. But like any drug that makes you "feel good"

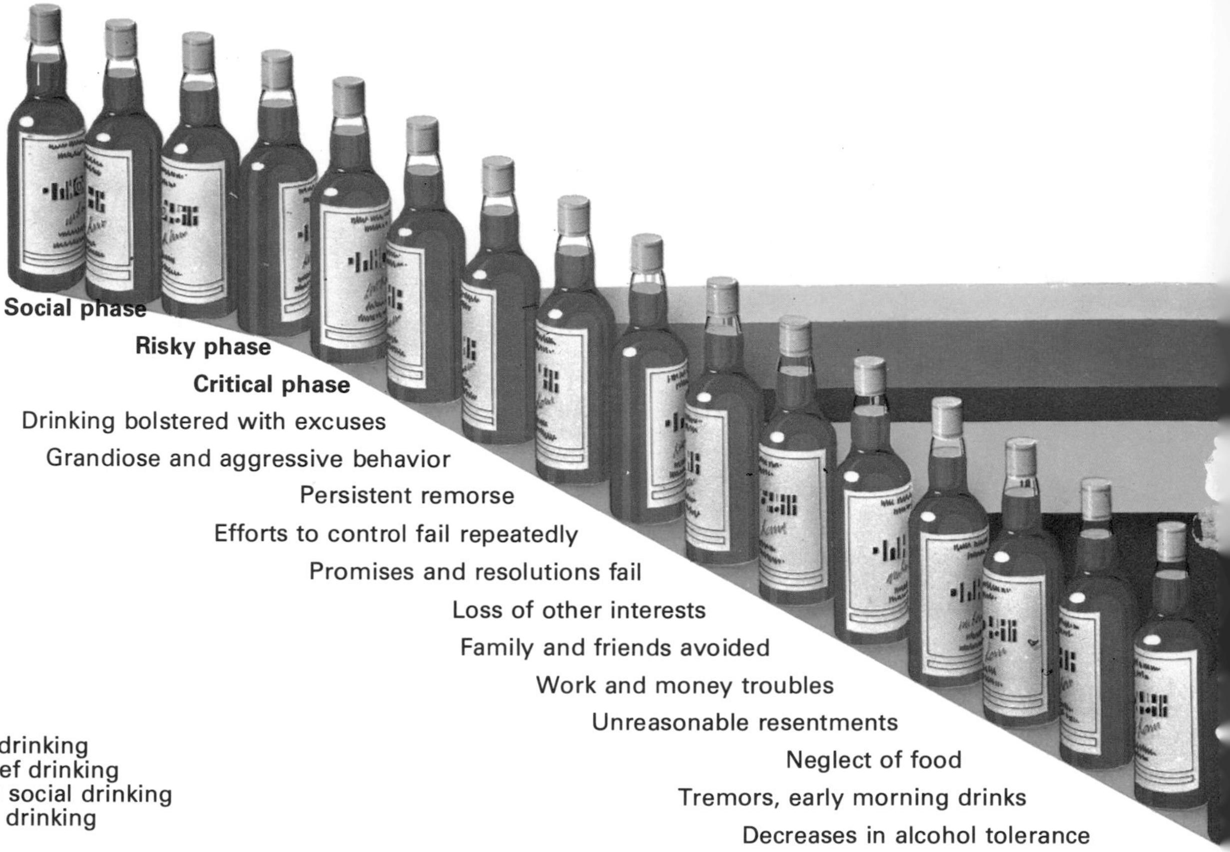

Social phase

Risky phase

Critical phase

Drinking bolstered with excuses

Grandiose and aggressive behavior

Persistent remorse

Efforts to control fail repeatedly

Promises and resolutions fail

Loss of other interests

Family and friends avoided

Work and money troubles

Unreasonable resentments

Neglect of food

Tremors, early morning drinks

Decreases in alcohol tolerance

Physical deterioration

Onset of lengthy intoxication

Alcoholic pha

Social phase
Normal social drinking
Occasional relief drinking
Heavy habitual social drinking
Constant relief drinking

Risky phase
Increase in alcohol tolerance
Onset of memory blackouts
Surreptitious drinking
Increasing dependence on alcohol
Repeated "under influence"
driving
Urgency of first drinks
Feelings of guilt about
drinking
Unable to discuss problem
Memory blackouts increase
Decrease of ability to stop
drinking when others do

alcohol can be addictive. Our diagram shows how this can lead to trouble. Occasional drinking, because it relaxes tensions, frequently becomes relief drinking. Because the body accommodates many of the burdens we thrust upon it, heavy drinkers grow tolerant of heavy amounts of drink. They then need more alcohol to get the effect they seek. The difference between a healthy drinker and a problem drinker is the element of compulsiveness, and the diagram shows how the compulsion develops.

ARE YOU A POTENTIAL ALCOHOLIC?

Some people are more at risk than others. Among national groups, the Irish have a high incidence of alcoholism, the Jews a very low one. Some professions are more renowned for being at risk than others: actors, officers in the Armed Forces, traveling salesmen, barmen, waiters, company

directors and journalists, for example. It is unlikely that these have some genetic characteristic in common, because drinking habits are characteristic of cultures rather than races. All evidence suggests alcoholism is avoidable.

The first problem in treating alcoholism is recognition. Potential victims are not easily recognized, least of all by themselves, while alcoholics are often as compulsive in their insistence on not being ill as they are in their drinking. The diagram should tell you your position – or that of a friend – in the alcoholism spiral.

The heavy drinker is in the interim phase when social drinking slips towards addiction. Judge if it applies to yourself or your nearest-and-dearest by answering honestly:
1. Do you slip away from work for a morning drink or drink at work before lunchtime?

The alcoholic abyss

The stages by which some heavy drinkers sink into alcoholism, and the possible escape routes.

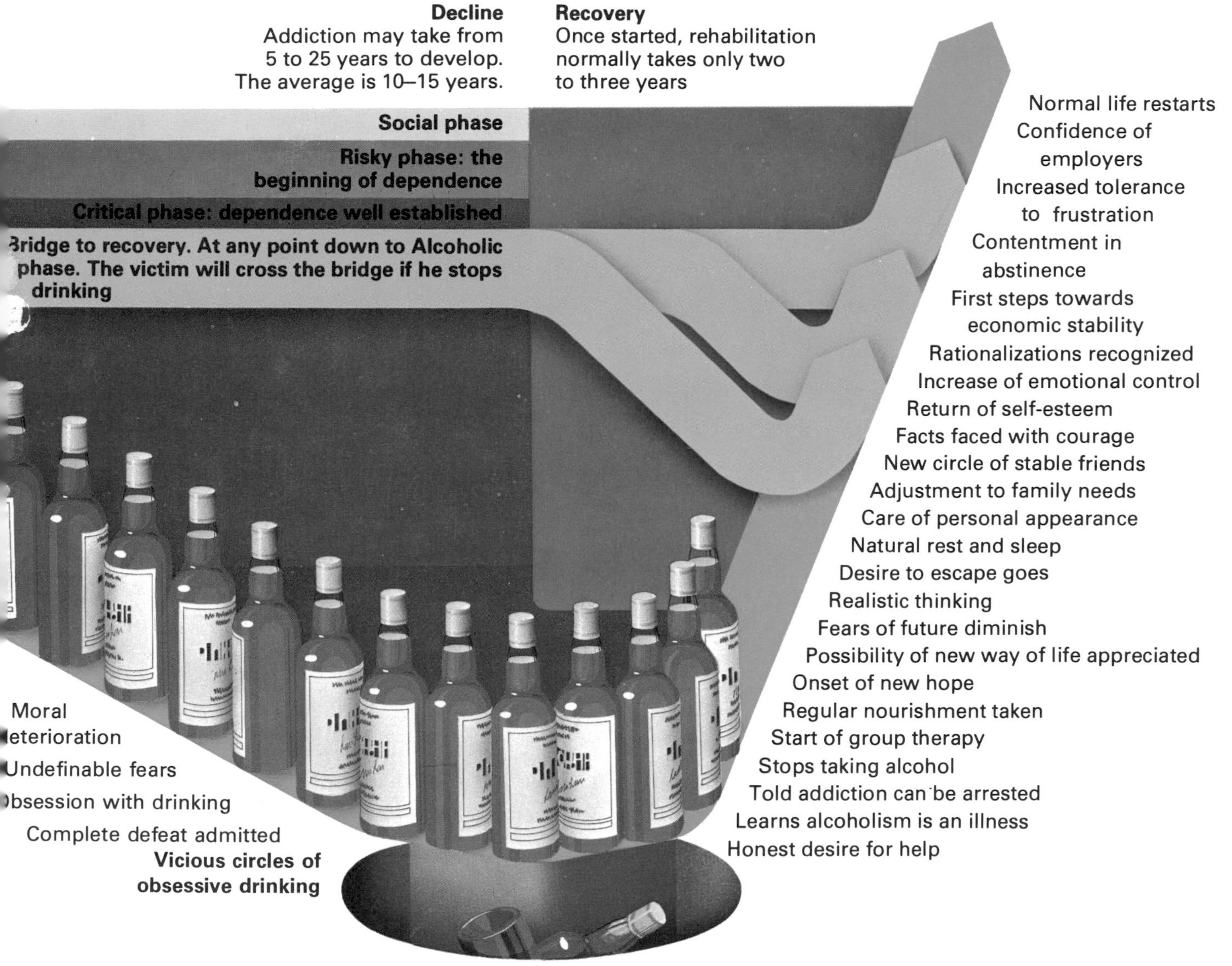

Decline
Addiction may take from
5 to 25 years to develop.
The average is 10–15 years.

Recovery
Once started, rehabilitation
normally takes only two
to three years

Social phase

**Risky phase: the
beginning of dependence**

Critical phase: dependence well established

Bridge to recovery. At any point down to Alcoholic
phase. The victim will cross the bridge if he stops
drinking

Normal life restarts
Confidence of
employers
Increased tolerance
to frustration
Contentment in
abstinence
First steps towards
economic stability
Rationalizations recognized
Increase of emotional control
Return of self-esteem
Facts faced with courage
New circle of stable friends
Adjustment to family needs
Care of personal appearance
Natural rest and sleep
Desire to escape goes
Realistic thinking
Fears of future diminish
Possibility of new way of life appreciated
Onset of new hope
Regular nourishment taken
Start of group therapy
Stops taking alcohol
Told addiction can be arrested
Learns alcoholism is an illness
Honest desire for help

Moral
deterioration
Undefinable fears
Obsession with drinking
Complete defeat admitted
**Vicious circles of
obsessive drinking**

2. Are you fairly frequently the worse for drink in mid-week?
3. Do you drink alone?
4. Do you have memory lapses about the time spent drinking?
5. Do you usually have at least a couple of drinks to help you face difficult problems?
6. Does your personality change for the worse after drinking?

If your answer is "yes" to more than one, beware. You are probably drinking too much and you now need that amount to be satisfied. But your body cannot adapt in the sense of resisting alcohol's attack on its vital organs. You must stop drinking for a longish period – say, six months – so that your body can unadapt, and you must never start drinking heavily again.

The alcoholic is someone with an illness that they are most unlikely to recover from alone. Yet no one can ever recover from alcoholism against their will, so it often falls to others to convince alcoholics they need help. Again, here are a series of questions to ask yourself and others to gauge the extent of alcoholism:
1. Do you need a drink first thing in the morning?
2. Do your hands tremble until you have a couple of stiff drinks?
3. Do your friends frequently joke about your drinking?
4. Have you started to drink in less pleasant bars than you once used to?
5. Do you get moody as you continue drinking?
6. Have you noticed over the last couple of years that you have become less ambitious?
7. Do people complain about the quality of your work?

Many affirmative answers indicate addiction. You *must* seek help: alcoholism is an illness. You may be lucky and find a patient and understanding doctor, or you may prefer to contact one of the organizations listed in Appendix 2. A person does not necessarily have to drink heavily to suffer serious ill-effects from alcohol. Some people only take one or two drinks, but that is enough to cause a serious change in personality which has ill-effects for their families. These people also need expert help.

Treatments. It may take an average of ten to fifteen years of drinking to become an alcoholic, but people who start to drink heavily in their teens may become alcoholics much more quickly. Once a person has admitted the need for treatment, the chances of recovery are good. People who have been heavy drinkers will always be at risk; there is no such thing as a cure. Treatment may differ in detail, and organizations may vary in their approach, but all those who treat alcoholism agree that a recovered alcoholic must never drink again. It is possible that there may be a few who can become controlled drinkers again, but this is a controversial point. No alcoholic should believe that he or she is one of them.

In almost every case, recovery begins with an immediate and complete end to drinking. This, and the subsequent treatment of malnutrition and other physical damage, needs expert supervision. The most immediate needs are usually vitamin supplements and tranquilizers to help through the initial difficulties of withdrawal. The long-term treatment must help the patient to live without seeking refuge in drink or, of course, in tranquilizers.

For more information about treatment and a list of organizations which can help, see Appendix 2.

DRINKING AND THE FAMILY

It is worth remembering that as alcoholism may start as a psychological attitude to drinking, so it is possible for children to learn this attitude from their parents: children of alcoholics have a higher risk than average of themselves developing the disease. Children naturally imitate the example set by their parents. If drinking is forbidden in the home and yet the children know that their parents go to drink in bars and clubs, then the children are likely to imitate this pattern as soon as they are able. The safest style of drinking is found among Italians and Jews, who introduce their children to alcohol in the home as part of normal family life. Children may then be taught by parents to enjoy alcoholic drinks in moderation. Teenage children may then cautiously learn the effects of alcohol in the safety of the home, and come to understand that alcoholic drinks must be treated with respect.

Recent findings also make it clear that even unborn children can suffer permanent damage from alcohol. They themselves consume none, of course, but it is the drinking mother who puts her baby at severe risk. Alcohol abuse is an important cause of damage to unborn babies. According to one estimate, one in three alcoholic mothers must expect her child to be born handicapped. (It is worth stressing that this applies to *alcoholic* mothers, not simply mothers who drink alcohol.)

Researchers in the United States, headed by Dr James Hanson of the University of Washington, put the figure still higher, at somewhere between 30 and 50 per cent. The blood of some babies is so rich in mother's alcohol that the child would fail a breathalyser test with his or her first breaths. And if they are born with the shakes, damage can prove to be permanent.

HOW TO DRINK HEALTHILY

To some extent society needs to change. Hostesses should perhaps offer more non-alcoholic drinks at parties, for instance. Missing out on a round in a bar or ordering a small glass or a non-alcoholic drink should not be regarded as a reflection on a man's virility. Alcohol itself should be deglamorized. But in the meantime:

1. Avoid drinking alone.
2. Do try to eat at the same time as you drink. Avoid eating salty snacks such as pretzels and nuts, which have no bulk and increase thirst. Eat bread, cheese, creamy spreads and dips, meatballs, blintzes.
3. Always provide such food for guests when offering drink. Serve food first, then drink.
4. Always measure the alcohol in a drink. Use the conventional size and shape of glass. Serve cocktails and spirits in small-diameter glasses. Only fill wineglasses half full.
5. Always dilute alcohol, preferably with water. Alternatively ask for a separate glass of water, so that you are not always sipping the alcoholic drink without thinking.
6. Avoid bars with loud music, which increases anxiety level (see Hangovers below), where you are likely to drink more before you begin to feel relaxed.
7. When hosting, limit drinking to one hour before serving the meal.
8. Try to limit wine to two half-filled glasses, and only serve brandy or other after-dinner drinks when the meal has lasted more than an hour and a half.
9. Serve your guests so that the pace of drinking is unhurried.
10. If a guest is drinking too much actively offer food and only top up the drink with half portions.
11. Do not thrust drinks on people. Make it easy for them to refuse by saying: "Would you like something to drink?" rather than "Come on, have a drink."
12. If you find it difficult to refuse a drink when you don't want one, or have had enough, ask for a drink which looks as if it is alcoholic. For example, a Virgin Mary, tonic water and lime, straight bitter lemon, or Piña colada without rum.

A safe level of drinking is not more than one-and-a-half ounces of alcohol a day; that is, about half a bottle of wine, or two pints of strong beer, or three-and-a-half measures of well-diluted spirits. This quantity was first recommended by a Scotsman, Dr Francis Anstie, in 1864 and is still known as "Anstie's limit". An official US Government report, *Alcohol and Health*, has since endorsed Anstie's advice.

ALCOHOL AND HANGOVERS

You get drunk when sufficient alcohol from the drink is transferred to the blood and carried to the brain, where the alcohol interferes with normal brain activity. First to go are the critical faculties, which is why everyone, including you, seems wittier as you drink. This is also why the drinker is the last person who should decide if he should drive; he isn't up to decision making. The rules that govern how quickly you get drunk are complex. If you want to relax, and lose your inhibitions quickly, the first essential is to join a group of people who have the same aim, because behavior is affected by atmosphere and suggestion. If you can arrange things so that your early party guests are lively extroverts, only a little alcohol will be needed, cutting back on your drinks bill and reducing the number of hangovers.

The effect of alcohol largely depends on the alcohol concentration in the blood stream. The basic rule is that the stronger the drink, the more quickly the blood stream takes up its load. Thus a glass of wine obviously gets you more drunk than the same sized glass of beer. However, drink stronger than about 18 per cent alcohol has less immediate effects than weaker drinks. It stays locked in the stomach and cannot pass into the duodenum and small intestine, where 80 per cent of alcohol absorption takes place, until it is diluted. The dangerously unexpected result of this quirk of physiology is that you can pour down a lot of brandy, say, at the end of a party, and feel much of the effects next day after your morning coffee.

Food in the stomach also helps to retain alcohol there, so that it is released slowly and more safely. You can reduce the risk of getting drunk by eating while, or shortly before, you drink. Nuts and snacks do not usually provide enough bulk; a good sandwich is more likely to help. Those who drink with meals are therefore less likely to get dangerously drunk than those who drink without eating anything.

Sobering up (removing alcohol from the blood stream) is done almost entirely by the liver. Only a small amount of alcohol is excreted in urine although, as a matter of all-too-frequent observation, some is also exhaled. The liver works steadily at its task, removing a single whisky or a large glass of wine an hour. The process is essential because even teetotallers have alcohol to the equivalent of a couple of pints of beer a day in their blood, as the result of fermentation in the gut. The liver's inexorable cleansing can be slightly speeded by taking fruit sugar (fructose), but not sufficiently for this to be a useful way of sobering up.

One of the main causes of a hangover is tiredness. Alcohol anesthetizes a part of our brains and prevents us from appreciating signals from our muscles and nerves which tell us we are exhausted. So we continue in a stressful way, and when the effect of the alcohol finally wears off we are left extremely tired. The nausea, stomach inflammation, headache and anxiety are extreme responses to stress which can be tolerated while the alcohol anesthetizes the body but are only felt with greater intensity when the alcohol wears off. A person who is tense and uptight and drinks at the same time is more disposed to have a hangover. Intense anxiety can cause a hangover the next day even if someone has not had anything to drink – combined with drink it is likely to be so much worse. If you find that anxiety combined with excessive drinking is your problem, try to learn a method of relaxation (see page 92) as well as changing your drinking habits. And those who eat rather fatty meals hinder the liver in its task.

Hangovers, although caused by the alcoholic content of the drink, can be made worse by other substances that are present. Of all spirits Bourbon whisky contains the largest quantity of these substances called *congeners*, and appears to give the worst hangover – according to a festive experiment undertaken by sixty students at the University of California. Half drank vodka and the other half Bourbon. The morning after having six doubles the night before, two-thirds of the Bourbon drinkers had hangovers compared with just over one-third of the vodka drinkers. Even more conclusively, one-third of the Bourbon drinkers had a severe hangover with nausea, malaise, headache and depression compared with one out of thirty of the vodka drinkers.

Congeners are the by-products of fermentation or distillation or both. Some congeners give different drinks their characteristic taste; the ones that produce hangovers are mainly amyl alcohol, methyl alcohol and acetaldehyde; a measure of only these congeners would give a direct "hangover index". Other congeners are contained in red wines (tannin) and beers (a rich variety of nutritious substances). This explains the apparent anomalies in our hangover chart.

Hangover chart

Drink	% Alcohol	Congeners ppm	Hangover index
Brandy and Bourbon	40	252	6.2
Red wine	8–12	400	5.9
Rum (red)	40	60	5.0
Sherry	20	350	4.9
Whisky (scotch)	40	4	3.0
Beers	3–6	380	3.0
White wine	8–12	350	2.2
Gin	40	3	1.9
Vodka	40	0–1	1.0

To avoid the worst after effects, therefore, stick to vodka, gin and white wines. Whatever you drink, keep track of what and how much you are drinking. There is a popular notion that hangovers are caused by mixing drinks. If this does often result in disaster, it may be because mixing happens most often when drinking is heavy anyway. A feeling of thirst may be part of a hangover, because alcohol is a diuretic: it encourages the removal of water from the body and the production of urine. The thirst can be simply cured by drinking water. Rest is the best cure for a hangover. A bad headache may be treated with acetaminophen, but not aspirin (acetyl salicylic acid) or tablets containing aspirin, which cause stomach irritation, particularly if the stomach is already irritated by alcohol. Occasionally the combination of alcohol and aspirin causes a dangerous bleeding of the stomach.

The "hair of the dog" remedy is not recommended Another drink is extremely risky; it is easy to spend two or three days in a rather drunken haze, during which time the drinker is a potential danger to others; on the roads, for example. Remember it is generally not safe to drive if you have had more than two or three small drinks. There is *no* way you can drink and drive safely.

An habitually heavy drinker has a hangover problem of his own. He may wake, suddenly, in the small hours, frightened by he knows not what. If this happens frequently it is a powerful danger sign: the wakening and the fright are withdrawal symptoms. The liver has reduced the blood stream's burden to an uncomfortable but still high level. Anyone who experiences this often should take warning: almost certainly, it is a sign of alcoholism and time for expert help.

STAYING HEALTHY AT WORK AND PLAY

Allergies

Do you feel ill when you smell paint, become breathless in front of a birdcage at the zoo, or develop severe stomach pains and wind on eating onions? The answer is that you are suffering from an allergy. Allergies can make people extremely ill with asthma, eczema or bowel troubles. In rare cases, allergies can be life-threatening. But they are also a form of illness which the patient can often avoid, once the allergy has been identified.

Allergies take so many unusual forms, however, that the causes often go unrecognized by those who suffer. Or if a person does recognize the substances which make them ill, they will frequently get little sympathy from friends who too often consider the story an unlikely one, like the girl who was allergic to beer and came out in spots if only a few drops were spilt on her feet. But if the cause of the allergy can be identified and the person can learn to avoid it, then the illness may miraculously end. Sometimes it is easy, sometimes very difficult, to identify the problem.

Allergies occur because in some people the body's defense against infection is over-sensitive. When foreign substances such as bacteria, dust or some foods enter the body they react by producing antibodies which attack the bacteria to prevent infection. Some unfortunate people make antibodies against normal, harmless substances in their environment like grass pollen. It is not surprising that when a mechanism evolved to protect us against a few bacteria reacts with the enormous quantities of pollen which we inhale, the body's response can be devastating.

When an allergic substance combines with antibodies in a person's body, excessive quantities of histamine and other irritating substances are released in the body, causing certain tissues to swell: especially vulnerable are the skin, the delicate lining of the nose, the windpipe and the intestines. This produces a spasmodic contraction of the tubes of the windpipe and bronchi, causing asthma in some people. But everyone produces their own type of antibody, which is located in different parts of the body so that the same substance from, say, cats might cause one person to develop asthma and another to develop a skin rash. Most people who are allergic to grass pollen suffer from hay fever in their eyes and nose, but in a few people only the chest reacts, causing asthma without any symptoms elsewhere.

The main types of allergy are discussed below.

Hay Fever only occurs when plant pollen and mold spores are present in the air in large numbers. There are about 15 million sufferers in the United States: most are sensitive to grass pollen. However, a wide variety of pollens may cause hay fever in some people.

Victims of hay fever suffer a running nose and sneezing, itching eyes and an itching throat. This dulls mental processes so that at times it becomes extremely difficult to concentrate. There is no easy escape from pollen. It is carried everywhere on the wind into the heart of cities and inside air-conditioned buildings. A modern building may provide the best respite because less pollen penetrates it.

People with mild hay fever may find that a drug prescribed by the doctor is sufficient to prevent the worst symptoms and they may then be able to play golf or watch a ball game. However, the severe sufferers must so far as possible stay indoors during the pollen season. They should keep doors and windows closed as much as possible. If extra air is needed in the room, then a frame covered with two or three layers of cheesecloth can be constructed to fit into a window. If the cloth is kept damp it acts as an excellent filter, but it must not be allowed to go moldy. Take care to avoid irritants such as dust, insect sprays, aerosols, tobacco smoke, air pollution, fresh paint and tar.

Perhaps the best cure is to go for a month's holiday at the start of the pollen season to an area where the pollen is out of season, either north where it has not started or south where it has finished. It is an advantage to go to the coast, where sea breezes are relatively free of pollen, or to the mountains where the air may again be clearer. For those who can afford it, a sea cruise is ideal (see Appendix 2).

If these measures do not work, the hay fever sufferer should try desensitizing injections of the pollen which is the cause of the allergy. The injections, which must be taken during the winter, cause the body to produce another antibody. This new antibody blocks the reaction of pollen with existing antibodies which are attracted to certain parts of the body, for example the nose or lungs, and cause the irritating symptoms of hay fever. It used to be necessary to have twenty injections, but now a modern injection is available which releases the pollen slowly in the body and has the same effect after nine injections. A newer "depot" formulation requires only three injections but it has not yet been proven to be equally effective.

Constantly runny nose and sneezing attacks (allergic rhinitis) may be caused by all sorts of things from cats to scrubbing *new* potatoes. Mice, monkeys, face powders,

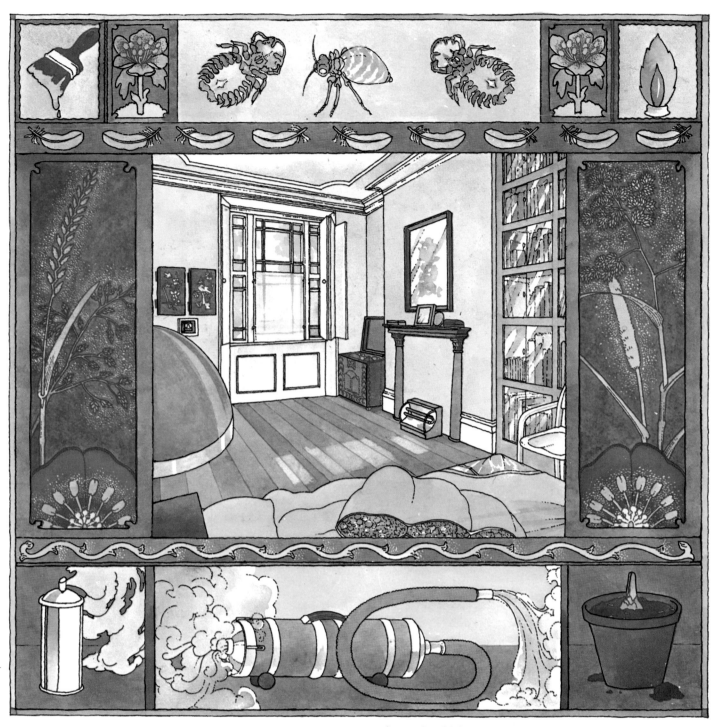

HOW TO MAKE AN ALLERGY-FREE HOME

If you want to try to make your house less likely to induce allergy, these are some of the things you might do, beginning with the bedroom.

First take out all unnecessary furniture to make the room as easy as possible to keep clean and dust-free. Remove all carpets and have a tiled, linoleum, or polished-wood floor. If you need a bedside rug, choose the washable type. Furniture should be plain wood, plastic or metal. If upholstered it should be plastic, cotton or nylon and the stuffing should be synthetic.

Walls should be plain wood or paint so that they can easily be wiped clean every two or three months. Windows should always be kept closed and should be covered by easily washable curtains. If windows need to be opened in the summer, then a filter frame consisting of several layers of cheesecloth can be made for placing in the window; moisten it for best results. All beds in the room must be fitted with a rubber mattress or the ordinary mattress covered with plastic sheeting, scotch-taped together to make it impenetrable to dust and mites. However, polyurethane and rubber can have an irritating smell for some asthma sufferers. The mattress can be covered with several cotton sheets to prevent the discomfort of sleeping on plastic. Box springs should also be entirely enclosed in plastic as this is a favorite place for house mites to live. However, another school of thought recommends *not* enclosing the mattress in plastic, which may make it damp and encourage the growth of

mites and mold, but alternatively vacuuming the mattress regularly to remove mites. Pillows should be made from synthetic material and washed every few weeks. Bed coverings should be made from cotton or synthetic material. Wool, hair, kapok or feathers should be avoided. Bookshelves should ideally be closed with a sliding-glass door. Toys should be kept in a box. Clothes and shoes should be stored outside the room.

The room should be cleaned from top to bottom every three months, as well as dusted, and the floor cleaned regularly. Dusting should be done with a wet or oiled duster, and floor cleaning should be done by a wet or polish method. If you use a vacuum cleaner, make sure that it is the type that is fitted with a special renewable filter and dust-collection bag. If possible the allergic person should not be present while the dusting is done, or for forty minutes afterwards while the dust settles. A nylon floor-duster is useful because it attracts dust electrostatically which must then be washed off.

Aerosols and strong-smelling substances should not be used when cleaning since these often cause irritation to the lungs of allergic people. Do not have any house plants in the room as these will contain fungi which shed spores. Even fresh flowers are best avoided, because they shed pollen.

Some people who suffer from allergies find that air-purifiers which remove dust-particles produce a dramatic improvement in their condition, while others find it makes them worse. Make sure you try before you buy. Air-conditioning does not always help hay-fever sufferers much, because they can be so loaded up with pollen while outside the house that it can take more than a week for it to be eliminated from the body.

feathers, certain fabrics and upholstery, fungal spores in damp houses, detergents and aerosols can all cause the condition. But the commonest cause is house dust. This consists of small pieces of dirt, fibres from material, hairs and minute scales of skin which have worn off the surface of the body. The skin scales are one rare cause of allergies but there is another cause which escaped detection until recently when it was discovered that house dust contained thousands of minute mites, about a third of a millimeter long, which are invisible to the naked eye. These mites live by eating the scales of human skin and are found everywhere that people are found. Bedding and upholstery are particularly full of them. They are quite harmless for people who are not allergic to them.

A great deal can be done to free a house from dust and mites (see page 143). Desensitizing injections to house dust are available but there is some controversy over how effective they are.

Intrinsic allergy. There is another type of allergic rhinitis which is not caused by inhaled particles. Some doctors call this "intrinsic" allergy. It usually affects people over thirty-five years old and is characterized by nasal obstruction and running of the nose, but not by sneezing. The patient loses his sense of smell and may develop polyps, which are small lumps of jelly-like material that hang in the nose. Food allergy is sometimes found to be the cause (see below). A few patients have nasal polyps and sneezing attacks as well. They are likely to sneeze because of allergy to inhaled particles, but if this is dealt with, the polyps will not disappear. Nasal polyps are usually treated by surgical removal – a minor operation – but it may have to be repeated every few years. Alternatively, a nasal spray containing a steroid drug may be found effective, but this must be used only under the supervision of a doctor.

Asthma, which simply means difficult breathing, can be a most serious complaint. There are nearly 9 million sufferers in the United States. It is most common in children. Although an allergy is often the main cause of asthma, infection and psychological stress are also important. However, it can be extremely difficult to sort out which factor is most important in an individual case.

The difficulty in breathing experienced during an asthmatic attack is the result of swelling of the membranes and constriction of the muscles in the breathing tubes, the bronchi, which leads to the lungs. The victim is then forced to wheeze, in attempts to get air into the lungs. The swollen membranes then produce a sticky liquid which further increases the difficulty in breathing.

Any of the dusts, odors or animals capable of causing hay fever or allergic rhinitis can also cause asthma. A great deal can be done to relieve the condition in some people by looking for the factor which triggers the attack and eliminating it from the house, or by general measures to make the house allergy proof (see page 143). Drugs such as aspirin can trigger asthma.

However, asthma does not always have an identifiable airborne cause. It is then called "intrinsic". The cause of most intrinsic asthma is unknown, but sometimes it may be caused by an allergy to food.

The psychological factor in asthma seems to be secondary; a child, for example, may find that it can manipulate its parents by having an attack. Stress makes any allergic

condition worse, but the most important factor is often simply fear of the asthma itself. But asthma should always be taken seriously because when it gets severe it can kill. Any attack which does not respond to the drugs which a person usually takes, requires medical attention. With modern drugs it is always possible to relieve asthma provided treatment is started early enough.

Asthmatics are also prone to bronchitis and should avoid people suffering from influenza or colds. These infections tend to aggravate the condition and set up a vicious cycle of repeating infections and asthmatic attacks. Asthmatics should avoid smoky rooms, as irritation from tobacco smoke usually makes asthma worse. Alcohol can also upset many people with asthma, and social drinking is likely to cause trouble from both smoke and alcohol.

The asthmatic may find it easier to breathe in bed if propped up on a lot of pillows. Most asthmatics are worse at night or in the early morning, even if the thing which caused the allergy was encountered many hours earlier. (For example, about one-third of hay-fever sufferers are at their worst when they wake up, although they encountered grass pollen the previous afternoon.) These night-time attacks often mislead people into concentrating on possible causes of allergy in the bedroom, when in fact the rest of their environment is equally important.

Asthma attacks often follow a definite pattern like this, and can be forestalled by taking an appropriate drug before the expected attack. A variety of different drugs and inhalers are available for asthmatics, and finding the right treatment is a matter for professional advice.

People who suffer from asthma will have to choose carefully the types of sports they pursue. Asthma is usually made worse by exercise, but movements which cause vibration in the chest like running, jumping, or boxing will provoke wheezing far more readily than "smooth" exercises such as swimming, cycling or even rowing. Many distinguished athletes have suffered from asthma, so someone who suffers from it should not necessarily curb their ambition to succeed in sport. Exercise, short of that which provokes wheezing, can do an asthmatic nothing but good.

Breathing exercises for asthma can help to teach an asthmatic to expel the air from his lungs and so be in a better position to take the next breath. These exercises should be done if an attack of asthma threatens, as well as first thing in the morning and last thing at night, in order to clear the chest.

Blow the nose to clear the upper passages as far as possible. If producing a lot of spit on coughing, do the following exercise to drain the lungs. Lie flat on the bed, with head and shoulders supported on a chair or stool at a lower level. Cough repeatedly to clear the passages. Then lie first on one side and then on the other, coughing again to clear each lung in turn. (Coughing can make asthma worse in some people, in which case this exercise should obviously be avoided.) When the breathing passages are clear, practice diaphragm breathing as follows: breathe in slowly without raising the chest, using the belly muscles and diaphragm; breathe out slowly, taking as long as possible and emptying the lungs as fully as possible. Children may be helped by being given candles to blow out or ping-pong balls to blow across a table.

Any asthmatic can bring on an attack voluntarily by increasing their rate of breathing, and the onset of many attacks is a consequence of an unconscious rise in the rate of breathing caused by emotion – often simple fear that an attack is developing. An exercise which controls the rate of breathing by humming while the breath is slowly exhaled may be practised and then used to nip an attack in the bud. A physiotherapist can give guidance on suitable exercises and can train a patient to perform them correctly.

Urticaria (hives) is an extremely itchy raised rash, very similar in type to the rash produced by nettle stings except that in some cases it may cover large parts of the body. Heat, cold or pressure of any kind makes the irritation worse. Certain foods, coloring matter or preservatives, and drugs, especially aspirin, laxatives, sleeping tablets and antibiotics are often responsible. Urticaria is also sometimes a reaction to vaginal candidosis (yeast infection).

To discover the cause, make a list of all the foods, drinks or medicines taken in the twenty-four hours preceding an attack. Foods commonly causing this allergy are: eggs, fish (especially shellfish), pork, strawberries and some other fruits, nuts and pips. After two or three attacks it should be possible to pinpoint the suspect substance or at least narrow it down to a short list, but identifying delayed food allergies of this kind is often not so simple (see below).

To complicate matters, many sufferers from urticaria will not develop their rash after they have been exposed to the thing to which they are allergic, unless a second factor is brought into play. This may be exercise, psychological stress, a hot bath, or pressure on the skin. One patient, for example, only developed his rash if he played tennis within twelve hours of swallowing aspirin.

It is not always possible to identify a definite cause. Psychological stress has been suggested as a cause in some cases. When no cause can be found, anti-histamine drugs can help to make an attack bearable, while rough or tight clothing, and overheating, should always be avoided.

Eczema is not always caused by an allergy, and expert help is needed in diagnosis. Eczema can be particularly distressing in childhood and it is often difficult to find any cause. If the baby is breast-fed, something in the mother's diet may be a cause and with careful observation it may be possible to eliminate it. Fish, eggs, citrus fruits or chocolate are possible causes and should be eliminated from the mother's diet for two weeks at a time to see if it makes any difference (see also under food allergies for further ideas).

If the baby is bottle-fed, it is possible that the eczema is caused by an allergy to cows' milk. Several artificial milks are available which either have allergic materials removed from the cows' milk or which are made from plant substances; ask your doctor or pharmacist for details. In severe cases of eczema children may have to wear gloves and face-masks to prevent them from scratching and making the condition worse. Bedclothes should be light to prevent overheating. Cotton should be worn next to the skin, and diapers should be washed in mild detergents or soap powders. Non-perfumed soap should be used sparingly, or an emulsifying ointment can be prescribed by the doctor for use in the bath. The child's skin should not be exposed to direct sunlight for any length of time. The child should not be vaccinated against smallpox because it may cause aggravation of the eczema.

Eczema in adults must be dealt with similarly. The cause may again be food or contact with some material (see below). Medical treatment with ointments and creams can often prevent the problem or at least control it. But care must be taken with the use of some creams, particularly those containing fluorinated corticosteroids, which may permanently thin the skin if used on the face.

Contact dermatitis is caused by some object or substance touching the skin and causing local allergy which may then spread. Detergents, for example, may start to cause an irritation on the hands which later spreads to other parts of the skin. Other common causes are metals, especially nickel and chrome, dyes and chemicals. The first clue to the cause usually comes from the part of the body affected. If, for example, it is the scalp, then the cause may be a shampoo or anti-dandruff lotion, hair dyes or rinses, curlers, combs, wigs or even a hatband. If it is the feet, then rubber or leather shoes may be responsible, or dyed socks. Once the cause has been found, a change of detergent or cosmetics may be all that is needed. Several firms now make cosmetics which are less likely to produce allergy.

Food allergy is much commoner than is realized because people simply learn to avoid foods which they know upset them. However, many people with chronic allergic diseases are suffering from unrecognized food allergy. It can cause urticaria, eczema, intrinsic asthma or rhinitis, diarrhoea, constipation, pains in the belly, swelling of a part of the face or tongue (so-called "angio-neurotic edema") and migraine. There is now a body of opinion which even attributes some forms of mental illness to food allergy, though this is still highly controversial.

A diet diary which records everything eaten and drunk sometimes helps to spot the offending food, but this simple system usually fails for two reasons: first, the allergic response to a food is frequently so delayed and prolonged that it is difficult to spot a relationship. Secondly, most people with delayed food allergy are sensitive to several different commonly eaten foods, and reactions overlap.

Most experts in the field agree that an "exclusion diet" restricted to foods which are less common causes of allergy offers the best chance of improvement. In extreme cases an artificial diet called "Vivonex" (made by Eaton Labs, Norwich, NY) may be used. This was developed for use on space flights, and is very unlikely to provoke allergy. The disadvantage is that it is so expensive that its widespread use is totally impracticable. Of course, after a person has lost their symptoms on an exclusion diet, all the foods which have been left out must be eaten one by one to see which causes symptoms.

Foods likely to cause allergy can be divided into groups. For instance, a person who is allergic to a nut such as hazel-nut is likely to be allergic to all the nuts, pits, peas and beans in their diet, even chocolate and coffee. However, the factory preparation of foods often in some degree destroys the allergy-causing part of the food, so that this person could probably drink powdered instant coffee (not the freeze-dried granules), and could also eat margarine made from nut-oil after it had been altered to make solid fat. Again, heat often destroys the allergy-producing chemicals in food, so that someone allergic to milk and yeast is likely to be able to eat bread (which may contain both).

Foods most likely to cause allergy, and those which are suggested as the basis of a simple but practical exclusion diet, are shown below. Remember, this diet is not intended to be nutritionally balanced, and once it has been tried for a month it should be abandoned if there is no improvement. If it is obvious that the allergy has disappeared when the exclusion diet alone is being eaten, then the other food groups should be started again, one by one, at weekly intervals. Any food which causes no ill effect can then be included in the diet while the next one is being tested.

Foods to avoid, one group at a time
1 Egg, chicken, sponge cake, mayonnaise
2 Milk, ice cream (but most milk-allergic patients can eat butter)
3 Nuts, pits and all fruit, peas and beans, cauliflower, chocolate, fresh coffee, tomatoes, candies, preserves, and drinks made from fruit or nuts (wines and cola), margarine, mustard, curry and all spices
4 Fish
5 Cheese (separate cause of allergy from milk)
6 Yeast in flavorings and drinks (most important are gravy browning and yeast extract spreads)
7 Onion
8 Mushroom
9 Pork and all liver
10 Wheat (bread, cookies, cakes, beer, and many other foods)
11 Processed foods containing artificial color (see tartrazine under drug allergies below) or flavor

Foods to eat on basic exclusion diet
1 Beef or lamb
2 Green vegetables (not cauliflower, which is a "pit" allergen). Potatoes.
3 Tea, sugar, but no milk or lemon
4 Gluten-free bread (buy it at the health food store)
5 Butter. Syrup for flavor but no jello
6 Rhubarb
7 Cook with lard or corn oil

Foods likely to cause attacks of migraine (see headaches, page 148) fall into two groups. First, the foods causing allergy – identify them as described. Second, there is a list of foods which contain a substance called tyramine which may provoke an attack of migraine without an allergic mechanism. These foods include: cheese, wine (especially red), chocolate, broad beans, yeast extract, bananas and canned fish.

Drug allergies are also quite common. There are two sorts. First, the true allergies: many drugs may cause a rash, some such as sleeping tablets may cause a sensitivity to sunlight. Sometimes drug allergy can cause other reactions such as asthma. Allergy to drugs, particularly penicillin, can be dangerous. If you change your doctor or go to hospital, do not forget to tell the doctor about your allergy. It is a good idea in such cases to wear a Medic-Alert bracelet or necklet (see Appendix 2) which warns of your allergy in case you should be taken to hospital unconscious.

The second sort of drug allergy can be equally serious: aspirin, for example, can make other allergies catastrophically worse. There need be no initial period of sensitization when the drug is being taken without causing a reaction. If a patient is aspirin sensitive, the very first dose of several chemically unrelated drugs used for rheumatism may provoke a severe attack of the patient's usual allergic disease. What is worse, tartrazine (FD & C Yellow no. 5), a yellow dye used in food manufacture, may do the same. Strangely, a number of anti-allergy tablets are colored with tartrazine – so beware. Tartrazine is the most widely used of all color additives for food in the US. It is commonly used to color orange drinks, as well as a wide variety of yellow and orange foods, and with other colors to produce various shades.

Cosmetic allergies. Deodorants, anti-perspirants, soaps, hair spray or lacquer are the commonest cause of cosmetic allergies. Hypoallergenic cosmetics may be better but can still cause problems. Read labels and avoid problem ingredients.

Occupational allergies. There are a great many allergies which are suffered by individuals as a result of exposure to particular substances at work. Bakers, for example, often become sensitive to flour or to weevils and molds which grow on the flour. These may cause eczema, a runny nose or asthma. Builders may become sensitive to sawdusts or cement which cause eczema or asthma. Paints and glues may cause a runny nose, asthma or eczema. Dry-cleaners and dyers often become sensitive to dyes. Cotton-mill workers often become sensitive to dust from the raw cotton which causes an allergic asthma. Farmers may become allergic to their animals, and moldy hay may give them a severe chest allergy called farmer's lung. Market gardeners may become sensitive to molds which grow readily in

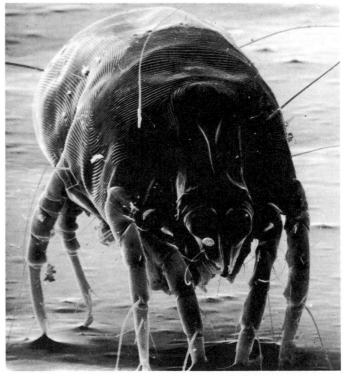

A scanning electron micrograph of the house dust-mite (*Dermatophagoides pteronyssinus*). The majority of beds contain some of these creatures.

greenhouses, causing asthma. Hairdressers and leather-workers often become sensitive to the dyes and chemicals they use in their work. Metal-workers may become sensitized to chrome, copper, nickel or oils which may all cause skin trouble. Even office workers may develop eczema, as a result of handling carbon paper or inks, or runny nose or asthma due to dust from old documents.

Colds and Flu

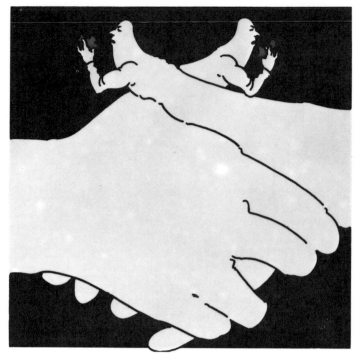

Few people escape colds. On average, an adult catches between two and five a year; teenagers catch more, and children most of all. As symptoms include coughing and sneezing, people correctly assume that colds are spread through the air to be inhaled by others. But recent research shows that in addition cold-bugs can survive for three hours on a variety of surfaces, including human skin. So they may also be transferred by touching or shaking hands.

The only efficient way to avoid spreading a cold is to isolate yourself. The best advice is to go to bed and keep away from others. Smoking may make people more vulnerable to colds and make colds – and particularly coughs – last longer.

What is certain is that there are hundreds of different viruses responsible. *Rhinoviruses* are the largest group and although scientists have identified more than 100 so far, there may be as many as 200. The other main group are the *Coronaviruses*, probably fewer in number but difficult to isolate in the laboratory. Despite the common belief that colds are caused by chilling of the body, scientists at the Common Cold Research Centre in Wiltshire, England, and elsewhere have been unable to induce colds in people by putting them in cold conditions with the minimum of clothes. However, these were healthy volunteers who may not be vulnerable to infection. Other experts who have studied sickness reports find that more people report sick after sudden snaps of cold, damp weather, probably because the virus survives better in the cold and damp.

There are very few drugs which are effective against viruses and none which are of any practical use against the cold viruses. Sometimes a cold may be made worse by a secondary infection with bacteria, in which case a doctor can usefully prescribe an antibiotic drug which will attack the bacteria. Other drugs may be prescribed to relieve the various symptoms of colds such as headache, fever, cough or blocked nasal passages. Doctors often do prescribe antibiotics for colds, partly due to pressure from patients, but this is bad practise since it may simply induce bacteria to become more resistant and put the patient in a worse position should they genuinely need antibiotics. However bothersome colds are, they rarely last more than seven to ten days, which is all the time required to produce enough antibodies to overpower the infecting virus.

Nevertheless, Dr Linus Pauling, with two Nobel prizes to his credit, suggests that vitamin C, in large doses, can prevent colds and, if caught early enough, cure them. He argues that early man lived on an entirely vegetable diet providing up to three grams of vitamin C a day, about three times the normally recommended daily intake today. Pauling suggests that we make up this deficiency, equivalent to around sixty oranges a day, but more easily consumed in the tablet form available at drugstores. However, several experiments have now shown that vitamin C does not prevent colds and may only ameliorate the symptoms. Large doses of vitamin C for short periods will do no harm, but are not advisable for a long period. The best way to take vitamin C is as fruit or vegetables, particularly oranges.

Influenza is also caused by a virus. There are two main types: *influenza A* which causes world-wide epidemics and *influenza B* which tends to cause more localized outbreaks in schools, factories or offices. *Influenza A* regularly changes its type and so evades the immunity which people develop against it. Many other viruses also cause flu-like illness. The flu virus is spread, like the cold virus, by contact and by coughs and sneezes. The virus concentrates its attack on the membranes of the nose, throat and lungs where it destroys cells. The destruction of the tissue causes a fever. The only protection against flu is vaccination. Vaccines are now available which are fairly effective. During any flu epidemic thousands of people die from the illness. The majority are old people who are in a poor state of health, people who suffer from heart and chest trouble, and especially those who suffer from chronic bronchitis, which is caused mostly by smoking. These are the people who stand to benefit most from vaccination against flu. Flu vaccination must be repeated every year. A vaccine against the common cold is not a feasible proposition because there are too many different types of cold viruses. Flu vaccination has been reported to have side effects. This risk is worth taking for people in poor health who are most vulnerable to the illness. However, the risk – although remote – may not be worth it for someone in good health.

What to do when you get a cold or flu

It is not necessary to see your doctor when you have an ordinary cold unless you have a persistent high temperature which lasts for several days, or if after three or four days you feel you are getting worse rather than better. Children who have a cold lasting more than five days should be taken to the doctor.

The best treatment for a cold is to go to bed early with a hot drink. An acetaminophen or aspirin tablet may help if you are suffering from a headache or pains. A little whisky or other spirits in the drink may help you sleep but *never* combine spirits with aspirin. If the nose or chest feel raw, sore or blocked, it may help to inhale steam from a bowl with a towel over the head. It can be more pleasant if you add drops of a menthol vapor rub to the water. Drink plenty of fluids, such as orange or apple juice.

Be careful when blowing the nose not to block off the nostrils, which may force infected mucus into the sinuses. And beware of medicines which are prescribed to shrink the blood-vessels of the nose or dry up secretions. They may have undesirable side-effects, particularly in old people. It is probably better to let the body fight the infection with as little interference as possible. Substances prescribed to curb a cough are also not generally a good idea, except perhaps to bring temporary relief. It is essential to cough so that infected mucus does not remain in the chest, where the infection will multiply.

Sore throats are often caused by virus infections which cannot be treated very effectively by drugs. However, a sore throat may also be caused by infection with bacteria called *streptococci*, in which case a doctor may prescribe antibiotics. If a sore throat is more than mild you should see your doctor. Gargling with plain water or an ordinary gargle mixture may bring some relief. Go to bed early, get plenty of rest and drink plenty of fluids. Soft foods and soups are best if there is discomfort or swelling.

Headaches

Headache is one of the commonest of all complaints, and may be caused by anything from bad lighting to conflict between people creating psychological tension. Sometimes a headache is simply an excuse for a dignified retreat from the scene, but it can also be a sign of serious illness. Whatever the cause, the pain is a biological sign compelling the person to withdraw, a warning that something is wrong. The pain of headache usually arises in the structures around the brain, not the brain itself which is insensitive to pain. The blood vessels that go to the brain, the membranes which cover it, and the muscles of the scalp are the usual source of pain. Any stretching in these structures will cause a pain which may be localized in one spot or spread to the whole head. In the worst cases it is a blinding pain which prevents the victim from doing anything.

Vascular headaches arise in the blood vessels which go to the brain and the muscles of the head. Arteries are sensitive to substances produced in the body which circulate in the blood stream. These substances, metabolites, may cause excessive dilation of the blood vessels in the brain in sensitive people; this stretches nerves in the blood vessels, causing pain. Vascular headaches generally throb in time with the heartbeat. The pain may seem to come from deep inside the head but more often comes from the front or back.

Muscular headaches are caused by pains developing in the muscles of the scalp and neck. These may be the result of having to hold the head in an awkward way while working or a result of bad lighting. But more often they are the result of spasms in the muscles caused by tension, and so are often called tension headaches. Anxiety is the basic cause. The pain which results is sometimes described as a vice-like grip on the head, or like pressure from a tight band. The intense contraction of the muscles compresses the blood vessels, so reducing the blood supply and causing metabolites to accumulate locally which dilate the blood

vessels, causing pain. Simple measures can be taken to avoid tension (see Relaxation, page 92).

"Eye strain" is sometimes the cause of headaches. You may need to have your eyes tested, or retested – see page 112.

Toxic headaches often occur when a person is ill with, for example, a cold or flu, but they can also be caused by food or alcohol. When too many toxic products are produced in the body, as in illness, and cannot be removed sufficiently quickly by the kidneys, then they may cause the blood vessels in the brain to expand, giving a vascular type of headache. Alcohol taken in quite small quantities can trigger appalling headaches in sensitive people. Migraine may also be caused by sensitivity to certain types of food such as cheese, chocolate, red wine, eggs, fish, salty foods such as cocktail snacks or salt meats, e.g., ham or corned beef, monosodium glutamate (which is the cause of "Chinese restaurant syndrome"), milk and milk products including ice cream, nuts including peanuts and coconut, and pineapple (see also Allergies, page 142).

Migraine headaches are particularly severe but only a minority of people suffer from them. The migraine attack usually consists of two phases. In the first phase the blood vessels in the brain constrict, and this may cause temporary disturbance of vision or, very occasionally, temporary weakness. Then the blood vessels dilate and severe headache follows, together with a feeling of nausea, vomiting and sometimes diarrhea. The person is quite unable to carry on normally while this is happening and must rest. Migraine headaches can be treated by a variety of drugs, so consult your doctor. By studying the pattern of your life you may also be able to identify something which triggers the migraine, such as an item of diet (see above). Other causes of migraine can include: bright or flashing lights; prolonged watching of television; dieting or going without food; fatigue; intense odors; the pill; sleeping tablets; anxiety; and even changes in the weather.

When to consult your doctor
Headache may also be a symptom of some underlying illness, such as high blood pressure and occasionally more serious conditions. If you suffer from frequent headaches or if any unusual headache persists, or recurs or rapidly becomes worse, see your doctor. Always consult a doctor about headaches which follow a blow to the head.

Treating your headache
If you have a severe headache, it may be best not to try and carry on bravely. People with headaches are hypersensitive to noise, more irritable and likely to be accident prone. If you are able to rest, that is the best thing to do. Aspirin is an extremely effective treatment for headache, although it can cause stomach irritation and should not be taken day after day without consulting your doctor. Aspirin also should not be taken with alcohol since this can irritate the stomach. Acetaminophen is an alternative to aspirin which seldom causes stomach irritation. Many proprietary preparations containing aspirin also contain caffeine, the active drug from coffee, which should be avoided if you wish to sleep your headache off but may otherwise help by causing the production of urine and the elimination of salts.

Hazards at Work

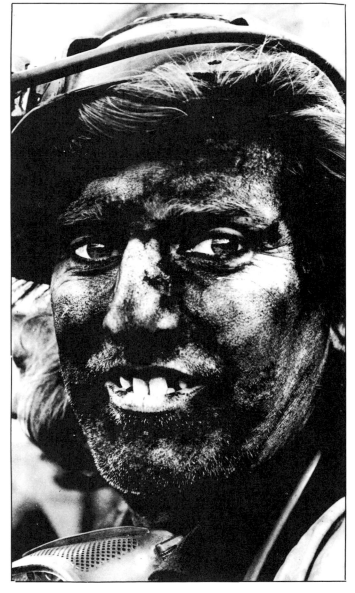

Each year in America about 5,000 people are killed in accidents at work. Another five million are injured – 40 per cent so seriously as to keep them away from work. Sometimes the deaths and injuries are dramatic and instantaneous, as in accidents; on other occasions death may be the result of long-lingering illnesses such as pneumoconiosis (black lungs) in coal miners. Some jobs are intrinsically more dangerous than others, notably coal mining, shipping and construction or demolition work. But accidents happen wherever people are working. Life down on the farm may be more peaceful than in the factories but it is not necessarily safer, as our league table of injuries shows on the following page. Even pedestrians are at risk as they walk under the scaffolding of construction sites.

Occupational hazards have become so much part of our everyday lives that the very phrase has become a cliché.

The worst conditions of the Industrial Revolution have generally been eradicated by tougher legislation and more sophisticated industrial processes. But some remaining old hazards, such as the dust that clogs the lungs of miners, quarrymen and cotton-workers have been joined by newer ones often involving chemicals which were unknown a few years ago. And there are always accidents. Yet now, at least, doctors and governments recognize the importance of occupational illnesses. It was not always the case. The only requirement for doctors under some early nineteenth-century legislation was to certify that children sent to work in factories *appeared* to be at least nine years old.

Nowadays, the USA, like most Western countries, has an elaborate hierarchy of committees and specialist bodies devoted to occupational safety. In a general book of this kind it is impossible to give detailed advice about every known hazard. The National Institute for Occupational Safety and Health (NIOSH), for instance, has identified no fewer than 4,400 potential hazards in 66 types of industries and 456 occupational groups. But before discussing the most common causes of occupational hazards it is important to stress that most illnesses and, indeed, most accidents can be prevented, although it usually costs money. So no matter what kind of work you do, whether it be indoor or outdoor, in a factory or in an office, be militant about your own health and safety:

1. Discover the potential hazards in your work.
2. Make sure all safety measures are enforced – and, of course, that you follow them yourself. More injuries are caused by a moment's forgetfulness – the safety hat left at home, the routine safety-check that is skipped – than occasional publicized disasters.
3. If you believe there is a health or safety risk, inform your safety representative, union official or management superior. Make sure that they then report it to the appropriate authorities.
If the hazard seems so serious or imminent that it would be dangerous to continue working, then stop work: the law protects workers acting "reasonably".
4. If you have to go to your doctor, tell him what kind of work you do and what materials you handle. They may be the cause of the problem.

The safety league table overleaf shows clearly the varying dangers of different occupations. Yet within these broad official categories variations are even more dramatic. Anthracite mining, for instance, has a serious injury rate of 11,100 per 100,000 workers compared with the overall average for mining of 5,800 injuries. Within the manufacturing sector logging suffers 14,000 serious injuries per 100,000 workers, sawmills 10,300 per 100,000. Shipping is the most hazardous form of work within transportation with 11,900 serious injuries per 100,000 workers. Even within relatively safe occupations such as finance and the service industries there are comparative black spots: real estate, for instance, has an injury rate of 1,800 per 100,000 compared with banking's 500 cases of serious injury per 100,000 workers.

All these figures cover both occupational injuries and illnesses. Overall illnesses comprise only 3 per cent of the total number of work-related injuries and illnesses. Of these illnesses, skin diseases and disorders are by far the most common, accounting for nearly half the total. But it would be unwise to minimize the dangers of occupational illnesses. Many take years to develop and may never be recognized as a consequence of work. Official figures thus certainly underestimate both the number and severity of occupational illnesses. However, the National Institute for Occupational Safety and Health (NIOSH) says that every year 400,000 people get sick from exposure to hazardous substances at work. Its leaflet, *Part of the Human Condition*, says that each year: "About 100,000 die prematurely as a result of those exposures. For some, the odds are overwhelming: of the one million current and former asbestos workers in the United States, between 300,000 and 400,000 can expect to die of cancer."

If you work in one of the high risk occupations at the top of our league table of injuries, then naturally take special care. The prime hazards for these occupations are:

Mining: Bronchitis; accidents; respiratory tuberculosis; and pneumoconiosis, a crippling and often fatal disease caused by the accumulation of mineral dust in the lungs.

Agriculture: Accidents involving tractors, falls and animals, notably bulls; infections such as anthrax, tetanus and brucellosis; farmer's lung, an allergy caused by inhaling moldy dust, usually from hay; and eye injuries.

Construction: Accidents, in particular falls from scaffolding or ladders and the collapse of foundations or other building materials. The machinery and transport vehicles associated with construction (and demolition) sites also cause innumerable accidents.

Shipping: Falls or blows from ship's tackle; accidents generally; skin diseases in fishermen, caused by allergies.

Such dangers are thankfully remote from most of us. The hazards below are less dramatic but far more common.

Noise. Damage to hearing is not only caused by loud bangs; most comes with prolonged exposure to noise which is not so loud that you cannot get used to it. This is now recognized as a major industrial health hazard. Noise is measured in decibels on a scale based on powers of ten: 10 decibels (dBAs) is ten times as intense as the quietest sound you can hear, 20 dBAs is a hundred times, 30 dBAs a thousand times as intense. Each increase of 3 dBAs doubles the sound intensity.

In the USA there are a series of legal limits reflecting both noise levels and the time people can be exposed to them. This ranges from eight hours at 90 dBAs to 15 minutes *per day* at 115 dBAs. If these levels are exceeded, protective equipment such as earplugs or helmets must be provided to reduce noise levels to within the legal limits.

Machinery. Hundreds of lives are lost and thousands of workers maimed every year because of faulty machine guarding. Safety laws are specific on guarding moving parts and inspecting unguarded machinery. Guards should provide positive protection without discomfort to the worker, and prevent all access to the danger areas during work. If they don't and are in need of replacement or repair, work should be stopped.

Ordinary hand tools also cause many accidents. Keep them in good repair, use the right kinds of tools and if necessary wear safety eye-goggles.

Lifting. Most spinal injuries result from incorrect lifting techniques and from carrying weights that are too heavy. The International Labor Office approves of 80 to 110 pounds, according to age and physique. Many labor unions have agreed limits between 45 and 60 pounds, but even this is far more than most men can manage. Damage may be cumulative and not necessarily immediate. As explained on page 102, the nearer the body is to an upright position when lifting, the less work is required from muscles and the less strain imposed on spinal discs. Keep arms close to the body, chin tucked in and place feet a hip-breadth apart to give a stronger base and balance. Most important of all, keep a straight back.

Chemical Hazards and Dusts. Almost every working process uses chemicals in the form of oils, solvents, metals, gases or resins. The *Registry of Toxic Effects of Chemical Substances* published by NIOSH lists the chemical data and known biological effects for no fewer than 22,000 substances. It has been estimated that anything between 3 and

THE SAFETY LEAGUE

Latest annual statistics for occupational injuries and illnesses per 100,000 workers

Industry	Fatal	Serious*
Mining	49	5800
Agriculture, Forestry, Fishing	28	4700
Construction	25	5500
Transportation and public utilities	19	5000
Manufacturing	6	4800
Services	5	2000
Wholesale and retail trade	4	2800
Finance, insurance and real estate	1	700

* accidents involving lost workdays

INTENSITIES OF TYPICAL NOISES

Approximate sound pressure level (in dBAs)	Source and location
200	Moon rocket at lift-off, 300m away
160	Peak level at the ear, of 0.303 rifle
140	Jet aircraft taking off at 25m
100	Very noisy factory
90	Heavy diesel truck at 7m
80	Ringing alarm clock at 1m
70	Inside compact-sized auto at 30mph approx 3m from domestic vacuum cleaner
65	Busy general office with typewriters Normal conversation at 1m
40	Quiet office
25	Still day in the country away from traffic

Source: Bureau of Labor Statistics, US Department of Labor.

Source: Noise, by Rupert Taylor, pages 55–6. Reprinted by permission of Penguin Books Ltd. Copyright © Rupert Taylor, 1970.

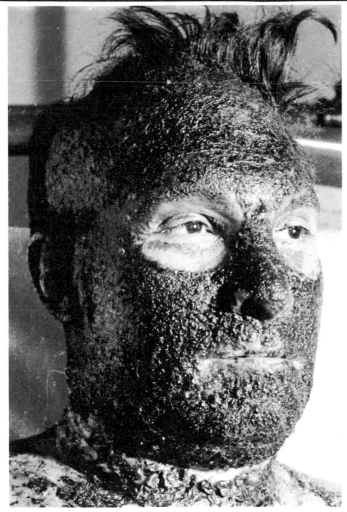

This worker's skin recovered – eventually. He would have been blinded had he not worn safety goggles.

25 per cent of the 600,000 new cancer cases which occur each year in the United States may be directly related to jobs. These particular cancer risks are discussed in more detail on page 136. But there are also non-malignant respiratory diseases. More than three million workers are exposed to asbestos, beryllium, coke oven emissions, cotton dust, silica, sulfur dioxide, sulfuric acid and toluene diisocynate.

Most diseases caused by chemicals in fact start with either their inhalation, which affects the lungs, or their ingestion through the skin and blood stream. Coal miner's pneumoconiosis is the best known, often fatal and caused by coal-dust clogging the lungs. Asbestosis is also particularly toxic and notorious but silicosis, byssinosis (from cotton, flax or hemp dust) and bagassosis (from sugar cane fibre) can all be fatal and cause chronic bronchitis and emphysema. Any kind of dust (including sawdust) is a potential hazard to health. Oil mist, caused by mineral oil vaporizing, can cause dermatitis and cancer; mercury and lead vapors are particularly dangerous. People working with fumes, gases or vapors in confined spaces *must* wear breathing apparatus.

Not all substances stop short at the lungs. Cadmium can affect both the liver and kidneys; vinyl chloride affects the bone structure – thickening the fingers, for instance – and can also affect the liver, causing cancer. Lead and benzene both affect bone marrow, and some substances affect the haemoglobin in the blood – carbon monoxide being the most lethal. Three particular substances cause the overwhelming majority of skin disorders: epoxy resins, mineral oils and solvents. They are widely used in industry. Protective clothing, thorough washing and medical attention for any skin rashes or injuries is essential. Chemicals should not be allowed to come into contact with the skin, because even if they do no immediate harm they can be absorbed through the skin into the body.

Radiation. There are several types of electromagnetic radiation, some harmless like radio waves, some lethal like gamma rays. Microwaves will "cook" any part of the body exposed to them with severe physical and possibly mental effects.

Infra red radiation can come from any red-hot material. Strong radiation produces burns, and long exposure can produce cataracts in the eye. This means the lens in the eye begins to go opaque and you start to go blind. Safety glasses with special filter lenses should therefore be worn and eyes examined regularly.

Ultraviolet radiation: the sun is the biggest source of this. Sun tanning is the skin trying to defend itself by developing brown pigmentation. Ultraviolet radiation can dry and wrinkle the skin, produce localized skin sores and – in certain rare cases where there has been years of open-air work on farms or building sites – skin cancer. The commonest occupational sources of this radiation are arc-welding and sterilizing units. Protective clothing and masks must be worn.

Radiation is one of the most insidious of all occupational hazards. Except in cases of severe over-exposure it can be neither seen or felt at the time, but its effects can include burns, cancer, leukcmia, sterility and infertility. The most commonly used are X-rays and gamma rays. Under US law the amount of such radiation to which anyone can be exposed is strictly limited, with equally stringent controls on radiation areas, protective clothing and monitoring equipment to measure radiation levels.

Accidents. Accidents are usually the result of lack of training – especially in the construction industry – and neglect. Noise, vibration, high and low temperatures, stress, fatigue and narcotic fumes can all increase accident-proneness. Usually, though, some additional hazard actually delivers the injury, such as poor lighting or oil on the floor causing someone to slip, or trip over some waste.

There are so many causes of occupational illness or injury that whole books have been written about them (see Appendix 2). Many, for instance, are forms of allergies which were covered earlier in the chapter. If you suspect that you may be suffering from an occupational disease, consult your doctor – both your family doctor and, if there is one, the works doctor, who may have more specialist knowledge. If the doctor confirms that you are suffering from such an illness, investigate your liability for compensation; labor unions are a great help here. But many diseases, such as asbestosis and scrotal cancer, are not sudden illnesses which the layman can easily detect; their incubation periods can take anything from ten to thirty years. So always be vigilant in taking all possible precautions all the time. In the US the Occupational Safety and Health Administration (OSHA) lays down safety standards and also undertakes workplace inspections. See Appendix 2 for more details of both OSHA and NIOSH.

Preventing Infections

Infections of the body are caused by many different types of organisms: viruses, bacteria, fungi and protozoa such as ameba. These infectious organisms enter the body in contaminated food or water; droplets carried in the air we breathe; direct contact on hands, lips, or in sexual intercourse; and as a result of animal or insect bites. It is common sense to avoid spreading infection by observing the usual rules of hygiene and by avoiding contact with people when they are ill. Also avoid using communal towels. Nevertheless, infectious organisms invade the body all the time and the body is equipped to defend itself against them.

The first line in the body's defense against infection is the skin itself, which is impervious to most assaults. Tears, saliva and the secretions of the stomach and the bowel all contain substances which attack stray bacteria, viruses or any foreign organisms. If an attacking organism does penetrate the body, then it will be attacked by antibodies and white blood cells which digest and kill any foreign substances they come across. These are the defenses of the body which are stimulated by vaccination in order to prepare the body in advance for a potential invasion.

Resistance to disease may be lowered by illness or the way we live. During convalescence, people are more vulnerable to disease, which is why they must rest. An inadequate diet with a shortage of essential vitamins will make a person more vulnerable to infection. So will smoking, excessive drinking, drug addiction, overwork, excessive worry, insufficient sleep and exercise. More information about most of these topics can be found elsewhere in this book.

An individual can protect him or herself from infection by high standards of hygiene (see page 57) and avoiding people who are ill, but also through vaccination (see page 170). Elsewhere in this book we advise readers on how to protect themselves against the cold, how to avoid sexually transmitted diseases and how to protect your health while on holiday abroad. But it is impossible to give detailed instructions on avoiding or preventing *all* diseases. Ask your doctor about quarantine measures which may be advisable in any individual case. In this section, however, we give the basic information about infectious conditions most common in temperate climates. Prompt recognition and careful quarantine measures can do much to prevent the spread of illness. Few drugs are effective against virus diseases, which are caused by germs which can only grow inside the living cell. Most, but not all, bacterial or fungal diseases can be treated effectively with antibiotic drugs

Brucellosis

Also called undulant fever, Malta fever and mountain fever.

Mode of infection: Caused by a bacterium, Brucella, transmitted by drinking or eating unpasteurized raw milk or dairy products, or by contact with infected cattle. Most common among farmers and butchers but rarely transmitted from one person to another.

Symptoms: Exhaustion and weakness at the least exertion, irritability, alternating chills and fever, headache and pains in joints and back. Glands may become enlarged in neck and armpit. May last for months but rarely fatal.

Treatment: Rest in bed. Vitamins and antibiotics.

Prevention: Never drink raw unpasteurized milk or eat raw cheese except from an attested Brucellosis-free (and tuberculin-tested) herd. Avoid contact with sick animals

Candidosis

Also called moniliasis, candidiasis.

Mode of infection: Caused by a yeast-like fungus called Candida albicans. Exacerbated by irritation. Diabetics are particularly vulnerable. The fungus often lives in the bowel and so infection does not necessarily come immediately from another person, but can come by contact.

Symptoms: A wet eruption of the skin with extremely unpleasant itching, which breaks out in any of the skin folds, the nails, the anus, vagina or the mouth, causing white patches inside the cheeks.

Treatment: Antibiotic drugs such as nystatin, tablets or vaginal suppositories. Also rinses and ointments.

Prevention: Scrupulous personal hygiene. Wash with soap and water only. Do not add perfume or bubble mixtures to baths which may cause irritation and provoke infection. Always wipe anus from front to back. Antibiotic treatment of bacterial infections may disturb the natural balance of bacteria in the body, leaving it vulnerable to fungus infection such as Candida. The pill also changes the metabolism and makes women vulnerable to vaginal conditions.

Chickenpox

Also called varicella.

Mode of infection: Caused by a virus, spread by contact or by breathing in droplets coughed out by infectious person. One infection usually gives lifelong immunity.

Symptoms: Symptoms appear ten to eighteen days after exposure to infection. Fever, discomfort, loss of appetite. Rash on back and chest spreading to face, scalp and arms. Rash consists of separate red spots which develop into a blister, fill with a clear liquid that becomes cloudy later, and finally forms crusts which fall off after about two weeks.

Treatment: Rest in bed while feeling ill. Personal hygiene is important to prevent secondary infection. Avoid scratching; cut fingernails and keep them clean to avoid secondary infection of spots. Use medicated shampoo for scalp.

Prevention: A person with the illness should be kept isolated until the crusts have gone, which is usually about twelve days from the start. The same virus which causes chickenpox also causes shingles (see below), so an adult with shingles can give a child chickenpox. Although the illness is generally not serious, special care should be taken to avoid exposing infants to infection.

Cystitis

Mode of infection: Bladder inflammation, often an infection caused by bacteria which may come from the kidney or, most often, travel up the urethra (the tube down which the urine passes). Most frequent in women.

Symptoms: Pain in the bladder area, tiredness, fever.

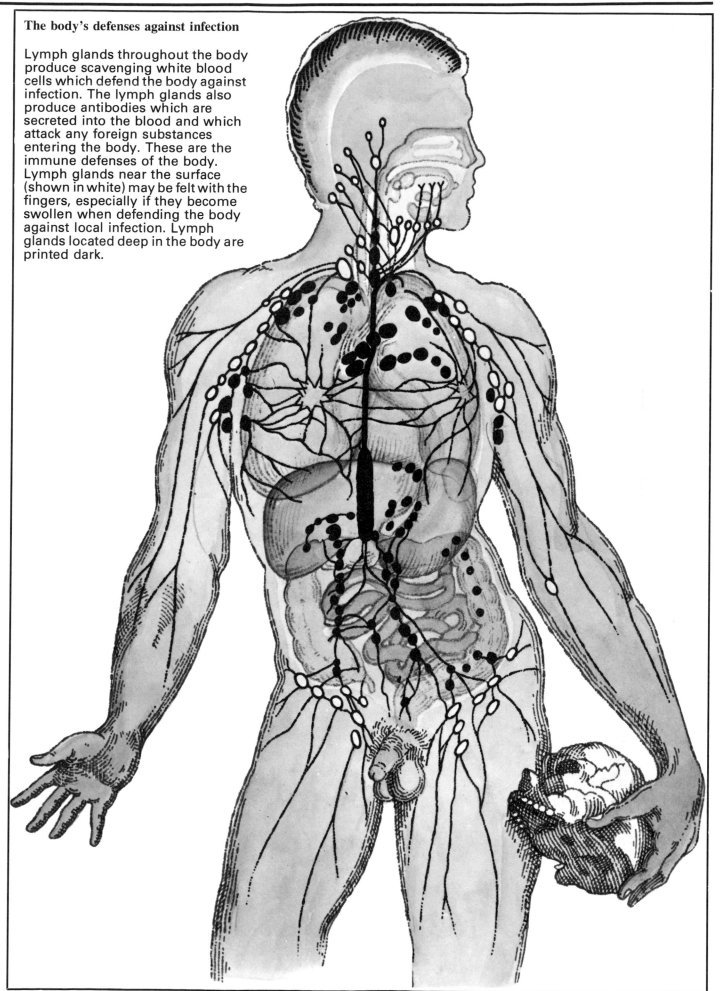

The body's defenses against infection

Lymph glands throughout the body produce scavenging white blood cells which defend the body against infection. The lymph glands also produce antibodies which are secreted into the blood and which attack any foreign substances entering the body. These are the immune defenses of the body. Lymph glands near the surface (shown in white) may be felt with the fingers, especially if they become swollen when defending the body against local infection. Lymph glands located deep in the body are printed dark.

Desire to pass urine frequently. Urination accompanied by burning sensation.

Treatment: Antibiotic drugs, rest, drinking large quantities of water – two or three times normal intake – which literally flushes the bacteria from the bladder.

Prevention: Keep the genitals clean. Wipe anus from front to back. Avoid alcoholic drinks and highly seasoned foods which may irritate the bladder. Refer to *You and Your Cystitis* by Angela Kilmartin (Warner Books, 1979).

Diphtheria

Mode of infection: Caused by a bacterium which enters the body through the windpipe or lungs. The bacterium is coughed into the air by an infectious person. Milk or other food may carry the infection.

Symptoms: These may appear within twelve hours of infection. Similar at first to those of common cold, sore throat, weakness and fever. But the illness rapidly becomes serious; breathing and swallowing become difficult. A poison produced by the bacterium paralyzes the heart and nerves. Untreated, the disease is often fatal. Medical help should be sought urgently.

Treatment: Antitoxin, penicillin and bed rest.

Prevention: Diphtheria is spread by apparently healthy people (carriers) as well as by those suffering from the illness. The disease is now rare because of vaccination. Ill people should be isolated until tests show that the infection has gone. Anyone exposed unwittingly to infection should seek vaccination, if not already vaccinated, and report any suspicious symptoms to a doctor at an early stage so that preventive treatment can be given.

Erysipelas

Mode of infection: Caused by a bacterium (Streptococcus) infecting the skin, and spread by contact or by touching some object which has been in contact with an infected person. Extremely infectious.

Symptoms: Inflammation of the skin appearing in dark red patches with swollen, raised border, particularly on the face and legs. Fever and headache. Commonest in middle and old age.

Treatment: Antibiotics. Acetaminophen for pain.

Prevention: Avoidance of contact with someone who has the disease. Bacteria may enter any small crack in the skin. If caring for someone with the illness, scrupulously wash with soap and water. Scrupulous personal hygiene and washing of food dishes.

Gastroenteritis

Also called food poisoning, gastritis, gastric flu.

Mode of infection: Stomach and bowel upsets with vomiting or diarrhea can have many causes – one of the commonest is over-indulgence in alcohol or food. They may also be caused by infection of bowel by viruses or bacteria, or by allergy or food poisoning. Food poisoning should be suspected when several people eating the same food all become ill at about the same time – usually within about twenty-four hours. Food poisoning has two common causes:

1. It is caused by eating food contaminated with bacteria called Salmonella which are common in sewage. If they enter the bowel they increase in number, causing infection.

2. Food poisoning is caused by eating food which has been spoiled through infection by Staphylococci, another type of

bacterium. These bacteria do not invade the bowel themselves but a poison (toxin) produced by them in the food causes the familiar symptoms. Another type of food poisoning, botulism, is caused by inadequate preservation of food. Food poisoning is also occasionally caused by eating poisonous plants.

Symptoms: Diarrhea, vomiting, nausea, pain and tenderness of bowel.

Treatment: Consult doctor; some drugs are available which may relieve symptoms but avoid unless prescribed by doctor. Most important, drink plenty of water, fruit juices or squash to restore fluids; add a level teaspoon of salt per pint and a generous teaspoon of honey or, if not available, sugar. Drink at least 2½ pints a day. Rest.

Prevention: Washing hands after going to toilet and before preparing or eating food. Do not store cooked food at room temperature. Avoidance of unhygienic eating places. Care in preparing and preservation of food. (See also Holiday Health, Chapter 9.)

German measles
See **Rubella**

Hepatitis

Mode of infection: Liver infection generally caused by a virus. Two main types: *infectious hepatitis*, spread by contaminated food or drink in areas where hygiene is poor. Symptoms of this illness appear two or three weeks after infection. *Serum hepatitis*, spread in blood from unsterilized syringes or by blood transfusion.

Symptoms: Headache, loss of appetite and fever. Followed by jaundice – that is, skin and whites of eyes become yellow. Liver and spleen enlarge and become tender; pain below right rib margin.

Treatment: Rest in bed while jaundiced. Convalesce for at least two weeks. Eat whatever food is most appetizing. Avoid alcohol, which may delay recovery of the liver, for at least a year after the illness. If jaundice does not clear up rapidly, a specialist opinion should be sought.

Prevention: Take care when traveling always to drink sterilized water. Passive immunity against hepatitis can be given by injection of an extract of blood serum – worth having if traveling in areas with primitive sanitation, or if someone in the family gets the illness. Isolate patient until one week after jaundice has disappeared. Take great care in disposal of wastes and in washing of clothes and dishes.

Impetigo

Mode of infection: Caused by bacteria – usually staphylococci but sometimes streptococci – which invade skin, particularly the face.

Symptoms: Skin turns red; pus blisters form which burst and make a weeping sore with yellowish, crusty scabs. Highly infectious, spreads quickly, especially to children.

Treatment: Application of antibiotic ointment, and antibiotics by mouth. Apply warm compresses of salt and permanganate solution to remove crusts.

Prevention: Anyone with the condition should have their own towels and avoid skin contact with others. Cut nails, scrupulous washing. Avoid scratching sores.

Influenza (see also page 147)

Mode of infection: Caused mainly by two different types of viruses. One of them regularly changes by mutation to new

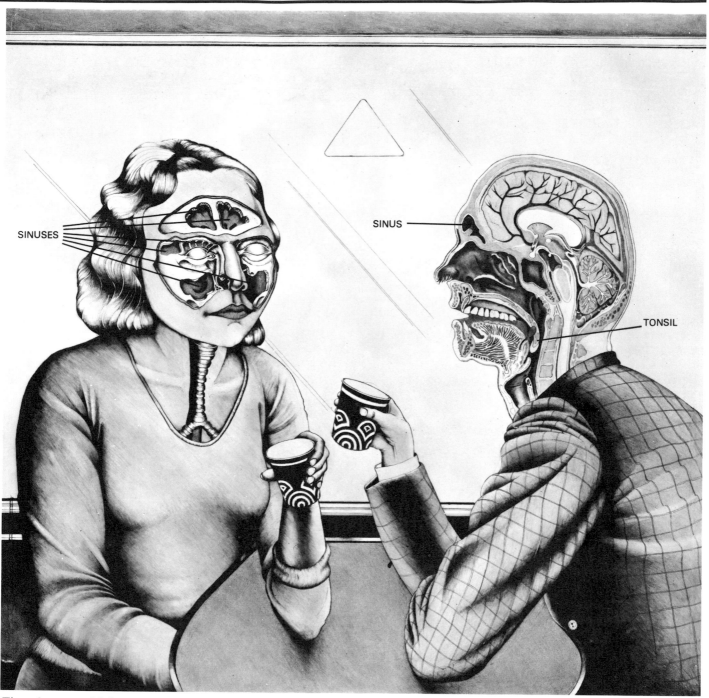

SINUSES

SINUS

TONSIL

The viruses which cause the common cold attack the passages of the nose and the sinuses shown in the illustration. When the passages and sinuses become inflamed they produce sticky mucus in an attempt to rid the body of infection. If sinuses become infected or blocked, then they may become painful – pain is felt above or below the eye.

varieties, causing widespread epidemics. Infection by inhaling airborne droplets.

Symptoms: Weakness, chills, fever, loss of appetite.

Treatment: Bed rest, plenty of fluids.

Prevention: Vaccination. Avoidance of people who have symptoms, avoidance of crowded places in winter.

Measles

Also called rubeola, morbilli.

Mode of infection: Caused by a virus spread by droplets in the air which are released when someone with the illness coughs or sneezes. One infection usually gives lifelong immunity.

Symptoms: First symptoms similar to cold: sore eyes, run-ning nose, coughing and sneezing. Raised temperature. Rash of many small red spots does not appear until three to five days after start of illness. Rash usually starts behind the ears and often spreads to whole body, disappearing after about a week. First signs of measles other than illness are Koplik's spots – red with white centers – which appear in the mouth and inside the cheeks about two days before the rash. Symptoms appear ten to fifteen days after exposure.

Treatment: Bed rest in well-ventilated room until temperature returns to normal. Avoidance of anyone with colds or other illness. Consult doctor, because complications – particularly infection of the ear – can occur.

Prevention: Vaccination. Avoidance of anyone with the illness until a week after disappearance of rash.

Meningitis

Mode of infection: Caused by several different types of bacteria, particularly the Meningococcus, which enter blood stream through nose or mouth and reach the nervous system. Also caused by viruses.

Symptoms: Shivering, temperature, severe headache, vomiting, fever, stiffness of muscles of neck and back, rash. Person may become unconscious.

Treatment: Prompt medical treatment vital. Antibiotics are effective against bacterial forms of illness. Some virus forms of the disease can also be treated with drugs.

Prevention: Close contacts of anyone who gets this illness should be observed for any early signs of the disease, and these should be reported to a doctor. Work is in progress on a vaccine. Patient should be isolated.

Mononucleosis

Mode of infection: Believed to be caused by the Epstein–Barr virus and to be transmitted by close contact such as kissing. Common in residential institutions such as colleges, military bases, etc.

Symptoms: Fatigue, fever, headache, sore throat, swollen glands in neck, armpit and groin. Blood test shows abnormal number of monocytes – large white blood cells. May last for weeks or months and is associated with depression.

Treatment: Rest and well-balanced diet. No drug treatment is available.

Prevention: Avoidance of close physical contact with anyone known to have the illness until symptoms have entirely cleared.

Mumps

Mode of infection: Caused by a virus which appears in saliva and is spread in air droplets. One attack usually gives lifelong immunity.

Symptoms: Headache, fever, vomiting, swelling of the salivary glands on one or both sides of the face just below the ear. In men, mumps sometimes also involves the testicles, and in women the ovaries, but seldom causes sterility. Illness appears two to three weeks after infection.

Treatment: Consult doctor, since similar symptoms are sometimes caused by other illnesses. Bed rest and plenty of fluids if feverish. In mild cases, rest at home until swelling goes down. A simple mouthwash occasionally, and acetaminophen tablets for pain.

Prevention: Avoidance of person with illness for three weeks after onset. Avoidance of towels, etc. used by infected person. Vaccination of young adults who have not had the disease.

Pneumonia

Mode of infection: Caused by bacterial infection, particularly by the pneumococcus which is present in all healthy mouths and throats. When resistance is lowered by colds, flu or ill health, then this or other bacteria may invade the lungs. Another type – viral pneumonia – is caused by a virus infection.

Symptoms: Sharp pains in the chest, a sharp dry cough, fever. Coughs up a rusty colored spit which may also contain blood or pus.

Treatment: Consult doctor. Antibiotic drugs and oxygen therapy.

Prevention: Proper convalescence after colds and flu. Avoidance of hurried eating, which results in inhalation of food. People who are bed-ridden should sit up as much as possible or change position frequently to prevent accumulation of fluid on lungs. Perform coughing and breathing exercises after an operation.

Poliomyelitis

Also called polio, infantile paralysis.

Mode of infection: Caused by a virus which enters the body through the nose or mouth and attacks nerves.

Symptoms: May be mild, resembling flu. Otherwise, headache, fever, vomiting, drowsiness, stiffness of head and back. Muscle weakness and paralysis of shoulder or hip may develop within a week.

Treatment: Skilled nursing in hospital. May spread to muscles controlling breathing so that a respirator may be necessary. Moist-packs relieve muscle spasms.

Prevention: Vaccination of people going abroad.

Psittacosis

Also called parrot fever, ornithosis.

Mode of infection: Caused by inhalation of a virus transmitted to people by birds such as pigeons, parrots, budgerigars, chickens and ducks.

Symptoms: Vary from mild flu-like illness to pneumonia.

Treatment: Antibiotic drugs.

Prevention: Avoid sick birds. Bird-fanciers should destroy sick birds.

Rabies

Mode of infection: Caused by a virus carried in animal saliva entering through a break in the skin. Commonly carried by dogs, cats, foxes, coyotes, skunks and bats, but can be transmitted to man by almost any animal – for example, a cow bitten by a fox may then bite a man, so transmitting the disease. The disease occurs in most parts of the world, including the Americas, and is increasingly common in Europe except for the British Isles, which remain free of it.

Symptoms: Convulsions, muscle spasms, hydrophobia – fear of water – develop because any attempt to swallow causes painful contractions of the larynx. Death inevitable if victim is not vaccinated after the bite. Symptoms first appear from a few days to months after a bite.

Treatment: When bitten by an animal, wash the wound with soap and warm water and go to a doctor. If possible the animal should be caught so that it can be tested for rabies. Immunization should begin immediately if the bite is on the face or neck; if the bite is further from the brain, then the animal may be tested for rabies first.

Prevention: Avoid any animal you do not know well. Do not let animal saliva enter any break in the skin. Avoid stroking or patting all stray animals.

Ringworm

Also called tinea.

Mode of infection: Caused by a fungus which is highly infectious. It may be spread by direct contact or by using infected linen, combs, etc.

Symptoms: An itchy eruption of the skin, especially of groin and toes, and scalp or nails.

Treatment: Antibiotic drugs such as griseofulvin. Must be taken by mouth until new nails have grown if nails affected, and anti-fungal ointment used.

Prevention: Prompt treatment of infection. Scrupulous hygienic measures, and avoid contact with victim.

Rubella

Also called German measles.

Mode of infection: Caused by a virus which gives rise to symptoms two to three weeks after infection. One infection usually gives immunity for life. Virus spread by infected droplets from coughs and sneezes.

Symptoms: Pink rash on face and body which fades after three or four days. Symptoms usually mild. Major risk is to fetus in the first three or four months of pregnancy.

Treatment: No special treatment necessary. If infection occurs in first four months of pregnancy, there is a possible ground for abortion.

Prevention: People with the illness should stay at home in order to minimize the risk of infecting a pregnant woman. Vaccination advisable for girls before puberty.

Scarlet fever

Also called scarlatina.

Mode of infection: Caused by the bacterium Streptococcus which also causes sore throats; close physical contact. Food contaminated with nose discharge. Infected droplets from sneezes etc.

Symptoms: Nausea, vomiting, headache, fever, sore throat and widespread red rash. Thickly coated tongue with raw red edges.

Treatment: Used to be a dreaded disease but can now be treated very effectively by antibiotics such as penicillin. Bed rest for ten days. Acetaminophen for pain relief.

Prevention: Isolation from family. All clothing, dishes must be disinfected. Patient no longer infectious when the rash fades and the skin starts to peel about two weeks after onset.

Shingles

Also called herpes zoster.

Mode of infection: Caused by the same virus as chickenpox.

Symptoms: Fever and pain for a few days. Many small blisters in lines along the back following the path of nerves, and extremely painful. The virus inflames the nerves, causing pain which may last for weeks or even months after the rash has cleared up.

Treatment: Pain-relieving drugs, drugs to prevent eye complication. Rest. Seek medical advice.

Prevention: Shingles is almost certainly caused by activation of viruses which have lain dormant in the body since a childhood infection with chickenpox. It does not seem to be caused by adults coming into contact with children with chickenpox. No means of prevention available.

Tetanus

Also called lockjaw.

Mode of infection: Caused by Clostridium bacteria from the soil and feces. The bacteria invade the body through wounds contaminated by dirt. Deep, dirty wounds caused by nails or bullets are particularly vulnerable.

Symptoms: Spasm of muscles, convulsions which may be so bad that the whole body arches backwards.

Treatment: Clean and dress wounds. Seek medical advice over any dirty wound. Antitoxin to counteract poison produced by bacteria, and penicillin to kill bacteria. Tranquilizing drugs. Muscle-relaxing drugs may be given and the patient put on a respirator.

Prevention: Vaccination, which gives protection lasting many years. Careful cleaning of wounds with soap and warm water. Professional care for deep wounds.

Tuberculosis

Mode of infection: Caused by a bacterium, Mycobacterium tuberculosis, which may be inhaled or swallowed in food. The bacteria most commonly invade the lungs but may attack many other parts of the body. The germs used to be spread in infected milk but this is now rare: most commercially available milk is pasteurized. However, certified raw milk may be commercially sold, unpasteurized, and milk which does not travel interstate is subject to state or local laws which may not require pasteurization.

Symptoms: Infection with tuberculosis often causes a mild illness which gives immunity to the disease. Pulmonary TB – that is, infection of the lungs – causes loss of weight, weakness, fever and bloodstained sputum. TB may also infect bones, joints, lymph glands, intestines, kidneys and the nerves.

Treatment: Drug treatments introduced in the 1950s have conquered what used to be a killer disease. The three most effective drugs are: Streptomycin, isoniazid and para-aminosalicylic acid.

Prevention: Vaccination. Never drink unpasteurized milk. Milk is likely to be safe in Western countries, but beware in less developed countries.

Whooping cough

Also called pertussis.

Mode of infection: Caused by bacterial infection, usually of a type called Bordetella pertussis, which infects the body in droplets entering the lungs. Highly infectious. One infection usually gives lifelong immunity.

Symptoms: Begins as a persistent cough and heavy cold with fever. This lasts a week and then for about another three weeks the victim suffers a barking cough which is very debilitating. This is an extremely serious illness in babies. Symptoms take up to two weeks to appear after infection.

Treatment: Rest. Food in small, frequent amounts if patient is liable to vomit. Drug treatment not very effective. Hospitalization is often necessary for infants.

Prevention: Vaccination, but this is controversial because it may cause damage. Avoid anyone who has had the illness for at least four weeks from the start of the illness or until the cough entirely subsides. Close contacts who were exposed before the illness was diagnosed should also be kept in quarantine for two weeks until it is known if they have caught the infection. Babies under one year who have been in close contact with someone who develops the illness may be given antibiotic drugs to prevent the infection developing – at an early stage drug treatment is much more effective.

SEX AND HEALTH

Introduction

A happy sex life is part of the enjoyment of good health. Enjoyable sex refreshes both the mind and body. It is both stimulating and relaxing. And not for nothing is sex so often called making love. Good sex often does just that. It would be false to pretend that sex between partners is necessary to health. It is not. For the body has worked out its own mechanisms to deal with the sexual feelings. So called "wet dreams" for men and erotic dreams for women can release sexual tensions – without need for either partners or masturbation.

But just as ill-health, tiredness and some forms of mental disease are likely to reduce the sex drive, so good health brings an appetite for sex to most people. One of the best things that has happened in the last thirty years or so is that nowadays sexual feelings are both accepted and enjoyed. Society's attitudes towards sex have undergone a great change. A generation ago sexual intercourse was only given official approval if it occurred within marriage. Today many kinds of other partnerships are increasingly accepted. Indeed, most people realize that even those with no partner can enjoy an active sex life.

A major influence for change came with the work of Dr Alfred C. Kinsey, who undertook a huge survey into the sex lives of 5,300 white American males and 5,940 American females. It was the first scientific attempt to discover what people actually did – rather than what others *thought* they did. *The Kinsey Reports*, as they were popularly known, were established in 1948 and 1953 and revolutionized our thinking.

Perhaps the main shock was how much sexual activity was going on. In theory marriage was the permitted place for sexual intercourse. Yet Dr Kinsey's statistics showed that large numbers of men, and more than a few women, were enjoying sex without marriage. In particular those who believed in female chastity before marriage were worried. For Dr Kinsey discovered that the woman who had premarital experience of orgasms was more likely to have orgasms in her married sex life.

Kinsey also discovered that sex inside marriage was not all that the romantic writers had suggested. For men, lovemaking resulted in orgasms. But women were not so lucky. Out of every four lovemaking sessions, only three produced an orgasm for the woman. (Kinsey did not ask exactly what sexual techniques were successful in producing the female orgasm.) Some women, indeed, never experienced orgasm at all, even after years of married life. In the first year of marriage, one in four wives had not had an orgasm. Even after ten years of marriage, about 12 per cent were still not having orgasms. For others, however, orgasms had come with marriage experience – suggesting that sexual results could be attained with practise.

Kinsey also asked about loveplay in sexual intercourse. Most married women reported somewhere between four to twenty minutes of loveplay before vaginal penetration. This usually included deep kissing, breast fondling and sucking, and manual stimulation of the genitals.

Just over half the women enjoyed cunnilingus or genital kissing by the man. Just under half had practiced fellatio, genital kissing by the female. Oral sex, in fact, was quite common, though less popular among older couples.

The next major piece of sex research came with the work of Dr William H. Masters and Virginia E. Johnson. Kinsey had *asked* what people did. Masters and Johnson studied sexual response in the laboratory, noting the exact bodily changes of both men and women in sexual activity.

For both male and female they charted a similar pattern of sexual response – excitement in which the penis becomes erect and the female clitoris and vagina enlarge; a plateau phase during which excitement increases; the orgasmic phase; the resolution phase in which bodies return to their previous non-excited state.

Their findings, first published in 1966, were particularly interesting for women. In the past, Freud and other psychiatrists had suggested that there were two kinds of orgasm – a clitoral orgasm and a vaginal orgasm. It was often suggested that the vaginal orgasm was the mature sexual response.

Masters and Johnson discovered that there was just the one orgasm. The physical changes were exactly the same, whether orgasm was produced by clitoral or vaginal stimulation. The center for sexual sensation, indeed, was the clitoris – whether that sensation was produced by the movement of the penis in the vagina, or by manual stimulation of the area round the clitoris.

Masters and Johnson also pointed out that many marriage manuals had been mistaken about clitoral stimulation. They had suggested direct manipulation of the clitoris, while the laboratory studies showed that this could quite often produce irritation rather than pleasure. Manual stimulation of the area *round* the clitoris was found to be the method used by most women.

This sex research changed attitudes, and some of the marriage manuals! Meanwhile the other major development was the discovery of the pill – a reliable and easy method of contraception. For the first time sex need not be linked with pregnancy for women. As all kinds of contraception became more widely available, unmarried men and women could enjoy sex without the fear of pregnancy.

Leading a Happy Sex Life

Today most of us are free to lead whatever kind of sex life we want. Any sexual activity which gives pleasure, and doesn't do harm, is increasingly and generally regarded as acceptable. But people's beliefs and feelings should be respected. Sex which harms or distresses another person is not ethical. It is not good to bully, nag or push somebody into doing what they do not want to do. Nor is it a good idea to distress yourself. Persisting in activities which worry you does not lead to happiness.

There is also such a thing as anti-social sex. Using force or fraud to have sex with people is anti-social. Having sex with people who cannot give proper consent is also anti-social. The young and the mentally ill need protection. The law usually steps in to make anti-social sex illegal. There are also some old laws lying around on the statute books of some states under which certain sexual techniques may be forbidden. Use discretion if you live in these states.

Sex is on the whole very safe indeed – although see the section on certain sexual diseases later in this chapter. Nor is there much that needs to be said about sexual hygiene. Ordinary soap and water will clean any part of the body – vaginal douches are neither necessary nor good for health. If you are sensitive about body odors, why not adopt a washing routine before sex as part of the loveplay?

There are some general suggestions which can help towards a rewarding sex life. Even the sexually experienced may find them worth thinking about, for one of the joys of sex is that it is never too late to make discoveries.

KNOW YOUR OWN BODY
Knowing your own bodily responses means that you must look, touch and feel. Men, since their genitals are within easy reach and vision, generally do this from an early age. Many women, however, are still amazingly ignorant.

Some women do not even know what their sexual organs look like. Spend some time with a small mirror, and a flashlight if necessary, looking at your own sex organs. Most sex books provide pictures of the female sex organs. Identify the various parts from this. If your own sex organs look slightly different from the ones in the picture, do not worry. Sexual features differ, just as facial features vary.

In particular it is important to identify the clitoris. This is the small hood at the top end of the space between the large lips. The clitoris is the center for sexual feeling. Directly touching it may not be pleasureable. But the area round it probably will.

Try touching it with your own fingers, and feel exactly which areas give the most pleasure – to what kind of touching. Until you, yourself, know what kind of touching gives pleasure, how can you expect your partner to know?

Most men will probably have done this kind of experimenting in youth. If not, they too can profitably spend some time looking, feeling, and touching. This same exercise can also be done together. It can be fun. As the military strategists say, time spent on reconnaissance is never wasted.

STOP MAKING RULES AND REGULATIONS FOR YOURSELF
There is a terrible human tendency to make up rules, regulations and categories. Consciously, or unconsciously, most of us have set ideas about how to make love and what our responses ought to be. When our personal performance does not conform to these rules, then we worry.

For instance, many people believe that sex between a man and a woman is made up of loveplay, followed by vaginal penetration by the penis, followed by the male (and possibly the female) orgasm. But this order is neither necessary nor even necessarily desirable. You can start with vaginal penetration and male orgasm, if you like, then follow it with oral sex, with the man stimulating the woman. Or you need not have vaginal penetration at all. The order in which you do things is up to you and your partner.

Another long-standing myth is that the woman's orgasm ought to be caused by the thrusting of the penis in the vagina. Many women whose orgasms instead come from manual stimulation in the area of the clitoris worry that they have not "achieved" vaginal orgasm. This goes back to the old idea that there were two different sorts of orgasm, clitoral and vaginal, and that the vaginal orgasm was somehow more mature. It is all nonsense. Anything that gives an orgasm is cause for pleasure and pride. *The Hite Report* showed that only 30 per cent of women have regular orgasms from penile thrusting. So, if you do not, you are in the majority. Just do a lot more of what turns you on.

Another belief is that simultaneous orgasm is somehow better than one partner's orgasm followed by the other partner's. This idea was started by an influential sex manual of the 1920s. Simultaneous orgasms are great – but so are sequential orgasms. Do not mess up your lovemaking by trying to time your orgasms. It usually gets in the way of spontaneous sex.

Men sometimes suffer from the idea that it is their *duty* to make sure a woman responds. Insecure men sometimes boast of their skill in this way. Of course, it is lovely to be a skilled and sensitive lover. But sex does not have to be started by the male, and kept under his control all the way. No woman wants her man to stop trying to give her pleasure. The push it in, poke it about and pull it out man is not much in demand. But neither is the man who feels it is all up to him. The lover who takes it as a personal reflection on his technique if his woman does not respond is a big bore.

Finally, orgasms are not the be-all and end-all of sex. It is not possible to measure people by their orgasmic capacity. If you start making love with the fixed idea that you *must* have an orgasm, or that your partner *must*, you are risking disappointment, guilt, anger and anxiety. All these emotions are very bad for sex.

What all these beliefs have in common is the way they impose an artificial pattern on sexual relations. Once you start measuring your own performance, or your partner's, against other people's or against some idea of what is "normal" or "sexy", you are just asking for problems.

SEX HAS TO BE LEARNED
The huge sale of sex manuals shows that most people agree that sex can be learned. Sexual techniques in books will also help make better lovers. But only if they are used intelligently. It is no good thinking that a sexual technique *must* work because a book says so.

Real sex is different from books. In 1977 *The Hite Report* indicated what 3,000 women felt about sex, what they enjoyed and what they did not enjoy. Perhaps the most interesting result of all was the variety of their response. What one woman enjoyed, another would loathe.

Sex, therefore, has to be an experience which is learned

anew for each different partner. You need to discover what your partner likes – not what you think they ought to like, what others have liked, or what some book says.

Indeed, this information needs constant updating. People's tastes change, with age, with mood, and with situations. The ideal lover doesn't simply apply a routine of so much foreplay, say, followed by so much sexual intercourse. He or she responds to what is desired by a particular person on a particular occasion.

SEX NEEDS COMMUNICATION

It sounds obvious to say that lovers must be able to communicate in order to have good sex. How, otherwise, are they going to be able to tell each other what they like doing, how, and exactly where? Yet thousands of couples cannot talk to each other in bed because they are too shy.

One problem is that the words are difficult. The official words sound too medical and a bit of a turn-off. The unofficial words sound obscene to many.

Non-verbal communication may be a solution. Be sensitive to responses such as "Umm" and "Ouch" from your partner. Listen – and try to remember. It is sometimes difficult to recall exactly what turned your partner on. But only by remembering the details of successful loveplay will you be a good lover.

Sex therapists Masters and Johnson acknowledge this problem. For some of their training, they suggest that one partner places his or her hand over the other's. By this means, the hand underneath can be guided to sensitive areas, lifted away from painful activities, and encouraged by pressure to continue pleasurable activities. No words are needed.

Words, however, will be a turn-on for some people. For some individuals this will mean the use of obscenities or slang which would otherwise be unacceptable. Others will enjoy verbalizing sex fantasies, or even running commentaries on what is going on. Try it. It can be both instructive and fun.

Masturbation

Nearly all men and about two-thirds of women have masturbated at some time in their lives. Some people continue to masturbate as well as enjoying sexual intercourse with a partner regularly. Others have recourse to masturbation when no partner is available. There is absolutely nothing wrong with masturbation. Ideas that it can cause ill-health, mental disorder or acne are nonsense. On the contrary, masturbation is a pleasurable habit which harms nobody, and it is a convenient source of enjoyment.

Most men and women masturbate with the help of sexual fantasies or sometimes pornographic literature. Both are good aids to masturbation. Sometimes fantasies (which may also be used to produce sexual pleasure during intercourse with a partner) are about behavior which would not be desired in reality. This is nothing to worry about. Sexual fantasies, whatever their content, do not have to be put into practise and are a good sex aid.

For men, it is obvious how to proceed with masturbation, since the genitals are outside the body and their response is visible. But for some women, it is not obvious how to masturbate because they are unsure how their genitals

work. Though clitoral manipulation of some kind is the most common form of female masturbation, some women use thigh pressure, muscular reactions and occasionally fantasies alone. *The Hite Report* (see Appendix 2) contains detailed examples of masturbation which will be useful for women who want to know how it can be done. The purchase of a vibrator will also help women who are finding it difficult to masturbate – and may enhance the pleasure of those who already know how.

For women, masturbation may be a worthwhile path to a better sex life with a partner. There is evidence which suggests that if a woman can produce an orgasm by masturbation, she is more likely to have one in sexual intercourse. Some sex therapists teach masturbation to non-orgasmic women, before trying to teach orgasm with a partner.

Common sense suggests that if a woman knows exactly what gives her pleasure, she can teach a man to do this, if he is willing to learn. Sometimes, of course, this does not work. *The Hite Report* suggests that, in this case, the woman may like to masturbate in the setting of sex with a partner – thus putting the pleasure into the context of mutual loveplay.

Homosexuality

About 20 million Americans are homosexual. Put another way, about one child in every five American families will be homosexual. The widely accepted estimate, based on The Kinsey Report and more recent researches, is that 10 per cent of men and women are basically homosexual.

But human sexuality does not fall neatly into categories. A much larger number of men and women have had a homosexual experience at some point in their lives. By their middle forties, 13 per cent of women and 37 per cent of men will have had a homosexual experience resulting in orgasm. The population, therefore, cannot be neatly divided into homosexual and heterosexual. There are many men and women who enjoy sexual contact with both sexes. Others will turn to heterosexuality, after a period of homosexuality – or vice versa. In single sex societies such as prisons and boarding schools, people who are normally heterosexual may turn to their own sex for sexual outlet.

Although many men and women will have had some homosexual experience, or at least feelings, many myths and prejudices remain. Most arise from fear or ignorance. A common slur on male homosexuals is that they are eager to seduce young boys. Yet statistics indicate that 90 per cent of sexual child abuse is committed by heterosexual men on young girls. Most homosexual relationships involve adults.

It is also often believed that all male homosexuals are effeminate in their appearance and manners, and that all lesbians are mannish. Neither belief is generally true, though individuals may sometimes conform to this pattern – as may heterosexuals. Most gay men and women look and behave like heterosexual members of the community – except in the sexual side of their lives.

In the past the law has often made the open expression of homosexual lovemaking illegal. Psychiatrists have treated it as a deviation from "normal" heterosexuality. Some therapists have offered "cures" for homosexuality.

Nowadays homosexuality is increasingly accepted. Although it may be associated with mental or emotional distress, it is not a *symptom* of such disorder. Many psychiatrists and therapists try to help the homosexual man or lesbian to come to terms with, and be happy about, their sexuality. Counseling can help with this. It can also aid relatives and spouses of homosexuals and bisexuals. A marriage need not break up because the husband or wife has homosexual relations: homosexuality is no more irrevocable than a previous state of heterosexuality. It is often simply a phase of a person's life, although it is one which can cause considerable emotional turmoil.

Relatives, marriage partners and close friends of gay people may find they need help in coping with their own feelings about homosexuality. There are organizations in America who can put them in touch with people in a similar position, and help them come to terms and accept their gay relatives or friends (see Appendix 2).

If you are worried by your own homosexual feelings, it will probably be worth contacting a homosexual organization which can offer advice and support. Finding others who share your feelings and experiences may calm your anxiety and help you to cope with social problems. Alternatively the organization may help you choose a sympathetic and up-to-date therapist or counselor (see Appendix 2).

Age and Sex

Growing old does not mean that sex has to come to a full stop. Elderly men and women can enjoy active lovemaking right into their seventies and eighties, if they desire to. Indeed, the occasional nonagenerian, according to a Danish survey, is still leading an active sex life.

Age, however, does affect sexual response. The process is not a sudden one, nor does it occur after a set number of years. It is rather a very slow decline over a long period. If men and women have led an active sex life for a long time, they will find this can continue right into old age.

The research of Masters and Johnson has shown the principles of sexual response are the same in youth and in old age. But age slows down sexual arousal in men, and may diminish the intensity of sexual response in both sexes. In particular, women may suffer from a lessening of vaginal lubrication. The vaginal walls thin with age, and the whole vagina can shrink. Sometimes the thrusting of the penis in the vagina irritates the bladder. Older women may find they have to urinate after sex, and that a long sex session can cause cystitis (see page 152).

The ageing male will probably find that it takes longer to get an erection, and that this erection is only at full height just before ejaculation. Intervals between erections will be longer, and ejaculation itself may be more of a leaking than a spurting sensation. But – as compensation – he will probably be able to hold his erection longer, and have better control of ejaculation.

If all this sounds rather gloomy, it need not be. Creams, jellies and hormonal creams can help women with lubrication and vaginal troubles. Estrogen replacement therapy (see Menopause, page 166) may also be of use.

A bit of imaginative thinking is also a very good idea. Old age may be the time to reconsider sexual patterns. Oral sex or manual stimulation by both partners may replace vaginal thrusting. A vibrator – useful for stimulation of both male and female – can be a good sex aid for the elderly.

If either lose the desire for sex, this may be the effect of ill-health. Similarly, many drugs given to combat disorders of the elderly can have this effect. Elderly men and women may also be more susceptible to alcohol.

If in doubt, check with your doctor. Sometimes people give up sex because they think it is dangerous – for instance, people with a heart condition. This is rarely so. Ask your doctor and insist on a detailed answer. If he or she still thinks that the elderly should not need sex, it is time to educate your medical adviser.

Sex Difficulties

Sexual difficulties will arise from time to time between the most well-matched partners. Tiredness, mental preoccupation, ill-health or just change of mood can produce occasional episodes of impotence in men, or orgasm problems in women. An occasional episode is nothing to worry about. But sometimes such difficulties become settled habits. Naturally they tend to arouse feelings of anxiety, guilt, or even anger, and these feelings in their turn can make the condition worse. Expert help and advice may be needed.

The most common problems in men are:
Impotence. This is failure to get an erection. When a man has *never* in his life had an erection, it is known as primary impotence. When a man has previously functioned, but has lost the ability, it is known as secondary impotence.
Premature ejaculation. The man ejaculates too soon for his partner – either just before or just after penetration of the vagina.
Ejaculatory incompetence. The man can have an erection, but cannot ejaculate into the vagina.

The most common female problems are:
Orgasmic dysfunction. Primary orgasmic dysfunction means that the woman has never had an orgasm. Secondary orgasmic dysfunction is used for women who have had orgasms by some method but cannot achieve orgasm in the way she wishes with her partner. Sometimes it is called situational orgasmic dysfunction. The exact definition of what constitutes orgasmic dysfunction varies.
Dyspareunia (painful intercourse). Physical problems may account for painful intercourse. There is also a condition known as vaginismus, in which the muscles round the entrance to the vagina go into spasm during penetration.

If any of these sexual difficulties occur regularly, then the first thing to do is check that there is not a physical cause. As well as tiredness and ill-health, sexual difficulties can also be caused by drugs prescribed for some other condition. Ask your doctor about the side effects of any drugs he is prescribing. A high alcohol intake can have the same effect. If intercourse is painful for the woman, it is worth checking to make sure there are no vaginal infections or other physical causes.

Having checked that there is no physical cause for your sex difficulties, you may wish to consider sex therapy. It can be expensive and for those who cannot afford it, it may be worth trying some of the do-it-yourself techniques now described in books (see Appendix 2). However, many people will find that these books do not produce results – probably because sex difficulties are likely to be surrounded by painful feelings and long-held attitudes. Dealing with these will probably need expert counseling.

If you decide that you need help, you will have to make a decision about what sort of help you need. Long-term psychotherapy of the traditional kind is expensive and drawn-out. Short-term sex therapy, often of the Masters and Johnson type, is probably a better bet if your problems are mainly sexual. Married or long-term partners may find that marriage guidance counseling can help. Women, particularly those without a regular partner, may find their local feminist group helpful.

If you decide to opt for sex therapy, you will have to avoid the thousands of quacks who have set themselves up in this field. Anybody can call themselves a sex therapist and many do. Some will be getting their thrills at your expense. Avoid anybody who offers "body therapy", nude counseling sessions, stimulates the erogenous zones under the pretext of "examining sexual response", or suggests intercourse with the therapist as therapy.

Anybody offering sex therapy should have a formal training in medicine, psychology or psychiatry. There is a special body called the American Association of Sex Educators, Counselors and Therapists, membership of which is a guarantee of training and ethical conduct. But some professionals do not belong. Your county Medical Society, State Psychological Association, or the Department of Psychology or Psychiatry at your local university or medical school, should be able to tell you the name of somebody specializing in sex therapy.

Having found the name of a qualified sex therapist, use the first session with him or her to make sure that it is the kind of therapy you want. Do you find the therapist sympathetic, easy to talk to, the sort of person you can trust? Ask about the cost and the likely length of treatment. Are you satisfied that everything will be confidential?

If all these aspects meet your approval (and the approval of your partner), then stick to the therapy. If you find that it is distressing you, discuss this with the therapist. Do not just quit. Therapy is a difficult and demanding process. If you just move from therapist to therapist shopping for an easy solution, you are not going to deal with your problems. Of course, if you have discussed it with the therapist, it may be that with their help you will choose to be referred to another practitioner.

Contraception

Birth control is now the rule rather than the exception. Yet many women – and most men – remain unaware of the relative merits and disadvantages of different methods. Which is best for your particular needs? What are the medical pros and cons of the various methods.

Using no birth control at all has risks. Out of every 100,000 women aged 25 to 29 who were taking no contraception measures at all, about 6 would die in childbirth every year. A similar number of women aged 40 to 44 would experience more than 22 deaths in childbirth yearly. So in theory the more effective birth control is, the safer it is. But unfortunately the most efficient methods of contraception – the pill, and to a lesser extent the IUD and female sterilization – carry health risks.

It is a matter therefore of balancing risks against efficiency. The pill is easy to take and by far the most efficient reversible method of contraception. But research has revealed that the pill makes the blood clot more easily, and makes older women more vulnerable to heart disease and strokes. But these dangers do not usually come into play until the age of 30. For women under 30, the pill is not significantly more dangerous than other contraceptive methods. But for women over 30, it begins to pose more serious health hazards. These dangers are striking when pill taking is combined with smoking. Women smokers on the pill face a sharp rise in the risk of death. By the age of 40, out of every 100,000 smokers on the pill about 59 will die yearly – more than four times the number dying in highway accidents. Even non-smokers face risks at this age, though only seven deaths per 100,000 would be expected.

One American contraception expert, Dr Christopher Tiezte, has shown from the statistics that the safest method of birth control for women of all ages would be the condom or diaphragm backed up by early abortion carried out under proper conditions. The problems occur with abortion, because some women do not believe in it, while others find it difficult to obtain. Also the efficiency of the condom and diaphragm varies with the users. Couples who find these methods work well should use them. But some couples will find them too difficult for use.

The pill, therefore, still has a place in the contraceptive strategy. It is most useful for the young, the unmarried girls or couples without a home for whom pregnancy would be a disaster. Couples starting a family, on the other hand, who would not mind the early arrival of a baby should think about using the condom or diaphragm.

All women in their thirties should reconsider their contraceptive strategy. From 30 onwards, women smokers are taking a frighteningly high risk if they continue on the pill without stopping smoking. Even non-smoking women after the age of 35 should consider using the condom or diaphragm, or trying the IUD. The IUD has side effects, but not ones that are likely to lead to death. Couples who have completed their family should think about vasectomy, which is a very efficient and safe method of contraception. Female sterilization is also a possibility, but it is a bigger and therefore riskier operation.

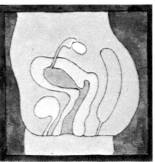

THE PILL
The pill is the most popular method of contraception in America. Although there are signs of a slight decline in its use, twenty-two out of every hundred married women under forty-five still use it.

History: The combined pill contains synthetic versions of the two female hormones – estrogen and progesterone – which control natural ovulation. These two hormones in combination manage to prevent the ripening of an egg in the woman's ovary. In the 1930s it was confirmed that injections of natural estrogen, progesterone or the male hormone testosterone would successfully prevent ovulation. But it was not until 1940 that a cheap and universally available oral contraceptive pill became a possibility. In 1955 a progesterone-only pill taken daily went on trial in

Puerto Rico, but it was soon decided that a "combined" pill was better for most women.

How it works: By altering the natural hormone balance of the body, the pill does three things. It alters the mucus at the neck of the womb, making it hostile to sperm; it prevents the ripening and release of the female egg; and it alters the lining of the womb so that a fertilized egg would not be accepted there.

Effectiveness: In theory the pill is 100 per cent effective. In practise, two out of a hundred women on the pill get pregnant in the first year of its use. These failures occur because women forget to take the pill, or because vomiting, diarrhea or interaction with some other drug means that the pill is not fully absorbed.

Advantages: It is the only completely reliable form of contraception which is easy to take and does not interfere with love-making. It helps menstrual disorders and premenstrual tension. Because it cuts down blood loss, it may help women with iron deficiency anemia. And it may modify acne, sebaceous and ovarian cysts, and prevent certain benign breast lumps.

Disadvantages: The serious side effects of the pill apply mainly to older women. It makes them more vulnerable to heart disease and strokes. The pill makes the blood clot more easily, and this in older women may produce a thrombosis or other circulation problems. Hypertension, or high blood pressure, can also be caused by the pill in some women. The statistics suggest that all these risks may increase with the number of years that a woman has been on the pill. Cigarette smoking is the other factor which combines with pill taking to produce a high death rate in older women. A few studies have suggested that women on the pill may be more vulnerable to cervical cancer, but these have not been confirmed. However, a barrier method such as the condom or diaphragm may protect against cervical cancer, because a virus may be involved (see page 134). Women who stop the pill to have a baby may find pregnancy delayed for a while. Mild side effects such as headaches, nausea and vaginal discharge occur with some women, but these may disappear after persisting or changing the brand. Depression can also be a side effect. There is an increased chance of chickenpox, some other virus infections, and infections in the urinary tract, but nothing too serious.

Advice: Women cannot conceive during the week in the monthly cycle that they are not taking the pill: it is perfectly safe to have sex then. If you do not want a period for some special reason, you can just keep taking the pills. (But make sure they are the right ones. Some brands of pill give you dummy tablets to take over the menstruation period; these will not stop a period.)

If you forget your pill, take it as soon as you can: twelve or even twenty-four hours late is certainly better than not at all. It is possible, however, that a delay of even twelve hours may lead to conception in highly fertile women, so take other precautions as well. If you have been vomiting or suffering from diarrhea, just take another pill, or use other precautions. If two or more of the following apply to you, you should think hard before going on the pill: age over thirty; overweight; smoker; anyone in the immediate family died of heart disease under the age of fifty-five (count father, mother, brother, sister); any personal history of heart disease, diabetes or blood pressure; on the pill for more than five years. If you are over thirty-five, the pill is a serious health risk, so consider other methods. Also tell your doctor if you suffer from epilepsy, jaundice or vaginal discharge. If you do go on the pill, stop smoking and have blood pressure check-ups yearly.

A progestogen-only pill, sometimes known as the mini-pill, is used for women breast-feeding and for others for whom the combined pill is not suitable.

THE CONDOM

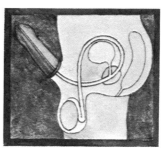

Well behind the pill in popularity comes the condom, which is used by seven out of a hundred married couples. The condom is declining in popularity, though more white couples use it than black couples.

History: The ancient Egyptians seem to have been the first to use some kind of condom. In Europe a linen version was in use in the sixteenth century, and in the next two hundred years it rapidly gained popularity. There were condoms made of gut and even of soft leather, decorated with ribbons. Not everybody was enthusiastic. Madame de Sevigny coined the famous remark that the condom was "armor against enjoyment and a spider's web against danger". Till the last century, however, condoms were used primarily as a protection against venereal disease, with birth control as only a secondary consideration.

How it works: The condom puts a barrier between sperm and female egg, and keeps all the sperms within itself. Leaving aside such curiosities as washable rubber condoms and odd designs to enhance sexual pleasure, condoms are mainly distinguished by shape and color. There are condoms made out of plastic or animal gut for those men and women who are allergic to rubber. Most condoms nowadays are also lubricated, though it should be remembered that this lubrication does not have any contraceptive effect. It merely makes for extra comfort.

Effectiveness: About ten out of a hundred women who are relying on their husband's use of the condom get pregnant in the first year of using this method. Regular and practiced use would mean a lower failure rate.

Advantages: There are no physical side effects. Condoms guard against veneral disease, and are useful for occasions when sex was not anticipated or planned. They can be obtained without a doctor's prescription in drugstores, barber's and sometimes from slot machines. It is sometimes claimed (but unproven) that they lower the risk of cervical cancer.

Disadvantages: They dull male enjoyment. Couples may find them off-putting in loveplay. They can be an expensive method of contraception.

Advice: Make sure you have a reputable brand. Do not use them after the date marked on the packet. Read the instructions, and use them before any genital contact. For extra protection against pregnancy, wear a condom in conjunction with contraceptive foam, cream or jelly used by the woman. But do not use Vaseline or grease as a lubricant, as these destroy the rubber.

THE DIAPHRAGM

Before the advent of the pill and the IUD, the only reliable method which allowed women themselves to control their fertility was the diaphragm. Today it is still used by about three in every hundred married women.

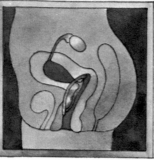

History: Although the ancient Egyptians may have used some kind of vaginal cap, it did not reach the USA until the nineteenth century. Before the diaphragm women had used vaginal sponges, tampons and douches. In the last century, spermicide creams, jellies and suppositories had also been invented, and with the diaphragm these proved efficient.

How it works: The diaphragm covers the cervix, reaching back to the end of the vagina and forwards towards the pubic bone, under which it lodges. It makes a barrier between the sperm and egg by covering the entrance to the womb. The spermicide which is used with the diaphragm kills the sperm.

Effectiveness: About thirteen out of a hundred women using a diaphragm get pregnant in the first year of using this method of contraception. Regular and practiced use would mean a lower failure rate.

Advantages: There are no physical side effects. It is often used as a stop-gap between the pill or the IUD. During menstruation it holds back the flow of blood, thus making intercourse less messy. By using a diaphragm with spermicidal cream or jelly, a woman gives herself some protection against venereal disease and sexually transmitted infections.

Disadvantages: They may be off putting in some forms of loveplay. Women who dislike touching their genitals may find them distasteful to insert. There is the danger that women in a hurry may insert them incorrectly. Diaphragms must be supplied with fresh spermicide after several hours, and care must be taken not to remove them for eight hours after sex.

Advice: Diaphragms must be carefully fitted by an expert and checked at regular intervals. Weight changes, or pregnancies, will usually mean a diaphragm of a different size is needed. Make sure the doctor or clinic you consult has the necessary expertise. Check that it remains in good condition, with the rubber still supple and shaped. Failures often occur because a diaphragm has become too old or misshapen. Do not use Vaseline or grease as a lubricant, because it destroys the rubber. Diaphragms must *always* be used with spermicides.

THE IUD

About six in every hundred married women relies upon an intra-uterine device (IUD) to prevent pregnancy. IUDs were once restricted to women who had children, but nowadays a growing number of women without children are wearing them.

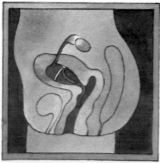

History: Sixteenth-century European doctors occasionally fitted women with intra-uterine devices. These were known as stem pessaries and they were aimed at improving fertility. The idea was that they opened up the entrance to the womb for the sperm. In the 1950s the IUD was rediscovered, this time as a contraceptive.

How it works: A foreign body in the womb usually prevents conception, probably because it affects the womb lining, so that the fertilized egg cannot implant itself there. Nowadays, some IUDs are coated with copper, which also seems to act against conception. Faint traces of copper are released into the blood stream, but nobody is absolutely sure why this helps stop pregnancy. A hormone-releasing IUD has also been produced. The most popular IUDs are the Lippes Loop, Saf-T-Coil, Copper 7 and Copper T.

Effectiveness: About four out of a hundred women using an IUD get pregnant within the first year of its insertion. British research has shown that the effectiveness of an IUD also depends on the skill of the doctor or nurse who inserts it.

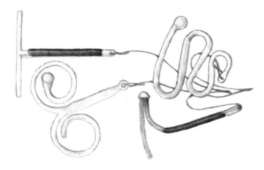

Advantages: Once inserted, an IUD can be left in place for two years or more. It is ideal for women who find other forms of contraception difficult to use. Smaller copper IUDs can be used for women who have not had children.

Disadvantages: Skill is necessary in fitting to avoid the possibility of perforation of the womb. Though pregnancy chances are small, once pregnancy has occurred there is a high risk of miscarriage. Some women find IUDs painful, or suffer heavy periods; some automatically expel the IUD from the womb, and occasionally women suffer from a discharge with copper IUDs.

Advice: Make sure you get your IUD inserted by a doctor or a nurse who is practiced in the technique. If you are doubtful whether your normal doctor is an expert, then it may be worth going to a Planned Parenthood Federation clinic instead. Have your IUD removed when your doctor suggests. Do not leave it for longer than he advises. If pregnancy must at all costs be avoided, use a spermicidal foam as a back-up.

WITHDRAWAL

About two in every hundred married couples rely on withdrawal, or coitus interruptus, to prevent pregnancy.

History: The Biblical story of Onan, who spilled his semen on the ground rather than impregnate his brother's wife, indicates its early origins.

How it works: The man withdraws his penis from the woman's vagina just before ejaculation, in an effort to keep sperm away from the female sex organs.

Effectiveness: There are no reliable figures for its efficiency, since so much depends on the individual self-control and skill of the man. But it is rarely efficient.

Advantages: It can be practiced when no other form of contraception is available. It has no physical side effects.

Disadvantages: Semen can be released into the vagina before ejaculation. Sexual satisfaction is often impaired.

Advice: Better than no precautions at all.

STERILIZATION

Nearly ten out of every hundred married women opt for sterilization to prevent further pregnancies. There are also about eight in every hundred who lose their reproductive powers as a by-product of such operations as hysterectomy.

How it works: The principle is to cut or block the Fallopian tubes through which the female eggs travel from the ovary to the womb. This can be done by tying, then cutting, the Fallopian tubes – called *tubal ligation* – or by simply putting clips, bands or even plugs on or into the tubes. These last methods allow the operation to be reversed. The most efficient method involves cauterizing and sealing the tubes irreversibly, but it carries a slightly higher risk than others. *Laparoscopy* is an operation which involves making a small incision below the navel, into which a laparoscope is inserted to view the internal organs. *Laparotomy* involves making another small incision through which the tubes are cut, clipped or sealed.

Effectiveness: In theory the operation is 100 per cent effective, but very rarely the Fallopian tubes rejoin automatically and the woman may become pregnant.

Advantages: It ends worry about pregnancy.

Disadvantages: The menstrual cycle may be disrupted, and for a time sexual intercourse may have to be avoided. Some disorders, possibly psychological, like backache, headache and depression have been reported. A woman opting for sterilization must assume that it will end all chance of bearing further children. Sterilization that involves opening up the abdomen carries the usual risks of such operations. When the sterilization is performed by laparoscopy, and the tubes are burned, there is the risk of burning a part of the intestine.

Advice: It is not a good idea to combine sterilization with abortion, because a woman wanting an abortion may be too upset to make a balanced decision about sterilization. If your doctor says he will only give you an abortion *on condition* you are also sterilized, contact another doctor or the Planned Parenthood Federation for help (see Appendix 2). Occasionally, old-fashioned doctors will recommend a hysterectomy (removal of the womb) for sterilization. Unless the operation is needed for some other reason, there is no need for such drastic measures.

VASECTOMY

Nearly ten out of every hundred married couples choose a male vasectomy as contraception. There are also a small number of men who are sterilized for other reasons.

History: Vasectomies only really became popular in America at the end of the sixties, though they had been available for some years before. India was the country which led the way in mass vasectomies for men. By 1970 vasectomies had become common in America too.

How it works: Vasectomy is the male equivalent of sterilization. The operation involves cutting and tying the two *vas deferens*, tubes which carry sperms from the testicles to the penis. Since these are just under the skin, usually only a local anaesthetic is needed. Vasectomies can sometimes be reversed by rejoining these tubes.

Effectiveness: In theory a properly performed vasectomy is 100 per cent effective. But very occasionally *vas deferens* rejoin of their own accord, or a third *vas deferens* is discovered and continues to let through the sperm. The other possible cause of post-vasectomy pregnancies is that it takes three or four months before the sperm-flow disappears. Sperm tests are necessary to check that all the sperms have disappeared.

Advantages: It does not in any way affect male virility. It does away with the need for troublesome forms of contraceptives. It is much easier and less serious an operation than female sterilization.

Disadvantages: It is not usually reversible and therefore a man opting for a vasectomy must assume it means an end to his chances of begetting children. It takes several months before infertility is ensured.

SAFE PERIOD

About three in every hundred married women practice the safe period method as a way of limiting their families. It is also called the rhythm method or natural family planning.

History: Up to the end of the nineteenth century, doctors remained ignorant about the female cycle. But a safe period was recommended by birth-control pioneers Charles Bradlaugh and Annie Besant.

How it works: All safe period methods are based on the principle that sexual intercourse must be avoided around the time when the female egg is released into the Fallopian tubes. This means a minimum period of four days, to cope with the 72-hour life of the sperm and the 24-hour life of the female egg.

With the *calendar method* the woman has to keep a record of her last twelve menstrual cycles. By deducting eighteen days from the number of days in the shortest cycle and eleven days in the longest cycle, it is possible to calculate when it is safe to have sex. If the woman's cycle varies from twenty-five to thirty-one days, the days that are reasonably safe are the first seven days $(25 - 18 + 7)$, and from day 21 onwards until six days after the next menstrual period $(31 - 11 = 20)$. This is a complicated and old-fashioned method. Far more effective is the *temperature method*. After ovulation, there is a slight rise in a woman's temperature, so that after three consecutive daily temperatures at the higher level it can be assumed sexual intercourse is safe. But to use the method effectively, sex in the time before ovulation must be avoided.

The *mucus method* is a new technique developed in Australia. Around the time of ovulation the cervical mucus changes in consistency. With proper training, women can detect this. The Human Life and Natural Family Planning Foundation exists to supply this training, which is best learned from an expert.

Effectiveness: About nineteen out of every hundred women using the safe period method of contraception get pregnant in the first year. Regular and practiced use would mean a lower failure rate.

Advantages: It is acceptable to the Catholic Church. There are no physical side effects.

Disadvantages: It prevents frequent sexual intercourse.

Women with irregular periods find the calendar method very difficult. A slight infection and a rise in body temperature can upset the temperature method. The mucus method involves study of body secretions, which some women would find distasteful.

Advice: Go to a specialist clinic or doctor for help. You need the best training you can get.

FOAM

About three in every hundred married women rely on contraceptive foam.

How it works: The foam forms a barrier at the cervix to stop sperms entering the womb. It also contains a spermicide which kills the sperm.

Effectiveness: The statistics put together all women who use either contraceptive foams, creams or jellies on their own. About fifteen in every hundred of these get pregnant in the first year of using these methods.

Advantages: Foam can be obtained without a doctor's prescription at drug stores. There are no physical side effects.

Disadvantages: It has a high failure rate. A new application must be made for each act of sexual intercourse.

Advice: Best used with either a condom or a diaphragm. Used on its own, it is better than nothing.

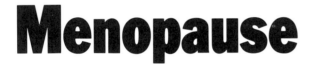

Menopause

Somewhere between the age of forty and sixty every woman faces the menopause, the time when periods stop and pregnancy is no longer possible. It is also known as the change of life or the climacteric, names redolent with the gloom and mystery with which it has been surrounded. But this need not be so. Indeed, one in four women experiences little or no difficulties at all.

The Symptoms: Strictly speaking, the menopause simply describes the end of a woman's periods, but it is often used loosely to cover the time before and after this event when some – but not all – women experience a range of symptoms which can occur either just before the periods begin to change their frequency, or for some years after. The menopause is such a variable phenomenon that as many as two dozen conditions, including irritability, tiredness, dizziness, pins and needles, constipation and flatulence, may be said to be symptoms. But seven are common, and more worrying than the others. These are: hot flashes; depression; vaginal dryness; insomnia; itching skin; aches and pains; and palpitations.

Unpleasant though they may be, these symptoms are not the sign of some dangerous affliction. The menopause is not such a fearful event. It need not just be endured; sensible health rules and a good doctor's help can reduce problems to a manageable minimum; and for some women it is a chance to rethink their lives and start a new career.

ESTROGEN REPLACEMENT THERAPY

Perhaps the single most important choice that faces the middle-aged woman is whether to ask for estrogen replacement therapy over the menopause. Doctors disagree fiercely over ERT (as it is known for short). Almost every article or book is either for or against it. But does it really work? And is it really safe?

Estrogen replacement therapy is based on the theory that during the menopause a woman's ovaries stop producing female eggs, and also stop making the female hormone estrogen. This lack of estrogen, so the argument runs, is the cause of many unpleasant menopausal symptoms. Give a woman estrogen pills to make up for the natural estrogen she has lost, and her symptoms will vanish.

Some doctors are so much in favour of ERT that they think of the menopause as "an estrogen deficiency disease". They have the idea that the menopause "castrates" women by cutting off their hormones. ERT is the means by which women can retain their femininity.

At the other extreme are those doctors, usually male, who believe that the menopause is a fuss about nothing. They give the impression that women who complain of menopausal symptoms are just neurotic or time-wasting. They point out, correctly, that ERT doesn't simply replace estrogen – it usually gives higher permanent levels than those occurring in nature.

The situation facing women is very confusing. The only point of agreement with everybody is that, despite years of use, nobody is really sure what the long-term effects of ERT may be. Women are likely to be offered ERT because a doctor believes in it, or refused it because a doctor opposes it. Rather than relying on just one doctor's advice, women should try to think for themselves, weighing up the risks against the advantages. For there definitely are risks. ERT produces hyperplasia, an abnormal thickening of the womb lining, in some women. The extent of this varies with the dose, and whether progestogen, as well as estrogen, is given. Hyperplasia, in its turn, can lead on to uterine cancer. ERT is definitely linked with womb cancer.

Other health risks are still controversial. Some evidence suggests that ERT may be linked with breast cancer, while other evidence suggests that it may guard against it. From studies on the pill we know that estrogen can lead to heart disease, strokes, high blood pressure and blood clotting troubles, and that these risks increase dramatically as women get older. Different kinds of estrogen are given in ERT, and the doses are smaller than the dose in the pill. It is possible therefore that some of the risks of the pill will not apply to ERT. But we still do not know for certain.

Just as there are risks from ERT, so there are undoubted benefits. ERT prevents, or at least delays, the bone thinning that in some middle-aged women can lead to "dowager's hump". ERT also restores the dry vagina to a moist texture. Hot flashes, which plague so many women, also respond well to ERT. Oddly enough they also respond well to placebos (mock pills containing no medicaments). But unlike placebos, ERT has a long-lasting effect.

One in four lucky women has little or no difficulties during the menopause, and for them there is no point at all in taking ERT. If you are having no trouble with the menopause, do not let an ERT-enthusiastic doctor persuade you into taking it. It would be absurd to take ERT like some kind of youth pill.

Three out of four women *do* experience trouble at the menopause. These women should at least try to cope with traditional remedies before going on to estrogen replacement. For there are other drugs which help, and about two out of these four women may find these are enough to make life tolerable. However, a short burst of ERT to cope with special occasions – a child's wedding or an important conference – can do no harm. So if some important occasion looms it is worth asking your doctor for temporary estrogen replacement to ward off hot flashes.

About half these women experience a truly unpleasant menopause with hot flashes crowding the day and night. The individual woman may well decide that it is worth taking the risks associated with ERT to have relief from these symptoms, bearing in mind that ERT only works directly on hot flashes and vaginal dryness.

Any woman going on ERT for some length of time should first have a thorough medical check-up. A history of diabetes, thrombosis, liver disease, breast lumps, womb trouble, high blood pressure or heart disease means that ERT is not a good idea. Make sure your doctor gives you a thorough examination and checks your blood pressure.

Having made a decision to go on ERT, there is quite a lot that women can do to minimize the risks they run. First of all, any woman on ERT should stop smoking. If she cannot do this, then she should not go on ERT. The combination of smoking and estrogen is very dangerous – as research on the pill has shown.

Secondly, she must insist on the right kind of ERT – estrogen *and* progestogen. Continuous doses of estrogen alone are now known to be dangerous. So is the so-called cyclical dose, in which three weeks of estrogen is given followed by a one-week gap with no pills. These forms of ERT offer considerable risk of hyperplasia.

The safest kind of ERT combines estrogen with progestogen, like the pill. Usually this means three weeks of estrogen followed by a week of progestogen pills. This produces a kind of mock menstruation, in which the lining of the womb is shed. Even so the risk of hyperplasia still occurs, and some doctors are now experimenting with a ten to fourteen day period of progestogen.

The major problem that remains is that the administration of hormones interferes with the body's responses. Normally vaginal bleeding would signal hyperplasia. On ERT there may be no sign, or breakthrough bleeding may occur for other reasons. Thus every woman on ERT should have regular endometrial biopsies, tests on the womb lining, about every twelve to fifteen months. It may also be necessary to have occasional scraping out of the womb.

These precautions mean that ERT is not going to be the simple easy treatment it was once presented as. Nor should it become a lifelong addiction. Ask for the pills to be tapered off every now and again to see if you can cope without it. The sooner you can, the better.

Women who have had early hysterectomies are an exception to some of these rules. If the womb has been removed there can be no risk of hyperplasia. If the ovaries, or part of them, have been removed, regular estrogen therapy may be necessary to guard, among other things, against bone thinning. Some women are particularly prone to this, and so may also benefit from estrogen replacement, regardless of a lack of other menopausal symptoms.

HOT FLASHES

Hot flashes are for some women the worst part of the menopause. In particular, night sweats, which produce insomnia, tiredness and make sleeping in a double bed difficult, can be horrible. There is no doubt that for severe and frequent flashes, estrogen replacement therapy is the most efficient treatment. But if you have only occasional flashes, there are other drugs that are worth trying first. Most of them are a mixture of mild tranquilizers with belladonna, a drug originally extracted from the juice of the deadly nightshade. The tranquilizer damps down the woman's nervous response, and the belladonna works on the blood vessels that produce the hot flashes. Many women find this adequate.

Flashes are made worse by alcohol, hot curries, lots of cups of tea and coffee, and embarrassment. Avoid these, and (in theory at least) the flashes should be reduced, although many women feel the morale building effect of a drink is worth the risk of a flash! The other simple help is some kind of top garment that can be easily taken on and off. Oddly enough, flashes also respond well to placebos, pills containing no drugs at all which the taker believes will cure her. So if you think something helps your flashes, the odds are that it will.

DEPRESSION

This hits many women during the years before and after the menopause. They feel weepy, lethargic, irritable, and unreasonably gloom-ridden. Indeed, because of old wives' tales about the climacteric, some women fear they may be heading for mental breakdown. In fact, this fear is exaggerated. Though many women feel depressed in middle age, there does not seem to be any greater risk of really serious mental illness. Those women who *are* admitted to mental hospital are usually the ones that have some kind of history of mental problems. The menopause has not caused their illness; it has just been the last straw.

Yet even a mild bout of depression is horrible for the sufferer and bad for her family. It is difficult to know how far, however, these feelings are due to the physical changes of the menopause, or how far they are due to the problems of middle age, "the empty nest syndrome" as it is sometimes called. At this time, children are leaving home, women are worried about growing old, and a marriage may be running into difficulties. If this is the case, a marriage counselor may be able to help as much as a doctor.

So women should possibly try to take a look at their lives to see if anything in them needs changing. Is this the moment to go back to work? Or to opt out of a tiring, boring job for something more fulfilling? Or might evening classes, voluntary work, or even a local political group help your morale? This advice sound trite, but it can work. Dr P.A. Van Keep, a Swiss gynecologist, surveyed a number of middle-aged working women. He found that for well-off women, a job seemed to ward off the unpleasant effects of the menopause. But it was just the opposite for the women at the other end of the social scale. For them a job, perhaps because it was boring, ill-paid and taken only because the money was needed, seemed to increase the unpleasant side effects of the change of life.

The other way to help depression is to make sure you are in good physical health. Put your eating habits right. Avoid getting overweight. Take regular exercise. Indulge in some morale-raising new clothes, hair-dos and other treats. Of course, depression can be helped a great deal by a sympathetic doctor who will take time to listen to your troubles. Tranquilizers, or possibly anti-depressants, may help, but don't let an overprescribing doctor give you bad habits:

make sure you can give them up every now and again. The aim is to manage without them. Severe depression needs more expert help, so ask your doctor to refer you for psychiatric help. The sooner you get expert attention the sooner you may get better.

SEX AND VAGINAL TROUBLES

Sexual and genital problems sometimes embarrass middle-aged women so much that they don't seek relief. Yet most of the complaints are easily cured. What is necessary, however, is that women should be frank and explicit with their doctor, who otherwise will probably be unable to diagnose what is wrong.

Dry vagina, also sometimes called vaginal atrophy, sometimes sets in at the menopause. The vagina loses its flexibility and usual moist surface. Try K-Y lubricating jelly round the vaginal opening. If this isn't sufficient help, your doctor may offer you an estrogen ointment, or suppositories. These work well, but their action is not just local. The hormone finds its way into the blood stream. Lavish and regular use of these creams may be the equivalent of taking estrogen replacement therapy – but without the safeguards. In this case, it is safer to opt for the real thing and ask for estrogen replacement therapy (see also page 186, Sex and Age).

There is no truth in the old wives' tale that your sex life has to decline in middle or even old age. Indeed, some doctors think a happy sex life helps keep the vagina in working order. Some women experience a new enthusiasm once the trouble of contraception is finished. So sex is probably good for you during the menopause.

Menstrual irregularities can be confusing during the menopause. Some women have increasingly heavy periods, or sudden floods. It is extremely upsetting, but not usually a sign that need worry you. There are drugs which cut down the flow of menstrual blood and which do not contain hormones: ask your doctor to recommend one. Check, also, that you are not anemic: look out for pale gums and pale corners of the eyes, as these could be a sign. Again, your doctor can test for anemia and prescribe iron tablets.

For most women, however, the periods phase themselves out by becoming either more scanty, or by occurring less frequently. This means that you may find it difficult to know whether bleeding from the vagina is an irregular period or a sign that you need a doctor's check-up. Keeping a record of your periods, to see what their pattern is, is a good idea. Any bleeding that does not seem to fit this pattern or that looks different in consistency, flow or color from normal menstrual bleeding, should be reported to your doctor. You are not wasting his time, but just making a reasonable check.

There is nothing particularly dangerous about the menopause itself, though cancer risks increase with age. Older women should remember to keep doing their regular breast examinations (see page 132) and they should also have a regular cervical smear taken. Doctors will do this, but so, too, will planned parenthood clinics. And don't forget that contraception should be continued for a year after the last period. If an unplanned pregnancy occurs at this stage and is unwanted, an abortion may be sought on the grounds that the risk of having a Mongol (Down's syndrome) baby is at its highest. The first step, though, would generally be an amniocentesis (see Chapter 1).

INSOMNIA

Not being able to sleep quite often causes a lot of unhappiness and worry, which in turn makes it more difficult to sleep! However, if you do find you have a sleep problem, it is worth analyzing why. If you are suffering from hot flashes, these probably include the so-called night sweats, when you wake up bathed in perspiration. In this case if you manage to deal with the hot flashes, either by estrogen replacement or by other treatment, the sweats will also go and your sleeping pattern should be restored.

If, however, your insomnia has nothing to do with sweats, it may be that you are one of those people who has always had a sleeping problem. The menopause, after all, is another stressful experience, like adolescence, illness, losing a job, and so forth. If you have had sleep problems before, you will probably have worked out your own system of coping by now. But before getting addicted to sleeping pills, don't despise the homely remedies of exhausting physical exercise and hot baths. It is also generally true that as we move towards old age, sleeping may become more difficult. However, we do not need that much sleep. Rig up a small lamp by the bedside (so as not to wake your sleeping mate) and if you cannot sleep, read, knit or do anything so that you do not get in the vicious circle of not sleeping, panicking and then being even more unable to relax. For some people, relaxation classes may help (see Chapter 4).

ITCHING SKIN

Itching in the genital area is probably a sign of vaginal dryness. For this and for any other skin irritations, consult your doctor. Skin irritations may be some form of disease, so it is worth making sure. Alternatively, it may just be one of the signs of menopausal "nerves". One form of this is the sensation that hundreds of ants are crawling about under the skin. This is extremely unpleasant, but do not panic. If you have checked with the doctor that it is not a skin disease, then it is just one of the eccentric ways in which the human system copes with the change. If you can cope with your other more serious physical and mental symptoms, this should go away too.

ACHES AND PAINS

If these are more than mild discomforts, check with your doctor to make sure it is not the onset of true arthritis or some other condition that needs treatment. If it is not, the aches and creaks may be a sign of distress at a difficult time of life, and part of the cluster of complaints that women suffer at this time. If you go on ERT, it will probably disappear. Otherwise, try regular exercise and possibly relaxation classes.

PALPITATIONS

This is another of the nervous symptoms women can experience. It is as if the heart beats like thunder or jumps out of the breast. Again, this is a symptom you should check with your doctor just in case there is a serious cause other than the menopause. But it is more likely that it will be simply due to the change, a nervous reaction which is frightening *but nothing else*. Alas, the more you worry about palpitations, the more likely they are to occur, so try not to panic. Mental quietness will help.

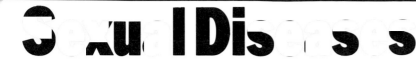

Sexual Diseases

More than a million American men and women are treated for gonorrhea every year, and a further 21,000 are diagnosed as having the first or second stage of syphilis. Yet sensible precautions could cut the incidence of venereal disease and reduce the number of sexually transmitted infections. There are only two major diseases which can be strictly defined as venereal: syphilis and gonorrhea. This is because they are always caught by sexual contact with an infected person. Exceptions are exceedingly rare. There are, however, several other illnesses and infections which are known as sexually transmitted infections, or STI for short. Some are not the result of sexual intercourse, but they are still treated by VD specialists. "I deal with anything between the hips and the knees," says one specialist.

Syphilis: The disease with all the horror stories. Fortunately it is still relatively rare. It *is* increasing, though, among homosexual men. It is easily cured at any stage with penicillin, but because it is such a serious disease doctors perform tests over several months to make sure it has really disappeared.

The first symptoms are sores, usually round the genitals, sometimes round the back passage or the mouth. They look like little craters, the size of a pinhead to a pea, with a shiny red center. They do not hurt and disappear without treatment. The second stage appears weeks or months later with a rash. This does not itch or hurt and indeed it can be confused with other illnesses. If in doubt seek advice; syphilis is extremely serious if untreated.

Gonorrhea is far more common than syphilis. It can be serious if untreated. Women, particularly, risk infertility. The cure is with antibiotics, but repeated tests may be needed. Doctors will probably want patients to take a syphilis blood test later, to check that they do not have both sorts of VD at the same time. Symptoms in men are easily recognized. There is a burning sensation during urination. There is also a greenish-yellow discharge from the tip of the penis. In women, symptoms are less obvious. It may hurt to pass water and there may be a vaginal discharge; but for almost four out of five women there are no symptoms at all, except an infected boyfriend.

Genital herpes is now the second most common sexually transmitted infection in the USA. It is caused by the herpes simplex viruses which also cause cold sores (often found around the mouth). Once infected, a person suffers repeated painful outbreaks. The virus retreats into the body between attacks when the victim is not infectious, and may reappear when the body is exposed to stress of some kind. There is no very effective treatment. Sexual abstinence during attacks may help to prevent spread. Infection in pregnancy puts the baby at risk (see page 16). Herpes is also linked with cervical cancer, so if you have had it get a regular Pap smear (see page 134).

Non-specific urethritis is the illness most on the increase. It is sometimes called non-specific vaginitis or non-gonococcal urethritis. Symptoms are as in gonorrhea: an inflamed urethra (the tube through which the urine passes); pain in passing water; and a discharge. Cures are not always easy; antibiotics are given, but relapses are common. Some men get Reiter's syndrome, which can cause the joints to be painful and swollen. Non-specific urethritis can occur without sex. But it is often sexually transmitted so doctors usually investigate partners, who might be carriers.

Trichomoniasis is caused by a single-celled organism in the female vagina. It has been found in virgins, but it can also be passed on by sex. Some men may be carriers. The cure is usually easy – metronidazole (Flagyl) tablets – but partners must be seen and checked to cut the risk of re-infection. Symptoms are a vaginal itch and sometimes a smelly discharge. In severe cases this can make the genital area red and sore. Occasionally, men have irritation in the penis from the same organism.

Venereal warts: These appear about three months after intercourse with an infected person, and tend to spread. They do not do any harm, except for looking unpleasant and itching slightly. But get them treated.

Other sexually transmitted infections include pubic lice ("crabs") and a skin rash called scabies. Scabies and crabs can be treated with lotion from a druggist, but it is best to check with a doctor to make sure there is nothing else wrong. Two rare infections occasionally turn up – chancroid, in which small ulcers appear on the genitals, and lymphogranuloma venereum, which is marked by sores and swollen glands in the groin. Candidosis (see page 152) is a vaginal infection which may be aggravated by sex and may cause irritation to the penis of the male partner.

CUTTING THE RISK

If you sleep with only one person and you are both faithful, you should avoid gonorrhea and syphilis. "A loving, caring partner is the best protection against VD," says one venereologist. Fidelity, however, does not rule out some of the less serious infections. If you get NSU, trichomoniasis or thrush, do not immediately assume your partner has been unfaithful. One-night stands or sex with strangers naturally carry a higher risk of infection. But it is wrong to assume you will only catch something from bums or prostitutes. Some very nice people have sex infections.

1. Use of a condom helps protect against gonorrhea and NSU, though not against syphilis. There is some evidence that copper IUDs may help protect women against gonorrhea. But the best protection for a woman is to make sure the man wears a condom even if he is vasectomized or she is on the pill.

2. Spermicidal foams, creams, and jellies give women some protection. Use these, particularly if you cannot persuade your male partners to wear condoms.

3. Talk about infection as well as contraception before having sex, say the health education experts. Confident men and women may be able to do this.

4. Urinate and wash after sexual intercourse. This is a way of flushing out germs. Nobody is sure if it works, but it is worth trying.

5. If you have any doubtful symptoms whatsoever, go to a VD clinic or a doctor. This is particularly important for women and homosexual men, who may have very few symptoms. If you are sleeping around a lot, it is worth considering having regular check-ups.

6. Finish any treatment. Many patients do not bother to get the final all-clear from the doctor. Because the symptoms have gone they think they are cured, but this is not always so.

HOLIDAY HEALTH

Vaccinations

We all take sensible measures to protect our health every day in our own familiar environment, but when we travel we are exposed to a new set of hazards. Wise travelers can do a great deal to protect their health. The necessary knowledge can either come from bitter experience or through careful planning. Here we examine the unfamiliar dangers of travel and foreign lands so that the traveler can take all precautions and enjoy the journey. Do not forget to insure yourself against medical expenses which may arise from illness or accident while abroad. It is also worth insuring for the increased air fare which you will have to pay if you have to return home as a stretcher-case occupying three aircraft seats, particularly if you are going on a skiing holiday. In a few countries such as Great Britain, insurance may not be necessary, since any serious illness or accident, and also minor emergencies, may be treated free.

If you fall ill *after* your return home, tell the doctor that you have been abroad and where you have been. Otherwise he is not likely to consider the possibility that you have contracted an unusual disease.

It is important to have the correct vaccinations for foreign travel not only in order to prevent ill-health but also to prevent a great deal of bureaucratic inconvenience. For instance, you might be diverted or have an unscheduled stop-over in a neighboring country. Cholera, smallpox and yellow fever are the subject of strict international regulations and the vaccinations which you are required to have depend on the country you arrive from, not your nationality. For detailed information, consult *Health Information for International Travel*, available from US Department of Health Education and Welfare, Center for Disease Control, Atlanta, Georgia 3033. Or ask the embassy of the country you are going to visit; do not rely on tourist offices, since they are likely to tell you only the minimum requirements.

The most important vaccinations for your personal safety are polio, typhoid and paratyphoid, tetanus and, if you are going to certain countries outside Europe, yellow fever, although others may be legally required in addition. Check that children are up-to-date with the usual childhood vaccinations. Diphtheria and whooping cough are very common in some African and other Third World countries. Vaccination against whooping cough may be advisable in these countries when the balance of risks does not make it automatically advisable in Western countries. **Polio:** Vaccination against polio is advisable for all holidays abroad except those in Northern Europe, Canada, Australia or New Zealand. People going to Spain, Turkey or North Africa are particularly advised to have polio vaccination. It is just as important for adults to be protected as children. Protection starts almost immediately and lasts for five years.

Typhoid and paratyphoid: Although these vaccinations are not required officially, they are the most important vaccinations for US tourists going abroad. They should be routine for all countries except North-West Europe, Canada, Australia or New Zealand. Protection lasts one to three years.

Tetanus: Vaccination is advisable for everyone except for children who are up-to-date with it. The booster for adults lasts five years.

Yellow fever: This disease occurs in parts of equatorial Africa and in Central and South America. Yellow fever is a mosquito-borne disease but vaccination against it is very effective. In the US vaccination may be obtained through the local office of the Public Health Service (listed in the telephone book under US Government, agencies of). This vaccination should not be done if possible at the same time as those for smallpox or polio.

Smallpox: Although this disease has been virtually wiped out, vaccination may still be required in a few countries during the early 1980s. In general, pregnant women, babies, and people who suffer from eczema and certain other diseases should not be vaccinated against smallpox – ask your doctor.

Cholera: Cholera outbreaks are likely in parts of West, Central and East Africa and in the Middle and Far East, and occasionally occur in some Mediterranean countries. However, there is still disagreement over the effectiveness of this vaccination and WHO has expressed no confidence in it. Nevertheless, vaccination may be required for entry into certain countries, although sensible hygienic precautions are the most important preventive measures. A certificate is valid for six months after a six-day waiting period.

Hepatitis: Passive immunity can be given against this disease, which can cause serious illness lasting several months, with an injection of human immunoglobulin (an extract of blood). This measure is well worth taking when traveling to Africa or the Middle or Far East or any country where sanitation is poor. It must be given after the other vaccinations, and lasts for up to five months, depending on the size of the dose given.

Rabies: This vaccine is only generally recommended for a person who has been bitten by an infected animal. Immediate treatment should then be sought.

Malaria: If you are going to a country where there is malaria (see page 175), you should make sure you obtain

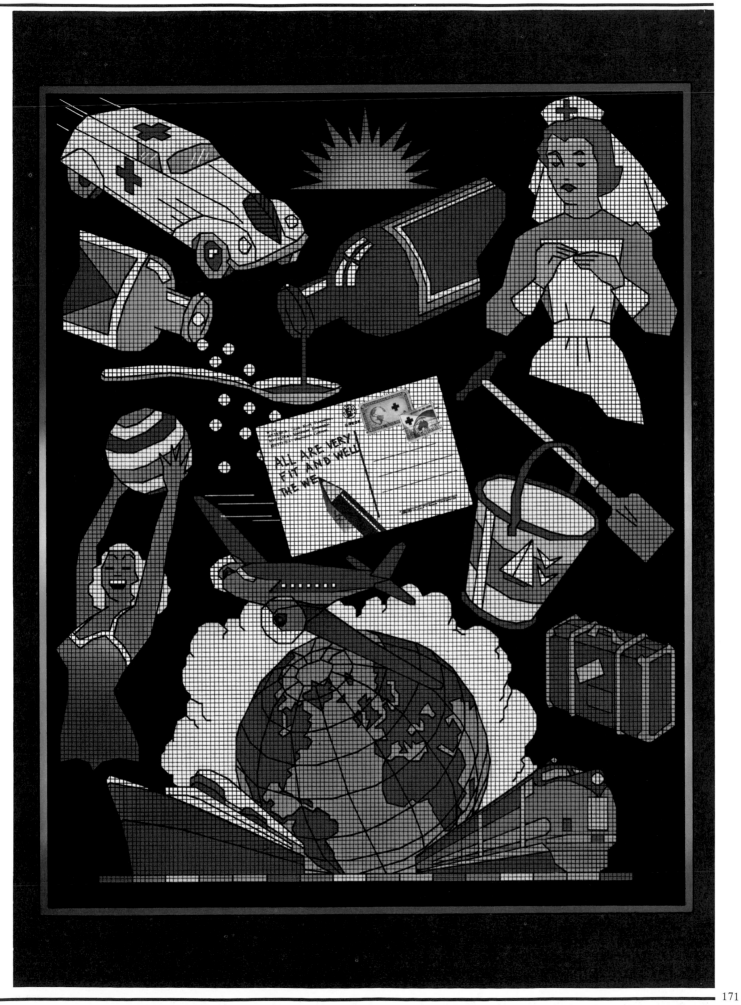

drugs to prevent the disease before you leave, and continue to take them for at least eight weeks after you have left the malarial area.

Smallpox, yellow fever and polio are live virus vaccines and ideally should be given with at least a three-week interval in between. If this is not possible, they can all be given on the same day, although the combination of smallpox and polio should be avoided if at all possible. Polio protection lasts five years, smallpox protection three years, and yellow fever protection ten years.

All vaccinations other than that for yellow fever can be given by a family doctor, but it is important that they are spaced out correctly for maximum benefit and minimum side effects. It is common to feel feverish after certain vaccinations and best to have an early night and avoid drinking alcohol, otherwise you may feel very ill.

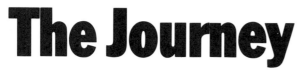

The Journey

MOTION SICKNESS

It has long been known that car drivers seldom suffer from motion sickness while passengers, especially those in the back seat, often do. This difference gives clues to the understanding of motion sickness and suggests ways in which we can control or prevent it. A person who is vulnerable should imitate the movements of the driver, even to the extent of pretending to drive with a toy steering wheel. However, it may not be necessary to go that far.

It appears that there is a natural position for the head when it is moving normally with the body, as in running around a bend: the head and body lean into the bend. This rule is broken when the body is moved artificially, and the head is thrown into unnatural positions. Drivers, or sailors occupied on the deck of a boat, are inclined to steady themselves by leaning into the motion and so maintain a more natural posture, while passengers are much more likely to allow their body to be moved passively and so are thrown into an unnatural posture. When the head is in an unnatural posture, there is a discrepancy between the information a person receives in the brain through the eyes about their bodily position and that received through the balance organs in the ear. This is what causes sickness. Doctors suggest two strategies for minimizing travel sickness:

Active strategy

A. If possible sit in the front seat and imitate the driver leaning into bends. If necessary use a toy steering wheel. Alternatively, restrict head movement by using a head rest.
B. Look ahead at the road. If forced to sit sideways, still look ahead and change seats from time to time to avoid a crick in the neck. Don't turn round to talk to passengers in the back seat.
C. Do not think about your stomach even if you start to get the first signs of queasiness. Talk or listen to talking on the radio (not music), or do mental arithmetic – anything to engage the mind.
D. Don't read, because this takes your eyes off the road. If you must read maps, ask the driver to slow down or better

still stop, especially if the road has many bends.
E. If badly affected, try drugs such as Marezine, though Marezine should not be taken in pregnancy. The Victorians believed that bubbly drinks such as champagne helped, but too much alcohol, which prevents the eyes from concentrating on the road ahead, is almost certainly self-defeating. Passengers going on a long journey are best advised to stick to the limit of one or two small drinks.
F. On boats, walk around on deck and scan the shore, the horizon or the sky – the only stable reference points – and lean into the motion of the ship. Do not watch seagulls or waves which are moving irregularly.
G. Provide children with special car seats so that they can see out of the window. These are also safer.

Passive strategy

This is the only possible strategy on airplanes, unless you have a window seat on a clear day, and the only strategy on ships at night, unless you want to stay on deck and look at the stars.
A. If possible, lie down on your back with face upwards. This limits head movement and puts your balance organ (otolith) in the most neutral position.
B. Shut your eyes: this reduces conflicting signals reaching the brain. Listen to the radio or talk if you cannot sleep.
C. Anxiety is often an additional cause of travel sickness. Yoga, meditation or other established methods of relaxation should help if you are familiar with them.

Especially for children

Children under twelve are particularly vulnerable to travel sickness, perhaps because they cannot so easily see out of the window and are not so interested in scenery. Get special car seats for young children. Play games such as counting horses or buses ahead (it does not count if it is behind). Open windows to provide some wind on the face: no one knows why this works but it may be by providing the body with another sense of movement, or by reducing the stuffy car smells which may cause nausea.

JET-LAG

The body has a regular daily rhythm in its temperature, sweating and pulse rate. When you fly north or south and do not change time zones, these rhythms are not interrupted; but when you travel east or west the rhythms of sleeping and waking are altered and it may take days for the body to adjust. After traveling across time zones, normally simple actions take place out of time: a person may want to empy their bladder several times during the night or move their bowels at a time they never would usually.

To minimize jet-lag try to have a good night's sleep before you go, and try to plan your journey so that you arrive near your normal bedtime and are able to sleep when you arrive. Keep alcohol down to a minimum while traveling, especially if you are traveling to a warm country, because it will delay your acclimatization. It is vital to allow time for rest after arrival and not attempt to go straight into an important meeting. If you do, you may make a wrong decision.

The pressure in the cabin is reduced during flight in even the most modern airplanes, and this often gives rise to a distended feeling as gases in the bowel expand. It may help to eat sparingly on the airplane. The atmosphere in an airplane is comparatively dry and people generally lose a

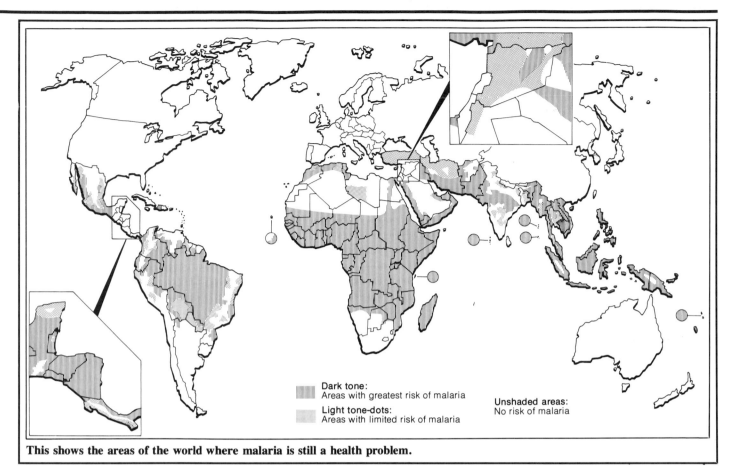

Dark tone: Areas with greatest risk of malaria	
Light tone-dots: Areas with limited risk of malaria	**Unshaded areas:** No risk of malaria

This shows the areas of the world where malaria is still a health problem.

lot of fluid. Soft drinks and water will help, but avoid fizzy drinks, which are likely to add to the distended feeling. Wear loose-fitting clothing and shoes, because the legs are likely to swell during the flight as a result of the restriction of movement, which prevents a full return of blood to the rest of the body.

Your ears

Diving under water, especially with an aqualung, and also high flying, may produce sharp changes of pressure in the ear. Anyone who has difficulty in equalizing the air pressure behind the drum should seek specialist advice before diving or flying. In flying, the main problem is coming down to land. Although all commercial flights have pressurized cabins, repressurization may happen quite sharply. When coming down in a plane it is always advisable to swallow at regular intervals, waggle the jaw, and if necessary pinch the nose and blow down it. This allows the air pressure to equalize in both sides of the eardrum by allowing the passage of air through the Eustachian tube, which connects the middle ear to the back of the throat. People who have special difficulty may find additional benefit from using decongestant nose drops or nasal sprays for two days before flying. Where possible, do not fly when you have a cold.

The commonest complication of air travel is a conductive deafness caused by blockage of the Eustachian tube, preventing pressure equalization. However, sudden changes in pressure may occasionally affect the inner ear as well, and cause rupture of a small membrane covering the entrance to the cochlea. Fluid may leak out, producing deafness and giddiness. As this condition is treatable by operation, it is vital to seek specialist advice as soon as possible. Delay may result in irreversible deafness.

When You Arrive

HYGIENE

The commonest source of illness among travelers is diarrhea caused by eating food contaminated by bacteria. Several more serious diseases, such as cholera, typhoid, paratyphoid, bacillary dysentery, hepatitis, amebic dysentery and other parasitic diseases, are caught from food prepared without sufficient regard to hygiene or from contaminated water. But most common of all is travelers' diarrhea, also known by picturesque names such as Montezuma's revenge, which is often caused by exotic local varieties of the common colon bacillus. People who come from Western countries with high standards of hygiene are vulnerable to these diseases, because they have not developed immunity over the years, unlike residents of countries where standards of hygiene are lower.

It is vital in countries where the general standard of hygiene is low to maintain the highest personal standard of hygiene, in order to avoid unpleasant and debilitating diarrhea. Vaccinations will protect against typhoid and paratyphoid but there are other serious diseases which can only be avoided by hygienic measures. And there seems to be an endless variety of travelers' diarrhea.

We recommend the following strict hygienic measures, which should be taken in any non-European, non-Western country. People going on package tours to Russia have contracted an unpleasant parasite called *Giardia* by simply brushing their teeth in tapwater. Care must also be taken in Mediterranean countries. The more insanitary the conditions in the country you are visiting, the stricter your personal hygienic measures must be.

1. Always boil or sterilize drinking water, including water used to clean teeth. Boiling is best but filtration with special equipment is effective and so is sterilization with chlorine tablets or iodine drops. Iodine tincture is more effective against ameba than chlorine tablets: add two drops of 2 per cent tincture of iodine to a quart of uncloudy water, and leave for half an hour. Remember that however high you are in mountain areas there is almost certainly someone else higher up putting their wastes into the water. If you have to drink unsterilized water, try to make sure it comes from a deep well with a wall around it to prevent surface water draining in.

2. Be cautious with shellfish – try to see them alive first. Avoid cold, cooked food.

3. Make sure food is well cooked and has not been left standing.

4. Make sure all fruits and tomatoes are peeled, or immerse in iodine water for half an hour.

5. Sterilize lettuce and unpeeled fruit with chemically treated water.

6. Only drink milk if it has been boiled, and do not eat raw cheese unless foreign residents tell you it is reliable. You can always cook it.

7. Do not eat leftovers or local ice creams.

8. Drink mineral waters made by reputable firms. Coca Cola, Pepsi Cola and other internationally licensed brand names can usually be relied upon and so can other soft drinks made in the same factories by the same local operator.

9. Avoid any food which may have been visited by flies.

10. If specially vulnerable to stomach complaints, consult your doctor about taking a sulphonamide-type drug, as a preventive but do not relax the hygienic measures. Enterovioform and other types of clioquinol drugs such as Mexaform have been suggested as the cause of extremely serious side effects on the nervous system. These drugs, which are also sold under many other names, have not been proven to be effective in treatment of diarrhea, and in the United States are only permitted by the FDA for treatment of amebiasis.

How to cope with diarrhea

Rest as much as you can and be sure to take plenty of fluids such as orange squash, soft drinks or fruit juice. Potassium is lost from the body when a person suffers diarrhea, and it is important to replace this as much as possible. It may be best to eat nothing for the first twenty-four hours, or if the attack is not too bad and you feel hungry eat a bland, starchy diet such as plain boiled rice which seems to help settle the stomach. It is best to avoid milk, which may make the bowel irritation worse. Diarrhea is the natural reaction of the bowel trying to expel invading organisms or irritating poisons, and so it is best not to try to prevent this with antispasmodic drugs such as Lomotil which paralyze the intestine.

If you do feel the need to treat the symptoms, an old-fashioned cure is still among the best; this is kaolin and morphine mixture, which relieves discomfort and slows the diarrhea. Drugs such as Streptotriad which attack the invading organisms may also help, although some diarrheas are caused by viruses which will not be stopped by any drugs. If diarrhea becomes acute, worsens or has not gone away after two or three days, then it is best to consult a doctor if you can. Stay indoors out of the sun if you have diarrhea, so that you avoid any unnecessary dehydration through sweating.

HEAT AND SUN

It takes a few days to acclimatize to a hot country, and some people may take a week or more. During this period the body increases the flow of blood through the skin, and more sweat with a lower salt content is produced. Sometimes the ankles swell up. It is important during this time to take things easily and rest indoors in the middle of the day, take plenty of fluids, eat extra salt, wear light clothing, and avoid drinking excessive amounts of alcohol.

If these precautions are not taken, you may suffer from heat exhaustion caused primarily by lack of salt and water in the body. The symptoms are lethargy, giddiness, headache, and sometimes muscle cramps and nausea. In some cases, a person may suffer from vomiting and collapse. The best treatment is rest in a cool room and plenty of fluids such as squash or fruit juice containing a small amount of salt.

In cases of severe exposure to heat, a person may suffer from heatstroke. Their temperature rapidly rises, their skin is dry, they vomit, collapse and go into a coma. This is caused by a failure of the body to control its temperature by sweating. The victim must be cooled by continuous spraying with cool water and vigorous fanning. Once the temperature is controlled, the victim can be treated as for heat exhaustion. Basic rules to avoid heat exhaustion are:

(a) avoid physical fatigue during the first few days in a hot climate;

(b) drink one pint of water for every ten degrees Fahrenheit outside temperature, or two liters of water plus another liter for every ten degrees centigrade:

(c) take extra salt with food.

Prickly heat: This is the name of an irritating rash which is common in hot climates. It is caused by the blocking of sweat glands through the formation of very itchy red pimples. It often occurs in the armpits, around the waist, and over the breastbone and forearms, where there are clefts in the skin and where clothes rub against the body. It can be prevented by wearing loose clothes which allow the sweat to evaporate more easily. Always wear cotton in hot climates; avoid nylon or any synthetic fibre. Wash frequently and apply talcum powder to the sore area. If the rash becomes infected, consult a doctor since an antibiotic cream may be necessary.

Sunburn: This can be extremely unpleasant but there is no need for anyone to suffer from it. In extreme cases, sunburn may cause a person to feel generally ill with headache, nausea and vomiting and high fever. But it is entirely preventable. Anyone going to the Mediterranean or Caribbean in the summertime should only spend half an hour in the sun on the first day, unless they have already had exposure to the sun at home, and not more than fifteen minutes in a tropical country. Each day the length of time in the sun can be roughly doubled, but be careful that areas such as shoulders and nose which tend to catch the sun do not burn. Products such as Pabonal or Pre-Sun, which block ultra violet radiation, are useful to protect exposed areas for sensitive people.

However, a cream does not give complete protection from exposure to the sun, and if you want to spend more time on a beach it is better to put on a shirt and wear a hat and thin trousers. It can also be a good idea to wear an old shirt while swimming and playing in the water. It is important not to forget the power of reflected light. People with fair skins need to be specially careful, since they may burn without even leaving the shade of a beach umbrella. Fair people are advised to take all precautions, and to wear long-sleeved clothing and use protective cream at least for the first few days of the holiday. Some doctors recommend vitamin A and calcium carbonate tablets to prevent burning, but trials showing them to be effective have not been controlled according to the strictest criteria and they may not be so effective as manufacturers claim.

If you do suffer from sunburn you may find that calamine lotion is soothing. Do not burst any blisters if you can help it. If blisters become infected, consult a doctor. Antihistamine tablets may help if irritation is intense.

It is best to get polaroid sunglasses because they cut down on light evenly across the spectrum; cheap sunglasses may let light in at some wavelength sufficient to damage the eyes.

SWIMMING

Two of the commonest hazards of the shore are sharp rocks and *sea-urchins*. It is good sense to wear sandals or sneakers while bathing in rocky areas frequented by sea urchins. If you stand on a sea urchin, remove as many of the spines as you can with your fingers and use tweezers (eyebrow tweezers are ideal) to remove any awkward ones. If you cannot remove a spine yourself, go to a doctor, who will do it for you. Leaving a spine in is sure to cause infection.

Jelly fish are another common hazard and are best given a wide berth. They can give an extremely unpleasant sting which can cause acute shock or collapse. The worst type is the Portuguese man-of-war, which is bluish-purple in color and has many tentacles. They go around in shoals and it is advisable to keep well out of their way. If stung by a jelly fish, apply soothing calamine lotion. If a fever follows or the pain is intense, consult a doctor. Sea anemones and sting rays can also give an unpleasant sting, and so can some fish if you stand on them when they are hiding in the sand. Treat them as for jellyfish stings.

OTHER HAZARDS

Insect-borne diseases: In many tropical and subtropical countries precautions must be taken to prevent malaria and other insect-borne diseases. Travelers are often given insufficient warning about these hazards, which are preventable if sensible precautions are taken. Malaria is caused by a parasite which is spread from one person to another by mosquitoes. The mosquitoes breed in wet, swampy areas and are active at night. Malaria is an extremely serious disease, killing more than one out of every hundred visiting Europeans who get it. However, it is possible to live perfectly safely in malarial areas if simple precautions are strictly adhered to.

The most important precaution against malaria is to take tablets of a drug which prevent the malaria parasite from growing in the blood if you are bitten by an infected mosquito. Obtain the drug from a doctor and if possible take it for two weeks before you go. The drug should be taken for two months after leaving the malarial area. Another drug (pyrimethamine) is available which is more suited to children because it does not have a bitter taste. In some areas (parts of Brazil, Southern Tanzania and around Vietnam, Laos and Cambodia) the parasite is resistant to these drugs and so special advice should be taken locally.

It is also important in malarial areas to take routine steps to avoid being bitten by mosquitoes. These are based on the knowledge that the malaria-carrying mosquitoes bite between dusk and dawn. After dusk, wear long trousers and long-sleeved shirts. Use an insect-repellent on the exposed skin areas. Those based on diethyl toluamide are probably more effective and are recommended by the Consumer's Union in New York. These applications only last up to about four hours, and less if you are sweating. If possible, make sure that all windows are covered with mosquitonetting, and use a mosquito-net over your bed. Check that there are no holes in the netting; if there are, the mosquitoes are sure to find them. Another useful measure is an aerosol spray to kill any stray mosquitoes which penetrate the room.

In Mediterranean countries, where malaria is not a threat but mosquitoes are still a nuisance, basic precautions can be simpler. Do not open the shutters at night until you have put the light out, and use the patent insect-repellent spiral taper – usually obtainable locally – which smolders through the night giving off smoke.

Other insect-borne and parasitic diseases: *Kala-azar* is an unpleasant and debilitating fever spread by sandflies. It occurs on some Mediterranean shores, including those of Greece, Yugoslavia, Southern Italy, Sicily, Spain and North Africa, and even on parts of the western end of the French Riviera. Fortunately, the disease is relatively rare. The sandfly is so small that a mosquito-net will not keep it out, and the only precaution is insect-repellent.

Filaria worms which cause *elephantiasis* – a gross swelling of the lymph glands – are carried by mosquitoes in various parts of the tropics. Other filaria worms which affect the eyes are carried by forest-flies and buffalo-gnats. These are rare in towns while nets and repellents will protect against them in the countryside.

Sleeping sickness is spread by the tsetse fly in Gambia, Sierra Leone, Ghana, Nigeria, Cameroon, Rhodesia and East Africa, but is only a serious hazard in rural areas. Several other diseases such as *dengue*, *yellow fever* are carried by insects, so it is worth taking precautions against insect bites in tropical and sub-tropical countries.

If you are traveling rough and staying in local houses, take insecticide powder to prevent attacks from fleas and ticks. Do not go about barefoot in underdeveloped countries, except on the beach, or you may be invaded by hookworms, which bore into the foot and then move to the bowel, causing debilitating disease.

A parasite called *bilharzia* – known to soldiers during the war as Bill Harry – lives in freshwater snails and as a parasite in man. It is most common in North, Central and parts of South Africa, but is also found in Brazil, Venezuela, the island of St Lucia, Iran, Iraq and isolated parts of Spain and Portugal. It can be completely avoided by not bathing in infected water, because the parasite can burrow into the skin, and by always drinking water that has been rendered clean – and therefore completely safe – through boiling.

A HEALTHY OLD AGE

Starting to Live

More people are living longer than ever before. In 1940 barely 7 per cent of the US population were over the age of sixty-five. Today the proportion is over 10 per cent and it is projected to rise beyond 12 per cent by the year 2000. The numbers and proportions of this elderly population will continue to grow as living conditions – notably sanitation and housing – and medical practise improve. This greater longevity will increase demands on medical and welfare services. It will also increase obligations for looking after ageing parents or other relatives. But growing old does not mean that people are unable to help themselves. Nor does it mean that people are inevitably condemned to poor health.

Few people in fact die of old age itself. A majority of even those who survive into their eighties or beyond still die of the same diseases as the rest of us: heart disease, cancer and strokes. Although older people become ill more easily than younger people and take longer to recover, generally they need to take the same measures to conserve and promote health as everyone else: eat a balanced diet, take regular exercise and stop or restrict smoking. It also helps to remain active mentally and maintain an active social life.

However, there are some health problems which are a particular consequence of growing older or, at least, more likely to occur among older people. There are also some universal problems which manifest themselves in different ways among the ageing. This chapter is devoted to these problems so that older people may help themselves – or children help their parents – to enjoy their later years.

Think of your life as having four distinct periods. The first twenty years or so are spent getting under way – childhood, schools, adolescence, further education and first jobs. During the next twenty years or so comes setting up homes, bringing up children, sorting out jobs and careers, deciding on what kind of life you want and doing something to try to achieve it. During the third twenty years or so, you consolidate and enjoy the pattern of your life; for most of the time, at least, your children have taken responsibility, or some responsibility, for their own lives. Then come twenty or thirty years or more of a new life, retired from the job that has occupied much of your attention and emotions for so long and with almost unrestricted possibilities of development. If you get it right, this can be the most satisfying period of all.

But if you are going to get it right you would do well to spend some time thinking about it before you reach it. If you look around, you will find plenty of examples of those who didn't get it right. They are probably no more numerous than those who have muddled their opportunities in earlier parts of life. If you intend to make the most of the opportunities in the last decades, however, it is worth looking at what produces unhappiness in this period.

The first cause of frequent rage and bafflement is that you should be retiring at all. People often work in large companies, see their seniors collect watches and retirement presents, and yet still manage to feel that an exception should be made for them. Sometimes, especially in small businesses, retiring ages can be more flexible so that people with healthy minds and bodies can stay at work. Yet it is as unreasonable to get too upset about retirement as to get irritated about a rainstorm: both will turn up at sometime or other. You need only to be ready, and what you need to avoid is a querulous, ill, self-pitying old age.

It is quite certain that shutting your mind to novelty is also bad, and so dismissing the modern social scene, the political parties and the lively arts should be avoided. What this means is that you must not choose your friends and companions from only your own age group. If you want to find what is novel, you are most likely to find it out from those younger than you.

The first decision, probably, that this affects is where you are to live. The choice is yours, but think very carefully indeed before you move. You may want to spend the rest of your life among those of your age and older, but be sure; leaving your old home can also mean leaving your old friends. It is usually best for elderly people to stay in their own community, where they are known. If you do move, make sure that your new home is reasonably accessible if you want people to visit you, especially your children and

Martha Leitch (*right*) was 66 when she first took up swimming. She learnt to swim on her second lesson, though she admits she has developed her own rather unusual style of breaststroke. Miss Leitch remembers when as a rather delicate child she was not even allowed to go in the sea with her brothers and sisters. Since she joined an old people's center nearly three years ago she has never been lonely and rarely inactive. She joined because she thought she would like to learn something such as painting. But there were so many other classes available that she has only just got around to joining the art class. She takes nine subjects – and is the star pupil in yoga.

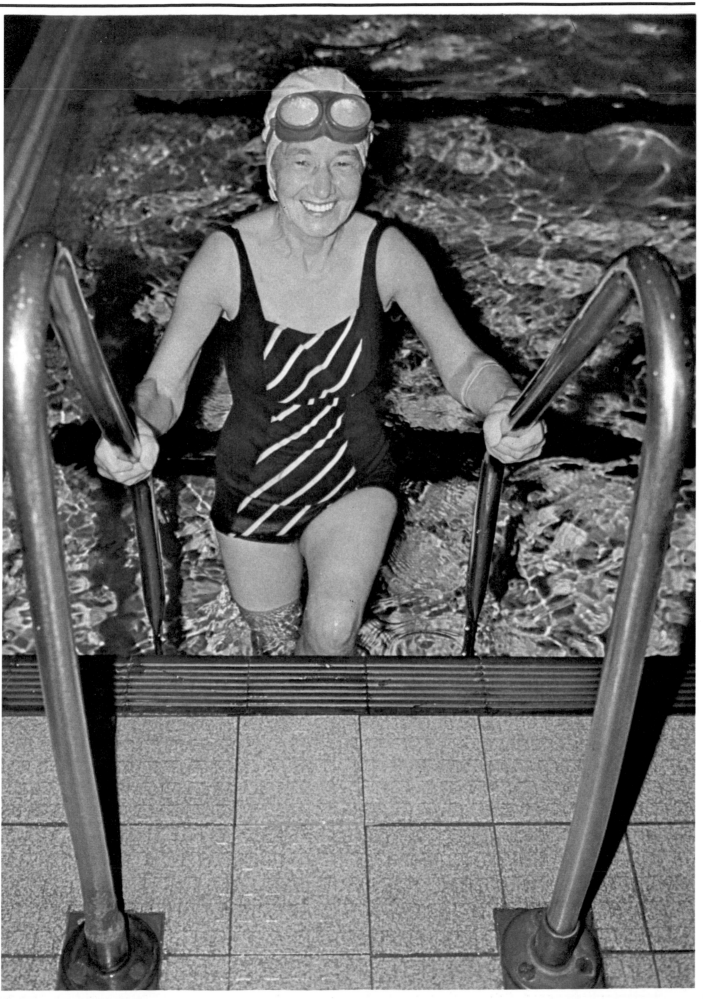

other relatives. The recreation may sometimes be better but a society formed merely of one age group can be not only confining but also more limited in the range and adequacy of its medical and welfare services. Consider, too, the availability of public transport; many old people have neither the money nor the health to drive their own cars for very long.

Planning for retirement has to involve some thought of money. The Social Security system is far too complex to be outlined in a general book of this kind, not least because individual circumstances do vary enormously. But many specialist organizations like the Social Security Agency, the Veterans' Bureau and regional offices of the Department of Health, Education and Welfare will be able to explain what it means for *you*. Your bank manager, insurance broker or accountant will be able to advise on saving and investment. Large businesses and labor unions are further sources of expertise and help about retirement.

Many senior citizens are content to spend their retirement pursuing hobbies for which there was previously no time. But considerable numbers still want to do some work, maybe voluntary work in community or church programs, maybe for extra money such as helping at the supermarket, but maybe something entirely different from earlier careers. Surprising numbers of people discover new talents in creative fields in their sixties and seventies. But always treat any investment with care. And married couples should always ensure that decisions are joint decisions – whatever they choose to do or not to do.

One very sharp change that the husband and wife should prepare for occurs when both spend the day about the house. For a long time one or both has been going out to work, and the effect on the household has been to allow them some relaxation from continuous company. Each has been able to meet others. With retirement, it suddenly becomes possible for them to spend a solid twenty-four hours cluttering up the house, creating an obligation to provide an extra meal a day, and quickly exhausting any repertoire of interesting events and people to talk about. It is extremely important to maintain a lively mind in retirement. Going out to work opens windows on what could otherwise be a claustrophobic world.

You can also use these retirement years to enrich your mind. A worryingly large number of people start, in old age, to regret the education they missed when young. Education the first time around, however, tends to lead to a career; the second time, it can really be for its own sake. There is a wide range of evening classes, week-end schools and summer schools, and they all have the advantage of mixed age groups and mixed social backgrounds. For the determinedly academic there is even university, and not necessarily at degree level either.

Naturally this advice applies throughout to men and women equally, and the choices made must allow for the preferences, or at least balance the preferences, of husbands and wives. Women have the advantage that if they have been "only" housewives the transition to pensioner status can be less abrupt.

The whole quality of your life will depend on your health. You are bound to suffer minor afflictions, and it is important to get advice from your doctor while they are still minor: don't put off the visit because you feel it is simply a matter of getting old. Many of the afflictions of old age are debilitating because the sufferers do not have much to do

except think about their health. Being busy in mind is, as ever, a good piece of preventive medicine. But make sure that you are also being practical about, for example, diet and avoiding accidents to which the old become increasingly liable. The following pages spell out in some detail how elderly people can help themselves, and how children can help their ageing parents.

CARING FOR AN ELDERLY PARENT: 11 RULES

1. **Loneliness.** One of the greatest problems of old age. Visit your parents regularly, and remember their anniversaries and special days. Try to get them out of the house for regular commitments such as a luncheon or social club. Do everything you can to keep them in touch with their own community where they have their friends. If possible, install a telephone and call them often.

2. **Warmth.** Help them to reorganize their house so that in the winter it is possible to live in one bed-sitting-room. Insulate the house and provide safe extra heating to protect them against hypothermia during a cold spell.

3. **Diet.** Make sure they are eating a varied diet and that they are not having having difficulty in shopping. Don't just ask them what they eat; look in the cupboard.

4. **Eyesight and hearing.** About one in seven people have such inadequate glasses that they cannot easily read the newspaper. Better lighting helps and large-type books are available from most libraries. Annual eye check-ups are advisable. Make sure your parents also have regular hearing tests.

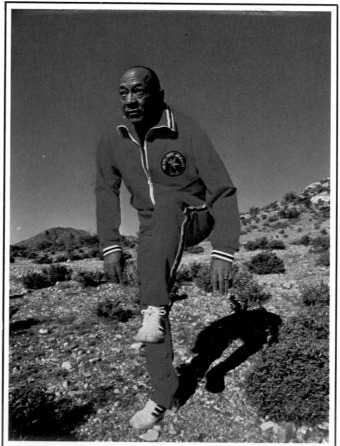

Jesse Owens exercises regularly to maintain his fitness in retirement in Phoenix, Arizona. At one time he held four world track and field records, including an Olympic broad jump record lasting twenty-four years. He is now active in community and youth work.

5. **Mobility.** It is vital for old people to keep moving and, if possible, to get out of the house every day. Make sure they are getting any chiropody they need – foot ailments, unlike routine foot care, is generally covered by medical insurance.

6. **Benefits.** Make sure the local welfare services knows about your parents and that they are taking advantage of any local facilities as well as Social Security benefits.

7. **Incontinence.** Look for any signs that your parents are having trouble with incontinence. Simple practical measures may solve the problem (see page 184), but don't be shy about seeking medical advice.

8. **Bereavement.** When one parent dies the other will need you to share their grief. It is necessary to work through grief before a new life can be started. Remember they will want to talk about the dead person: this is natural and healthy. Tranquilizers cannot do more than provide a temporary solution, and are probably best avoided because they interfere with the normal process of sorting out and understanding of feelings. Try not to let the surviving parent make any irrevocable decisions such as moving house until a year has passed.

9. **Drugs.** Many old people have trouble with their medicines. Make sure they understand when each tablet has to be taken, and help them work out a timetable system. If in doubt, do not hesitate to telephone the doctor or the druggist to check. Make sure that your parent asks to see the doctor when he or she gets a repeat prescription.

10. **Depression.** Watch for the following signs: loss of appetite, disturbed sleep, and general loss of vigor and interest in life. Depression can often be successfully treated with drugs, so take your parent to the doctor.

11. **Accidents.** Do all you can to make the house secure against accidents (see page 180). Secure loose carpets, avoid long electrical cords, make sure these is lighting in cupboards and dark passages, provide bannisters on both sides of the stairs.

LONG LIFE AND HEALTH

Although few people die of old age itself, there are medical consequences of the ageing process. The arteries slowly harden in old age and this process is aggravated by atheroma, which causes blood vessels to silt up and can lead to strokes and heart disease. Cells throughout the body are replaced by inactive supporting tissue. Specialized cells slowly die in various organs of the body, making the body much less adaptable to sudden stresses. The cells of the skin, the intestine and the blood usually continue to be replaced in the normal way, but the fibrous tissue supporting the skin changes so that skin wrinkles and becomes less elastic. The skin is likely to become covered with areas of pigment and the flesh is easily bruised, particularly the backs of hands. Muscles waste slowly and bones become thinner and more brittle. An old person often shrinks in height because of thinning bones and permanent changes in posture. The brain itself also loses cells which are irreplaceable. This may affect an old person's intellectual powers but most commonly affects their ability to remember recent events. The older person should feel fit and happy, and only under the stress of sudden physical exertion should there be any difference between an old person and a younger. The body's ability to adapt to ageing is remarkable.

Because old people become ill more easily than young people and take longer to recover, they often suffer from

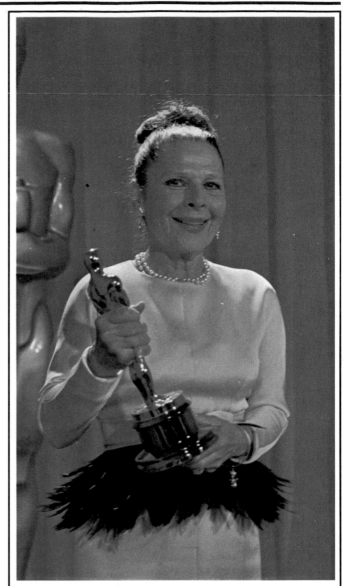

Ruth Gordon was in her seventies when she won an Academy Award for her role in the movie *Rosemary's Baby*. Born in 1896 she wrote plays as well as acting in them, and marked her eightieth birthday by starting a new book. "Stay up to date," she says "and people want to hang in with you."

several disabilities or illnesses at once. This creates special difficulties for doctors in diagnosing their illness and in treating it. Old people are often slow to recognize the importance of symptoms of illness in old age and too ready to put up with them, partly because they attribute these symptoms to ageing. In the checklist at the end of this chapter we list a number of important symptoms which should lead old people to consult their doctor.

Do not, however, be unduly depressed by this recital of the consequences of ageing. Innumerable men and women remain vigorous, active and healthy through their seventies, eighties and even nineties. In our researches for this book we met an 87-year-old cyclist, an 85-year-old dancer, a 92-year-old runner and a 67-year-old swimmer. But you do not have to be particularly athletic to enjoy your later years. At evening classes throughout the country old people are learning new skills and hobbies. Some are even studying for university degrees. Should anyone discount the qualitative contribution of older people to our way of life, they should re-read their history books.

Conserve Health and Fitness

Old people, as has been said earlier, need to take the same measures to conserve health as younger people. You must take care to eat a balanced diet, take exercise and stop or at least cut down on smoking. It also helps to remain active mentally, socially and sexually. But here, in alphabetical order, is more specific advice.

Accidents

A major threat to the aged, but a great deal can be done to make an old person's house safer and to prevent falls and burns. More accidents to old people in the home occur on the stairs than any other place in the house. Make sure that the carpets are securely fixed on the stairs and that corridors and stairs are well lit. Remove clutter. If there is a step in a difficult place, mark it with bright paint and a special light. Carpets and rugs should have non-slip backs and floors should not be polished underneath them. Put a non-slip mat in the bath and install a grab-handle. For someone who is very infirm, a walk-in shower with a flexible shower hose and a stool to sit on will be much easier than a bath. If possible, obtain a non-slip bathroom floor covering. Try to get rid of uneven surfaces and replace any defective tiles or linoleum.

To avoid burns, the most important measures are not to smoke in bed and to make sure that any paraffin heater is one of the modern self-extinguishing kind which can be tipped over with safety. Be sure to use a fire guard around an open fire or the electric type with a red-hot element; many old people suffer dreadful burns from night-clothing catching fire. Woolen, nylon and terylene fabrics are safest. Hot water bags should be renewed regularly because an old bag can split and cause a bad scald. Electric blankets should be serviced annually; remember there is a danger if they get wet. For old people, electric stoves are safest.

Bed

It is best for old people not to spend too much time in bed as this can cause muscle wastage, bedsores, congestion of lungs and the clotting of blood in leg veins. Simply the weight of blankets on the feet over long periods can cause foot-drop. If you have to spend a long time in bed, obtain a cradle to lift the weight of the blankets off the feet and provide bedclothes which are as light as possible yet provide all necessary warmth. To prevent bedsores, don't stay in one position all the time in bed as the pressure on the skin cuts off the blood supply and damages the skin by pressing it against the bone. Also, lie propped up with pillows, with a protective pad under the legs to take the weight off the heels. Sheepskin bootees are an alternative way of protecting the heels from bedsores. If a person cannot move they should be lifted into another position once every hour. If an old person is bedridden, it is advisable to ask the doctor what home nursing services are available locally.

Bowels

It is not necessary to have a bowel motion every day. Some people go on average every three days and are still not constipated. A person is only constipated if the feces are hard, not simply if the bowels have not moved for forty-eight hours. To prevent constipation, eat a diet with plenty of roughage, whole wheat bread and whole wheat breakfast cereal, and drink at least four or five pints of liquid a day (more in hot weather). It is also important to go to the toilet when the need is first felt and not delay. Regular exercise helps to strengthen the abdominal muscles which help in bowel movement. Constipation can have serious consequences in old people by interfering with the emptying of the bladder and causing mental confusion. If it does not respond to increased roughage in the diet or mild laxatives, it should be treated by the family doctor.

Deafness

This is extremely common in old age but often goes unnoticed or is accepted because it comes on so gradually. Loss of hearing should be reported to the doctor. Quite often it is simply due to an accumulation of wax which can be syringed out. If this is not the explanation it may be necessary to see a specialist. Many people who would benefit from a hearing aid do not have one simply because they have not had their hearing investigated. When talking to deaf people, do not automatically shout. It may be that their problem is in interpreting the sounds they hear rather than in actually hearing them. Try to talk slowly and distinctly, accentuating consonants. Talk face to face so that they can lip-read or at least get clues by watching your mouth, and make sure that your face is in a good light.

Diet

Eat a varied diet to ensure that you get all the necessary vitamins and minerals (see Chapter 2 for fuller details). Old people often become deficient in certain vitamins or minerals, simply because they lose interest in food. If this happens, ask yourself why. Is it because of illness, loneliness, unhappiness, depression? The solution may be to seek medical treatment, to go out once a week to a luncheon club, to cook for a friend now and again, or to find someone who will help with the shopping. Keep an emergency store of favorite and staple foods, including cans of fruit and vegetables, so that you do not have to worry if you cannot get to the shops for a few days in bad weather or when feeling low.

Watch your weight. It is important to keep weight within the normal range in old age. Excess weight puts more of a strain on joints, reduces mobility and makes operations more of a hazard. If weight is a problem, cut down on sugary foods, cakes and cookies, rather than bread and potatoes, which contain vitamins and minerals.

Drugs

Old people respond more idiosyncratically to drugs than younger people; sometimes very small quantities which would have no effect on a younger person are too powerful for an old person. Do not hesitate to report any disturbing symptoms which start after taking a new set of tablets. The doctor may then adjust the dose or perhaps prescribe a

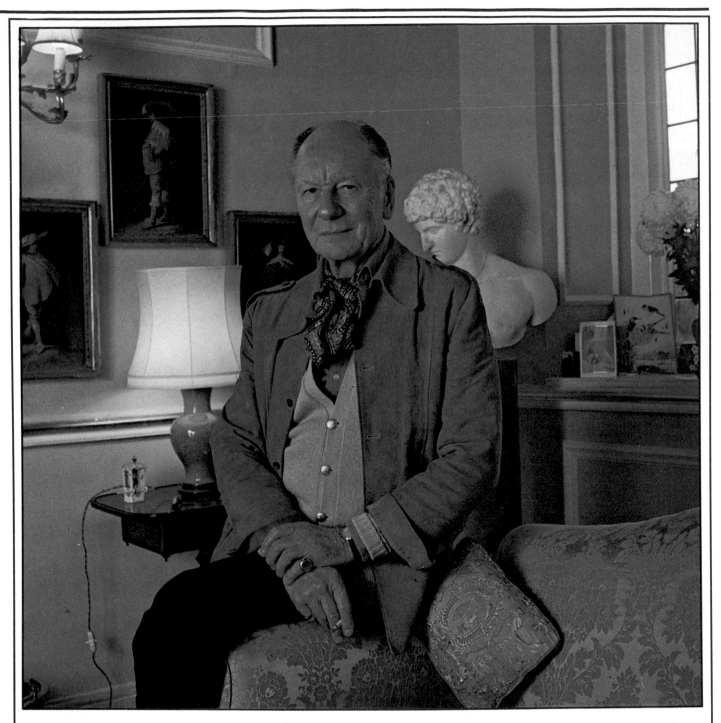

Sir John Gielgud. Still a star of theater and movies in his seventies. The variety of his career is undiminished by age – movies, Shakespearean parts, modern drama, directing. One month in Pinter's *No Man's Land*; the next in *Julius Caesar*. Has age had any effect at all? "I find that you are treated very politely and called 'Sir' rather than 'John'," he says. "I also think one can interfere with a little more authority at my age and with a little more tact." The cigarette, however, is not recommended.

different drug. Quite often, old people are given too many drugs which make them confused and ill. Then when another doctor takes them off all the drugs they show a miraculous cure. But more frequently, old people are to blame for not taking the tablets prescribed for them or not taking them according to instructions. Many old people have to take four or five tablets at various times of the day. It may help to work out a drug time table, or to put aside all the tablets to be taken each day in a separate container. Sleeping tablets should not be kept beside the bed, because an old person may easily wake in the night and think they have not taken their tablets and by mistake take another dose. If they have difficulty in understanding the instructions on a bottle, they should ask the druggist to repeat them or to write them out on a separate sheet of paper in large letters. Some older people are incapable of taking their own medicines by themselves, and an informed relative or neighbor, or perhaps a health worker from a community or voluntary welfare agency may have to give the drugs. Old medicines should not be kept but given back to the doctor, and the doctor seen every month or two rather than taking repeat prescriptions automatically.

Exercise

Old people do not have the same reserves of strength as younger people and so cannot take the same forms of exercise. Yet it is possible that a significant amount of physical deterioration arises from decreasing activity rather than advancing years. It has been shown many times that the capacity of elderly people for physical exercise can be improved with training just as with young people – in muscle strength and cardiovascular efficiency, for instance. And the amount of exercise necessary to have this "training effect" is within the reach of most senior citizens. Simply walking at 3 to 3.5 mph will produce improvement except in those already used to walking a great deal.

Failure to maintain fitness may mean that the capacity to maintain an independent lifestyle is otherwise in jeopardy. Elderly people also need some specific forms of exercises, notably those to maintain the mobility of joints of the body, which tend to become less mobile with the advancing years.

Walking, as has been stated, is excellent. If you find it difficult to walk far, go for several short walks with rests in between, to help maintain or improve mobility. Swimming, cycling, dancing and yoga are also excellent exercise, but old people should always avoid violent or prolonged exercise and should not continue if it is unduly painful. Gardening is a good way to combine exercise and enjoyment – many gadgets avoid the need for heavy digging – while even a rocking chair helps to prevent stiffening up and maintains the circulation.

No age is too old to begin gentle and cautious exercise. A comprehensive program designed for senior citizens has been devised by the President's Council on Physical Fitness and Sports. *The Fitness Challenge in the Later Years* offers three series of exercises graded according to difficulty or stress (see Appendix 2).

Falls

A serious matter in old age when bones do not mend so easily as in younger people, and the person may find it difficult to move normally afterwards. Older people have inefficient postural mechanisms, and are liable to be unsteady. Once they start to fall they are often unable to correct their balance. Even getting out of a chair can sometimes be hard and often leads to falls. This is the recommended technique: first, sit on the edge of the chair, rest a moment then hold on to the arms of the chair. Then, tightening stomach muscles and keeping head in the air, rise to the standing position. On rising, old people often feel light-headed as the blood supply to the brain is temporarily diminished. After a few moments, though, this feeling should wear off.

Some old people suffer from drop attacks, in which they fall suddenly to the ground. The attacks have many causes, one being a sudden drop in blood pressure similar to that commonly experienced by other old people on rising from a chair or when a person of any age gets quickly out of a hot bath. These can be very frightening and give an old person a fear of going out alone. Drop attacks are sometimes caused by a certain type of neck movement and it is possible to get a special collar from the doctor to prevent this happening. If it does happen you may have difficulty in finding your feet again once you have lost the normal standing posture. It may be helpful to wriggle around until the feet can be placed against some solid object; when pressure is felt on them again it should be possible to rise. It is best to rest

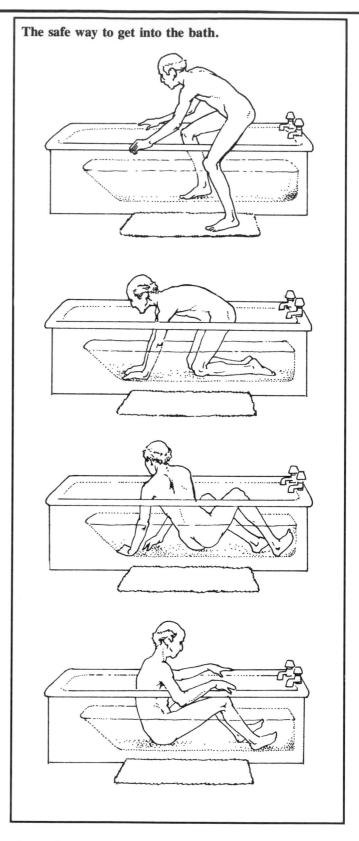

The safe way to get into the bath.

after a drop attack, and it is essential to notify the doctor and be checked up after this experience.

Eyes

Many old people have sight problems, which can be put right by the correct glasses. Eyes should therefore be examined annually by an optician. Specialist advice from hospital eye departments is available for the partially blind. Much can be done to help partially blind people with magnifiers, correct lighting and large-type books.

The Heart and Blood Vessels

These are neither so strong nor so adaptable in old age. To keep them working well it is necessary to continue with regular exercise and as far as possible avoid smoking or eating a fatty diet. However, it is also wise to avoid putting sudden strains on the heart and circulation. For example, it is unwise to take either vigorous exercise or a hot bath after a meal because the heart must then circulate blood to the muscles or skin as well as the digestive organs. It is not good to sit for long periods with crossed legs because this presses the knee into the back of the other leg, interfering with the flow of blood. You must also be careful to wear shoes which do not pinch the feet and restrict circulation, because this can cause injury to the tissues, particularly around the toenails. Thick woolen socks and soft shoes keep the feet warm and encourage the circulation.

Old people are particularly vulnerable to angina, coronary artery disease and heart failure. A severe pain in the chest when exercising should be reported to the doctor; similar pain which cannot be relieved by rest may be the sign of coronary heart disease but may only be a form of indigestion. In old people, heart disease is not always signaled by this type of pain but any discomfort in the chest indicates the need for consultation with a doctor. Shortness of breath, palpitations, mental disorientation or physical collapse can also be signs. If you suffer such an attack, lie down and move as little as possible until the doctor comes, and loosen tight clothing around the head and waist. Do not attempt to go upstairs to bed.

Although a heart attack need not be fatal, it is a warning that too much strain is being put on the heart. Readjustment to life by improving diet, reducing stress and taking moderate exercise often makes people who have had a heart attack feel much better afterwards than they did before.

In old age the heart sometimes becomes less able to pump blood around the body and begins to fail; when this begins to happen a person usually feels a shortness of breath and a feeling of fatigue. The ankles also begin to swell, particularly at the end of the day, and the person often feels the need to pass water once or twice during the night. The seriousness of these symptoms may not be realized until the person wakes up in the middle of the night gasping for breath and coughing. The condition – called heart failure – can be treated by drugs, so consult a doctor. However, rest is also important. It may therefore help to have your bed brought downstairs so that you can easily rest during the day and not have the difficulty of stairs. It is also important to give up smoking, reduce the amount of salt taken with food and to eat a light diet. Similar symptoms may be due to anemia, and so the advice of the doctor is necessary to exclude this illness.

Hypothermia

Old people are much more vulnerable to cold than young people because their appreciation of the temperature of their surroundings is less accurate and their thermostatic control less reliable. This makes old people vulnerable to hypothermia, a gradual cooling of the body below normal temperature. Surveys in major cities have shown that as many as one in ten people over sixty-five can have deep body temperatures at least one and a half degrees centigrade below normal – that is, on the borders of hypothermia. A cold spell together with a failure of the heating would put

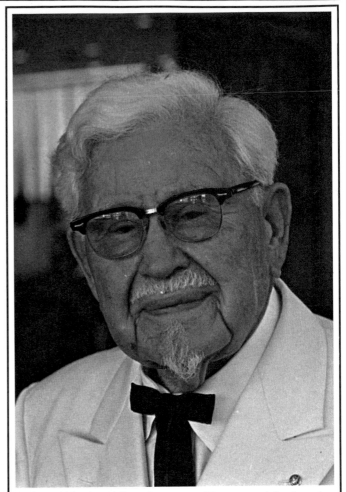

Colonel Harland Sanders was 66 years old when he founded his Kentucky Fried Chicken restaurant chain in 1956. He had previously run his own restaurant for twenty-seven years, but had to sell after the interstate highway bypassed it. Now there are more than 6,000 Kentucky Chicken diners in nearly fifty countries serving a billion meals a year. Well into his eighties he traveled around 250,000 miles a year to promote the enterprise. "We are wasting a lot of brain power and energy by making retirement compulsory. For a lot of folks like me, working is their hobby. They like staying active, facing challenges."

their lives in danger. In very cold weather an old person with inadequate heating will gradually cool down, and when their temperature goes below 32.5° C (90° F). their body movements and speech become slow. They usually do not realize what is happening, become drowsy and finally unconscious. You can tell when anyone is suffering from hypothermia because the whole body is cold, even their armpits and their abdomen. Hypothermia sufferers should be taken to hospital. But treatment of a mild case can be started at home by slow warming. Wrap the person in blankets, warm the room, provide well-wrapped hot water bags and warm (but not hot) sweet drinks. Investigation into the cause of hypothermia is essential, as it is commonly associated with other diseases which should be treated.

Try to avoid becoming a victim in the first place by keeping one room of the house really warm. It is often quite easy to turn one room into a mini-apartment. If your children or relatives cannot help in the task, ask your local social welfare organization or one of the organizations listed in Appendix 2 for advice.

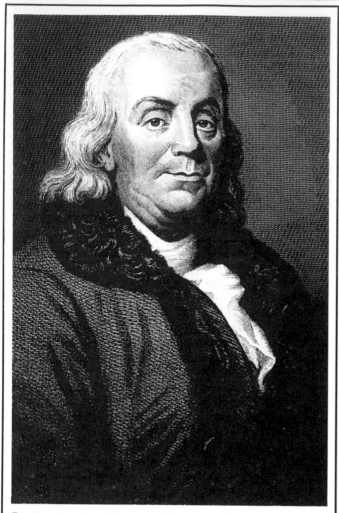

Benjamin Franklin was 70 years old when he was appointed to the committee that wrote the Declaration of Independence, and eighty-one when he played a crucial role in persuading Congress to agree to the terms of the Constitution.

Incontinence

One of the commonest reasons why elderly people have to go into hospital wards is incontinence of urine – the inability to manage the bladder adequately. It is a problem fraught with such shame and embarrassment for the sufferer that people won't ask for help. Yet much can be done either to cure or to control incontinence in a way that means sufferers can continue to lead an independent life.

The word incontinence covers a lot of different problems, but all have in common urinating at unexpected or inconvenient times. Rather than total loss of control, it can be a series of sudden leaks, the need to go frequently by day or night, the urge to go immediately, or just a problem about getting to the lavatory easily. Other symptoms which should lead to a medical consultation are dribbling after urination, leakage when coughing or laughing, pain or burning while urinating, difficulty in starting, dribbling or difficulty in forcing the urine out, blood in the urine or bad-smelling urine.

At the first sign of any of these it is crucial you should see your doctor. Even though it is an embarrassing subject to mention, it is worth acting fast. Incontinence is more easily helped at its onset, while delay often exacerbates problems. Explain in detail to the doctor exactly how, when, how often, and with what physical sensations the attacks of incontinence occur. Mention, too, if there is any change in your life which you think might have brought it on. The doctor will probably want to examine you.

Sometimes incontinence in women occurs because the muscular valve which controls the flow of urine fails to work. Your doctor may think this could be cured by a local operation, or he may decide a physical therapist could help with exercises. This is a topic where increased knowledge is constantly being gathered, and if you feel that your own doctor's advice and treatment is not helping, then it is worthwhile to ask for a specialist opinion by either a urologist, a gynecologist or a physician practicing geriatric medicine.

The essential problem in urinary incontinence is for an exact diagnosis to be made of the cause of the trouble. Once this is done, many methods of treatment are available, for example a course of drugs like antibiotics for cystitis or specialized drugs to control urination.

Drugs need your doctor's prescription, but there are things you can do to help yourself. It is important, first of all, to keep on drinking normally. Some people hope they can beat their problem by drastically reducing their liquid intake. That only increases the chance of complications. However, you may find it is worthwhile to drink more in the morning and less in the evening, so as to have less need to pass water during the night.

Keep your bowels moving regularly. This is extremely important, since constipation alone can create incontinence of the bladder, and occasionally of the bowel, too. A doctor will treat this with enemas, but a healthy diet with lots of roughage such as bran is needed to make sure it does not recur. Sedentary people are more likely to get constipation, so do take exercise.

One in three women, either when elderly or before, suffers at some point in their lives from "stress incontinence" – they leak at physical moments such as lifting, coughing, sneezing, or sometimes just turning over in bed. See a doctor about this. It is also worth seeing whether exercises worked out by a physiotherapist might help. Here are some you can do by yourself at home.

1. Sit or stand comfortably without tensing the muscles of the bottom, tummy or legs. Imagine you are trying to control the onset of diarrhea by tightening the ring of muscle round the back passage. Do this several times until you can make the correct movement.
2. Sit on the lavatory and start to pass water. Try to stop the flow in mid-stream by tightening the muscles round this front passage. Do this on several occasions until you get the feeling of conscious control.
3. Now that you have identified the muscles, do the following exercise: you can do it quite unobtrusively sitting, standing, or lying down. Tighten first one set of muscles, then the other; then both together. Count four slowly, then relax. Do this four times. Repeat the sequence every hour you are awake, if possible, and keep it up over a three-month period.

How people cope with incontinence depends on the way it affects them. For instance, many elderly people who are slow or handicapped in their movements wet themselves just because they cannot get to the lavatory in time. A commode, disguised as an armchair in the living room or in the bedroom, may cut accidents like this to the minimum. There are also heightened lavatory seats and grab-rails available for people who find using a lavatory difficult. The problem of dribbling can often be made tolerable for men by gadgets that fit on to the penis with a bag concealed in the trouser-leg. Bedridden people can be helped by special easy-to-use urinals or bottles.

There are protective pants, pads, mattress covers, bed-pans, special clothes, neutralizing deodorants and various other gadgets. There is a much wider choice than is generally known, so if one idea is not effective, ask for something different. A bit of persistent self-help – instead of giving up in despair – can make the management of incontinence much easier.

Before you spend a fortune on aids, make sure you are getting what is available from your doctor and community or voluntary services. You must overcome your reluctance to ask for help; it is nothing to be ashamed about. Incontinence is a difficult and complex problem and very occasionally is a cry for help when people are in situations which have become unpleasant or intolerable for them. It often happens when a person is moved from one institution to another, or from their own home to a hospital.

Joints

These begin to wear out as people get older and are subject to attacks of osteo-arthritis, rheumatoid arthritis and gout. A doctor should be consulted about painful and swollen joints. Tendons and ligaments become weaker in old age and old people easily damage them, possibly by a sudden movement. This can cause a complete break such as commonly occurs in the Achilles' tendon, or it may cause an incomplete tear which is the cause of tennis elbow or frozen shoulder. These conditions usually cure themselves in the end but medical treatment can speed it up.

The cause of *osteo-arthritis* is not known. It often develops in the joints which do most of the weight-bearing – that is, the knees and the hips. The lining of the joints becomes worn away and they can be felt grating together. Reduction in weight can help halt further damage. It is also important to exercise the muscles around the joint to maintain strength. Physical therapists will advise the correct exercises, but a lot more can be done by choosing forms of exercise which do not involve putting all the weight on the legs. For an old person who is otherwise fit, swimming, cycling, rowing and horse-riding are possibilities. A walking stick held on the opposite side to an affected limb can also be a great help and reduce the weight on the limb to a quarter. For a person who is generally infirm, a tripod stick or walking frame is the best aid, and a rocking chair can be a great help in keeping limbs mobile while keeping weight off them.

Rheumatoid arthritis is a different illness from osteo-arthritis, and may actually be caused by an infection, although researchers have so far failed to identify an organism causing it. A person may suffer from rheumatoid arthritis at any age but it is most common in late middle age and after. Sometimes an attack starts with a fever but more often it begins insidiously. Pains in the joints may begin first or the initial signs may be a loss of appetite, loss of weight and tiredness. Inflamed joints should be rested as much as possible and the doctor may decide that it is best to splint them. It is important to seek medical treatment at the beginning of the illness. Drug treatment is available which controls pain and reduces inflammation. In severe cases of either type of arthritis, an operation to replace a knee or hip-joint may ultimately be the best answer. Such operations have a very high success rate (more than 90 per cent) and the new joint is absolutely pain-free and as good as new. There are many gadgets such as raised lavatory and bath seats which can make an enormous difference to everyday life for people disabled by arthritis.

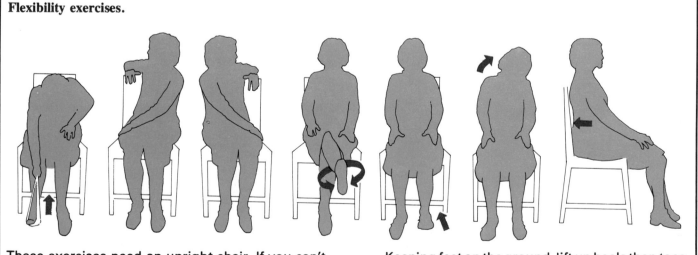

Flexibility exercises.

These exercises need an upright chair. If you can't make a movement, don't. Never strain yourself.

With a scarf under the shoe, using it as a lever, gently pull each toe up several times.

For waist mobility, start with your hands on either side of the chair and swivel round.

For swollen ankles, hook or cross one leg over the other. Press toes up, down, out, in, then circle round one way and the other.

Keeping feet on the ground, lift up heels then toes. Do with each foot, then both together.

For neck flexibility, let the head sag forward (don't push), then lift it up. Let it fall to the side, then bring it up. Do this both sides.

Sit in the chair, bottom right at the back and spine touching the chairback all the way up. Draw yourself up – chest out, head up.

Mobility

Mobility is the key to staying young, or, to put it another way, nothing makes you grow older faster than immobility. So the rule is to keep moving. This applies as much to the bedridden or partly-immobilized as to the really fit. There is a widespread assumption that as you grow older, the less physical activity you should take. Often without any prompting either from people or from illness, older people start cutting down on their activities. But when you stop doing something, you soon find that you *cannot* do it. A vicious circle sets in.

The other assumption is that physical fitness will decline with age, and that therefore it cannot be improved – only, as it were, kept at a static level. One ten-year study of a group of elderly people, however, showed that an extensive program of physical exercise left them fitter aged seventy than at the start of the experiment a decade earlier; physically they had improved and were "younger" at seventy than at sixty.

Even a little movement helps. Another experiment involved twenty-five elderly men and women doing exercise for just twelve weeks. They only exercised twice a week, with fairly gentle exercises worked out under medical supervision. After this twelve weeks, they were examined again by a heart consultant. He found that their blood pressure had dropped, their resting pulse rate was lower, and their blood fat levels had improved.

In order to keep mobile, it is important to use all the limbs that can be used. "Use it or lose it" is not far from the truth. Even if you are in a wheelchair, you can do arm-and-shoulder exercises. In general though, it is wise to check with your doctor before taking up a new kind of exercise. And don't push yourself to the limit. "If you ache the following day, it's a sign you have worked too hard" is the rule that many physical fitness specialists or teachers lay down for their keep-fit classes.

Elderly people with severe handicaps, of course, will need more than a few exercises. The important thing is not to assume that a physical disability puts an end to mobility. There is always something that can be done to make life easier. Nowadays there is a wide range of disablement aids, ranging from the simple walking stick to elaborate electronic wheelchairs. For example, an elderly woman with a severely arthritic hip could get either crutches or a walking-frame to help her get about. Inside the home, grab-rails at various important junctions would help her move from room to room, and work in the kitchen. The bathroom could be fitted with a specially high lavatory seat and a shower with a seat, instead of a bath.

One warning: do take expert advice on what aids to get. Doctors or welfare workers will be able to advise you about what is available from community welfare services. Occupational therapists can advise you about what aids you need. Never buy elaborate and expensive equipment without taking this advice first. You may be buying what you could get free, or it simply may not be the right aid for your particular disability. Unfortunately, there are a few unscrupulous operators about who will try to sell you costly hearing aids, elaborate armchairs, or expensive walking devices. If you really think it might be worth it, take the literature to an expert for advice. Never, never let a salesman talk you into buying without doing this, and be especially wary of salesmen who visit you at home. The best way to choose disablement aids is to go, preferably with an

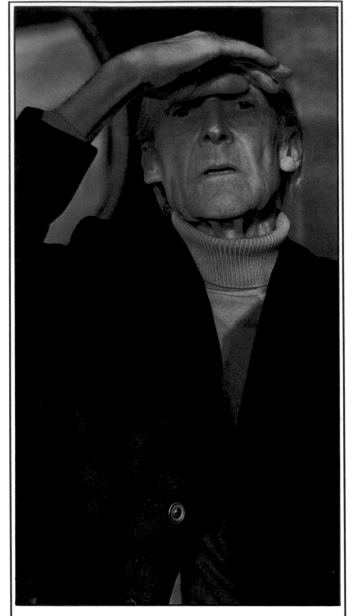

Bill Brandt, the photographer who recorded the social contrasts of the Thirties, was still working in the Seventies. In the Fifties he began producing startlingly original nude studies, while in his seventies he began branching out again to make collages of driftwood and jetsam.

expert, to a center where several can be tried and tested.

Finally, you can increase your mobility by changing your house or where you live. If you do not have a car or find you cannot afford one, move house to wherever there is a good bus service. In the same way, moving from a large house with many stairs into a one-level apartment or bungalow might help – bearing in mind that for some people stairs provide good exercise!

Sex

Many old people continue to enjoy sex in their eighties and there is often no reason why sex life should not continue at this age. The exercise is good for the heart and lungs, quite apart from the pleasure which sex itself brings. However, interest in sex naturally declines in both men and women. Women sometimes get a dry vagina after the menopause, although this can be considerably helped by the use of jelly or cream and sometimes by hormone treatment (see section on the menopause, Chapter 8).

Sleep

Old people often require less sleep at night but worry when they cannot get it. The sleep-rhythm becomes upset, and frequently an older person tends to have little cat-naps during the day. If you do doze after lunch you cannot expect to sleep as long or perhaps as deeply during the night. If you take too little exercise you may not be sufficiently tired to sleep well at night; it can be a good idea to take a walk before retiring to bed. Other important factors are:

1. A comfortable mattress: some old people continue to use broken mattresses on which anyone would find it difficult to sleep.
2. Do not drink tea or coffee late at night as they are stimulants which keep you awake. A warm milky drink, a glass of wine or a drop of brandy are excellent ways of promoting sleep.
3. Try to avoid worrying about problems just before going to bed, because you may stay awake all night thinking about them.

If sleep is impossible it is probably best to walk about or read a book to try to break the train of thought. But do try to avoid sleeping tablets. They interfere with normal sleep and dreaming and sometimes make older people confused. The effects of the drugs may persist the next day, and getting up in the middle of the night when under the influence of the drug may lead to a fall. Sleeping tablets may also prevent an old person from getting up in the night to pass water, thus making them wet the bed. If failure to sleep is due to pain or depression, a doctor may be able to help by relieving these causes.

Stroke

This occurs when the blood supply to the brain is interrupted by a blood clot in a vessel, or by the rupture of a blood vessel. The result is damage to the brain which may result in paralysis of half of the body or in loss of some faculty such as speech. Old people often have little strokes which are sometimes barely noticeable except to someone who knows the person well. Minor strokes may impair mental ability or ability to walk or talk. They may even produce an apparent alteration in character such as loss of interest in life or in personal appearance. When a person ages rapidly, begins to walk unsteadily or develops a slight droop at the corner of the mouth they may have had a minor stroke. A person may suffer many minor strokes over a number of years. These should always be reported to the doctor.

Major strokes are much more serious and can involve paralysis or loss of speech. If a right-handed person has a stroke which paralyzes their right side, they also lose the ability to speak; and for a left-handed person paralysis on the left side also goes with loss of speech. But a great deal can be done to rehabilitate a person who has had a stroke, by the doctor working in co-operation with a speech therapist, occupational therapist and physiotherapist. Remember, though, that someone who has had a stroke and cannot speak can often hear perfectly well and can be extremely upset when friends fail to realize that they can

understand everything that is being said. Communicate by asking questions which can be answered by yes or no, and by saying squeeze my hand or blink once for yes. The brain in any case has surprising powers of recovery. Old people are often able to relearn how to feed themselves, to walk and to speak. Again, the specialist senior citizen and welfare organizations will be able to advise.

Check Your Symptoms

If an elderly person has the symptoms below, they should see their doctor. The cause will often be simple and put right quickly, but it might be serious.

Eyes: Flashes of light before the eyes; seeing double; failing sight; seeing haloes around objects; pain in the eye or above the eye.
Hearing: Loss of hearing; reduced effectiveness of hearing aid; ringing in ears.
Skin: Spots or sores on skin which enlarge or bleed; irritation or sudden dryness of skin; a lump anywhere, particularly in the breast; widespread itching.
Feet: Pain or discoloration of the toes or forefoot; pins and needles or numbness.
Legs and arms: Loss of power in an arm or leg; persistent trembling or shaking; pain, swelling or stiffness in a joint or bone; pain in the calf.
Chest: Breathlessness; pain in the chest, arm or throat; persistent cough or hoarseness; coughing blood.
Bowels: Loss of appetite; difficulty in swallowing; dry cough or excessive thirst; unexplained loss of weight; persistent indigestion; vomiting blood; altered bowel habit; persistent constipation or diarrhea; passing blood from the bowel; black feces.
Bladder: Blood in urine; difficulty in urinating; increased frequency and urgency of urination.
Genitals: Itching around genitals; bleeding from vagina.
Feelings and behavior: Falling or unsteadiness; giddiness, unnatural tiredness, marked deterioration of memory; feelings of despondency, hopelessness or persecution.

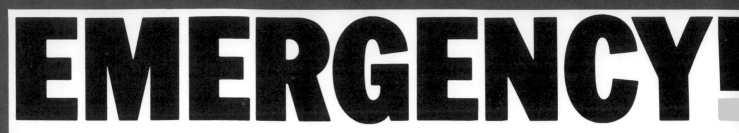

EMERGENCY!

When to Call the Doctor

Whenever possible, go to see your doctor in his office. But do not hesitate to call a doctor in the evening or at night if someone is obviously seriously ill or there has been a serious accident. In an emergency you can call on any doctor, but try your own doctor first. Or you can take the ill person to a hospital emergency room.

It is impossible to give a comprehensive list of circumstances when a doctor should be called in an emergency at night. A high temperature or fever is not normally sufficient reason to worry the doctor. However, if the fever is accompanied by other symptoms such as a severe headache it may be wise to call the doctor, even though all that he may be able to do is to give advice on the telephone. Coughing a small amount of blood, blood in feces or urine are not usually sufficient reason to call a doctor at night unless accompanied by severe pains or other symptoms. However, a doctor should be called when a woman bleeds from the vagina during pregnancy, especially if it is accompanied by pain.

A doctor should be called if someone has difficulty in breathing, or has an unexplained severe and continuous pain in the abdomen – or anywhere else – which does not go away after half an hour, or has a severe, constricting chest pain, especially if accompanied by sweating, or when someone collapses or loses the ability to move limbs or to speak.

Parents should call a doctor to their child if the child suddenly becomes ill or feverish and lies still without the energy to move. Children cry differently when ill and a mother usually knows when something is seriously wrong; if the child does not have the energy to respond in the normal way, then that is a good indication that something is wrong and the doctor should be called.

Copious diarrhea in babies is an emergency when the doctor should be called. An epileptic attack in a child lasting more than ten minutes, or recurring attacks, should be treated as an emergency. Rashes are hardly ever an emergency and are best taken to the doctor the next day so that the rash may be examined in daylight.

There is no need to call the doctor if your child vomits once, cries for half an hour or so, or misses a meal, provided that they are otherwise happy and gaining weight and sleeping well. Call your doctor if the child looks odd – pale, blue or yellow; if the child appears to be in pain and will not be comforted – the legs may be drawn up and fists clenched; if the child has a persistent cough, persistent diarrhea, or persistent vomiting; if a baby misses two or more feeds or a child does not eat for twenty-four hours; if the child has convulsions; if there is blood in the urine, feces or vomit; if there is any injury to the head and the child does not recover in fifteen minutes. Odd behavior such as drowsiness, listlessness or irritability may also be reasons for seeking medical advice.

Earache is a common cause of doctors being called by parents at night but there is not much that can be done until morning, when a course of antibiotic drugs may be started. The best remedy for earache or any pain is a small dose of acetaminophen or other simple pain killer. Panic or conflict in the family when illness is recognized is often the reason for calling the doctor. Pause for a moment to ask yourself if it is a genuine emergency: if you are really worried, especially in the case of a child, do not hesitate to call the doctor.

Alphabetical Guide to Emergencies

These guidelines tell you what to do in a crisis when someone may be seriously ill or hurt. If in doubt, always call a doctor. They will decide if medical treatment is necessary and may give advice over the telephone. However, it may save vital time to take the injured person to the nearest major hospital emergency room. It may help if someone else can telephone the hospital to say that you are coming – do not waste time doing this yourself. Remember, the injured person will be less frightened if you remain outwardly calm. Reassurance is important, as it will reduce the physical and emotional shock. This is especially important with children.

Artificial Respiration

Mouth to mouth (mouth to nose)
This is the most effective method and should be used except where there is severe injury to the face and mouth; where the casualty is trapped face downwards; or if the casualty is vomiting.

Positioning the head
(tilted back) to open
airways
closed airways

1

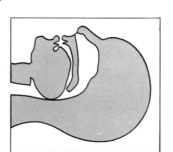

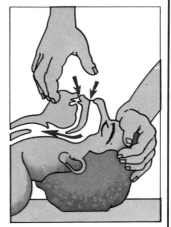

1. Lay casualty on his back. Extend head backwards. Remove obvious obstructions from the mouth. Loosen clothing.

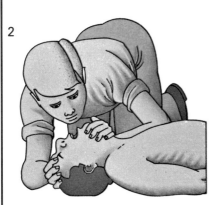

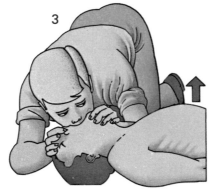

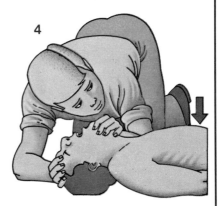

2. Position of head and hands.

3. Seal nose by pinching, blow into mouth and watch chest rise.

4. Remove your mouth, watch chest fall.

With a baby or young child, seal lips round mouth and nose and blow gently into lungs until chest rises.

Continue to give artificial respiration until natural breathing is restored and then place casualty in recovery position (p.196). Send for medical aid.

Revised Holger Nielson
This should be used if the face is damaged or the jaw fractured, making mouth to mouth resuscitation impossible.

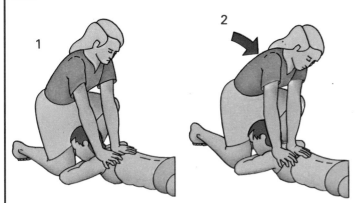

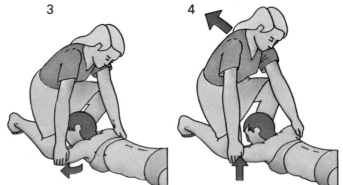

The casualty lies on his front with head facing forwards, hands under his chin and his elbows out. The mouth and nose must be clear of obstruction. Loosen clothing.

1. Kneel in front of casualty with hands flat on his back just below shoulder blades.
2. Rock forwards, keeping your arms straight until they are vertical over the body.

Let the weight of your body be the force.
3. Slide your hands past his armpits and along arms to grasp them firmly just above elbows. Rock backwards until body is vertical, raising elbows until resistance and tension are felt.
4. Drop elbows and return to picture 1 position.

Repeat as necessary. Keeping all movements continous and smooth.

Bandaging
Slings: to support and protect the arm

1. arm sling.

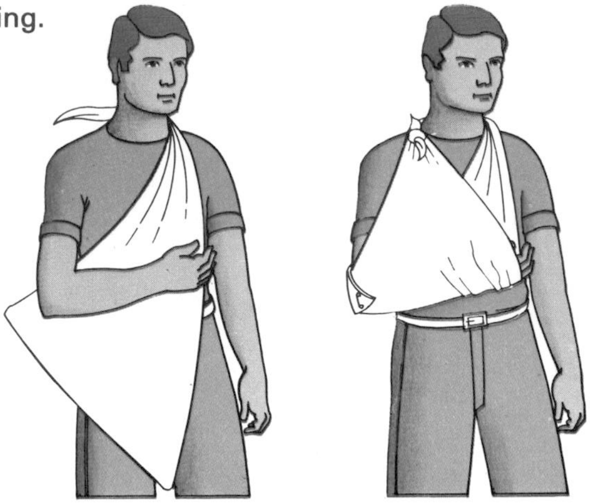

2. triangular sling – supports hand and forearm in raised position. Particularly in case of hand injury, badly fractured ribs or on a rough journey.

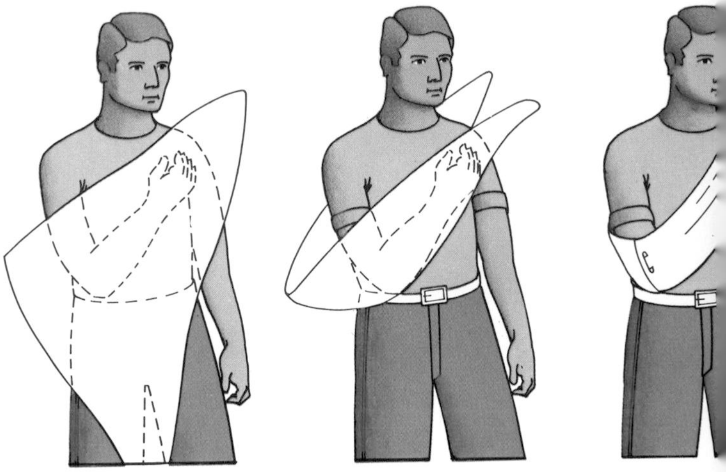

Roller bandages

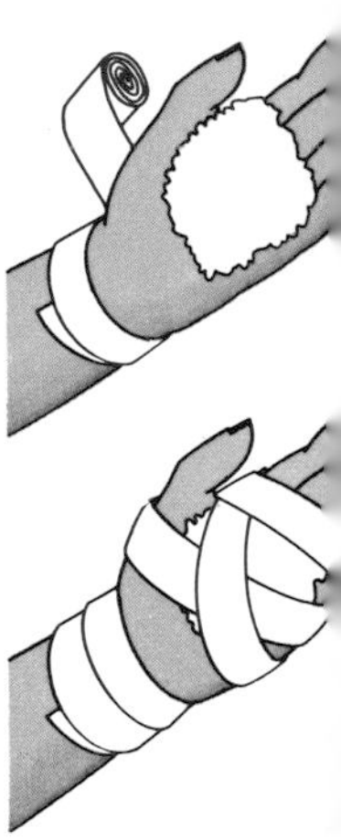

A two-inch b

Fractures

Do not move unless absolutely necessary. If the injured person must be moved, immobilize the injured part as shown below but do not attempt to correct any deformity. Treat for shock. Check bandages every half hour, and loosen if the limb is swelling. Seek expert help.

Broken finger

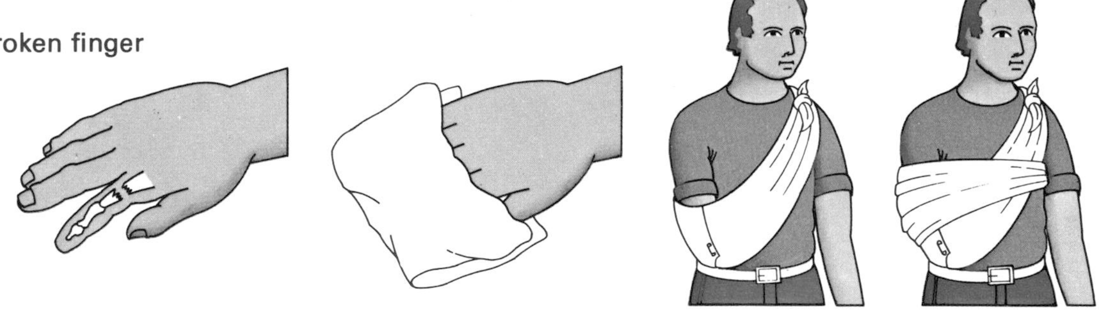

Fractured wrist: make sure wrist is supported by the casualty or by the first-aider *at all times*.

Fractured wrist

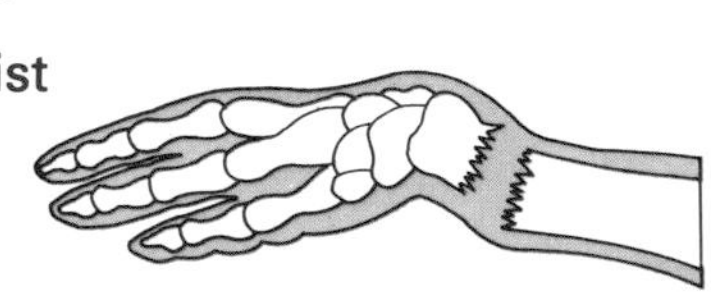

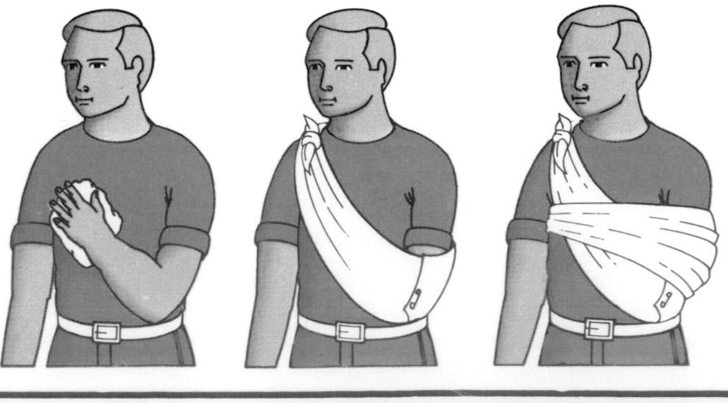

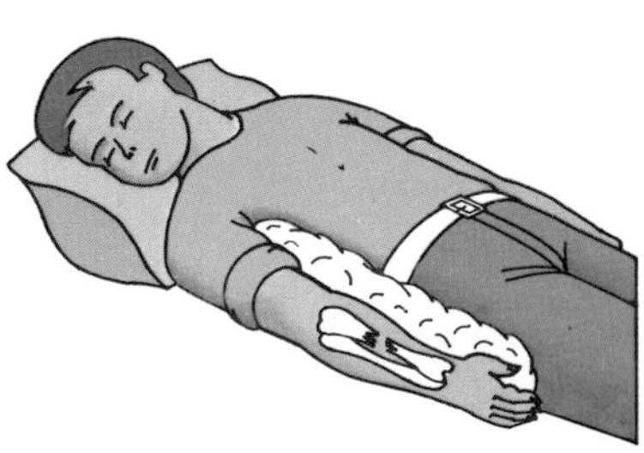

Broken arm

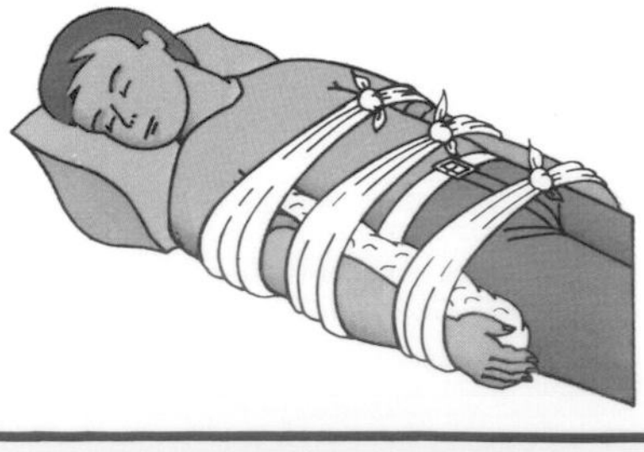

Bites and stings

Snakebite

What to look for:

The majority of snakebites come from non-poisonous types and even if the bite is from a poisonous snake, poison may not have been effectively injected. When a poisonous snake does bite effectively, severe pain occurs immediately followed by swelling and discoloration of the skin.

What to do:

If no immediate symptoms develop:

- Calm the victim and keep him or her from moving around unnecessarily.
- Immobilize the bitten limb and keep below heart level.
- Take victim to hospital or doctor as soon as possible.

If symptoms are mild or moderate, i.e., mild swelling, discoloration, moderate pain, weakness, nausea, vomiting, shortness of breath.

- With victim lying down, put a constricting band above the wound tightly enough to prevent blood returning to the body via the veins but not tight enough to prevent flow of blood in arteries – check that there is a pulse in the limb below the band. Use belt, necktie or shirt for band. Wash surface of the wound. Keep victim still with affected limb below heart level. The band must be slackened for 90 seconds every 15 minutes. Get to hospital or professional help quickly.

If symptoms become severe, i.e., rapid swelling and numbness, severe pain in wound, and possibly in addition slurred speech, drowsiness, convulsions, shock, pinpoint pupils, twitching, unconsciousness.

- Apply band as above. Make two to four incisions through the full thickness of the skin (about ¼ inch deep and ½ inch long) at or near the fang marks. Make the cuts along the long axis of the limb and use a knife or razor blade which has been sterilized in a flame. Now suck out the blood and lymph containing the poison and spit it out. (The poison will do no harm to the person who sucks provided they have no large open sores in the mouth.) If a small blood vessel is cut while removing venom, stop the bleeding with pressure and continue. But DO NOT make cross cuts and DO NOT make cuts on head, neck or trunk.
- This process may be repeated as the swelling grows and spreads. If necessary, apply another constricting band higher up and remove one lower down.
- DO NOT give alcohol or any kind of stimulating drink such as tea, coffee or cola, which will cause blood vessels to dilate and spread poison. DO NOT give sedatives or aspirin.
- Get victim to hospital as soon as possible where antivenom is available and supportive treatment can be given. Move victim with as little exertion on his part as possible.
- If necessary, treat for shock or stupor (see below) and if necessary give artificial respiration until help can be obtained.

The majority of venomous snakebites in the US are caused by rattlesnakes, moccasins and copperheads. These are called pit vipers because of a sunken pit extending from the eye to the nostril. Less than two per cent of venomous bites are caused by coral snakes, which are only found in the South from North Carolina to Florida and from Louisiana to central Texas, Arizona and southwestern New Mexico. It is important to distinguish the type of snake

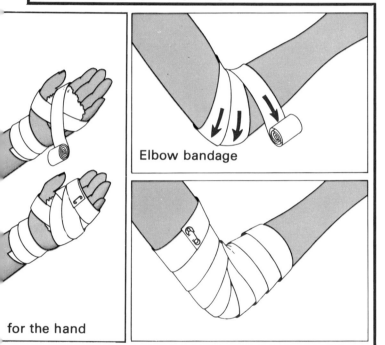

Elbow bandage

for the hand

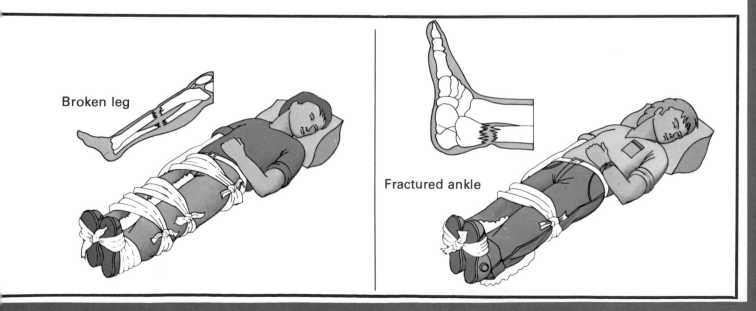

Broken leg

Fractured ankle

which caused the bite, because treatment differs. The pit vipers strike and rapidly try to escape, whereas the coral snakes hang on sinking in their fangs with a chewing action. However, the bite of the pit viper leaves a more conspicuous injury which swells. Non-poisonous snakes have six rows of teeth, four in the upper jaw and two in the lower jaw. If this pattern of teeth marks is seen, then the wound may simply be treated as a dog or cat bite (see below). Most snakebites occur on the legs; strong boots and trousers provide the best protection.

Poisonous lizards: The gila monster of Arizona and small areas of adjoining states and the beaded lizard of Mexico are poisonous. Symptoms similar to snakebite. Treat as for snakebite. No antivenom available.

Insect bites and stings are not often serious. Very rarely, a person may have a severe allergic reaction, go into shock, and possibly have difficulty in breathing, or the heart may stop. If this happens it will develop over the first one to twenty minutes following the sting; seek medical help and give artificial respiration and heart massage if necessary. Normally, bites and stings are only serious when received in large numbers or are in awkward places such as the mouth. Remove stings if left in the skin and soothe with surgical spirit or a *weak* ammonia solution or a solution of bicarbonate of soda. If the sting is in the mouth, give a mouthwash of one teaspoonful of bicarbonate of soda to a tumbler of water. Apply ice packs to relieve pain and take antihistamines to relieve itching if necessary.

Spiders: Only the bite of the widow and recluse spiders may occasionally prove fatal. Attempts to remove the venom by suction are generally ineffective and unnecessary. Make victim comfortable and obtain professional advice.

Centipedes: Large species in southern and western USA inflict a most painful bite which may be accompanied by swollen lymph glands and local swelling. Treat as for insect bites.

Scorpions: Treat as for wasps and bees. Only two species of bark scorpions from Arizona and New Mexico inflict stings which may occasionally be fatal, especially in children under three. In such cases seek expert help. Antivenom is available.

Dog or cat bites. Treat as for a wound. Tincture of iodine is recommended for cleansing bite wounds. An anti-tetanus injection is advisable. If the animal is behaving oddly in any way suggestive of rabies, report it to the police and seek expert advice as quickly as possible. The animal should be shot and examined for rabies infection; if positive, anyone who has been in any physical contact with the animal should be given anti-rabies vaccine.

Bleeding

Press the edges of the wound together firmly for a few minutes, put on a sterilized dressing, then pad and bandage. If the bleeding continues, raise the limb, if possible, and put on more pads and bandages. Never remove the bandages; if bleeding continues, add more. Do not use a tourniquet to restrict the artery. If there is a foreign body in the wound, only remove it if it is obviously on the surface. Otherwise, cover a wound containing a foreign body lightly and bandage firmly *around* the area, being careful not to press on the foreign body. Seek expert help. Small wounds should be washed before bandaging. Stab wounds may cause

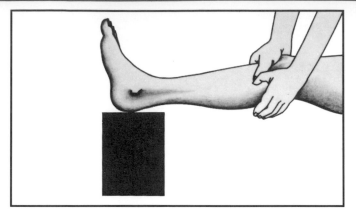

internal damage even if the actual entry is small and should always be taken to a doctor.

Varicose veins. Bleeding from burst varicose veins is serious and you should act quickly to prevent the rapid loss of blood. Apply immediate, direct pressure with the hand to the bleeding point. Remove anything from the leg which could impede circulation. Lay casualty flat on their back and raise the leg up. Seek medical aid.

Internal bleeding. If internal bleeding is suspected it is important to get medical help immediately. Meanwhile, make casualty lie down with legs raised. He should be kept quite still. Loosen all clothing, and check for other injuries. Keep him warm and watch his breathing and pulse rate.

Burns or scalds

Fire. Smother flames with a coat or blanket. Cool the burnt area with cold water for at least ten minutes. Cover with dry, clean dressing. If large areas are burnt, wrap the person in a sheet and take him to hospital emergency room. Do not use creams or ointments and do not remove burnt clothing next to the skin.

Corrosive chemicals. Speed is essential. Flood the affected part with running water for at least ten minutes to dilute the chemical. Remove contaminated clothing under the water if possible. Seek medical attention.

Eye injury from chemical: urgent treatment required to prevent permanent damage. Flood eye immediately and copiously with nearest available bland liquid – water or clean milk. Continue for at least ten minutes. Take the casualty quickly to hospital.

Chemical taken by mouth see Poisoning.

Sunburn. Rest in the shade. Give cold drink. If sunburn is severe, seek medical help. (Skin lotions are available for mild sunburn.)

Scalds. Caused by moist heat such as boiling water, steam, hot oil. Place affected part under slowly running water or immerse in cold water for at least ten minutes. Reduction of heat is essential. Remove anything of a constricting nature (rings, belts, etc.). Treat as for a burn and take to hospital if badly scalded.

Remember:

DO NOT burst or break blisters.

DO NOT apply any lotions or grease.

DO NOT breathe over burnt area.

DO NOT touch the burnt area, as this will spread germs.

DO NOT remove clothing or handle the casualty more than necessary.

DO NOT remove dressings once they have been applied.

DO NOT put fluffy or hair materials (.e.g., cotton wool) on to burnt area.

Choking

If the victim is still able to breathe effectively do not interfere with his attempts to remove the foreign body. The symptoms of choking are readily confused with heart attack or stroke but can be distinguished in the following way:

(a) The victim will usually have been eating immediately prior to the incident and suddenly is unable to breathe or speak, and unable to answer questions.

(b) The victim may make the distress signal of choking: holding the hand to the throat.

(c) the victim may turn a bluish color and make exaggerated breathing movements.

If the victim is conscious but unable to breathe at all:

● Rapidly strike the back with the heal of the hand four times with the victim bending over. If the victim is lying down roll him onto his side facing you and, supporting his chest with your knee, deliver rapid blows to the back between the shoulder blades. In the case of an **infant or child** place over the knee or down the forearm and deliver sharp blows to the back.

● Perform manual thrusts (Heimlich maneuver). Stand behind the victim and join hands round the waist (or chest in the case of a fat or pregnant person). Place the fist slightly above the belt but below the ribs. Rapidly thrust into the abdomen with a forceful movement. If the victim is lying down: place him on his back, kneel astride the hips, place hands one on top of the other just above the navel and below rib cage. Thrust into the abdomen with hands forcesfully. In the case of an **infant or small child**: place over forearm with head down. Place fingertips on the child's abdomen just above the navel and below ribs. Press fingertips into abdomen with a quick upward thrust.

● If these actions do not work repeat until they do.

If the victim is unconscious:

● If it is possible to give mouth to mouth respiration do so – see the instructions above. If there is no pulse give heart massage – see instructions page 195. Forceful respiration may keep the victim alive if the foreign body is partially dislodged.

● If it is impossible to give artificial respiration then roll victim onto his side and, supporting his chest with your knee, deliver rapid blows to the back between the shoulder blades. In the case of a child place over arm or knee.

● Perform manual thrusts. With victim lying on back, kneel astride the hips. Place hands one on top of the other just above the navel and below the rib cage. Thrust into the abdomen forcefully. In the case of a small child place over forearm or knee with head down. Press fingertips into abdomen with a quick thrust at a point between navel and ribs.

● If a foreign body can be seen in the mouth and it is possible to grasp it easily then remove it. But beware of pushing the object further into the throat especially in the case of a small child. That is why other procedures are recommended first. Finger probing should only be attempted when the victim is unconscious and other attempts have failed. This is what to do:

● With the victim on his back grasp the tongue and lower jaw between the thumb and fingers and lift. This draws the tongue away from the back of the throat and may help to relieve the obstruction. Insert the index finger down the inside of the cheek into the back of the throat and attempt to hook out the foreign body or ease it into the mouth by pushing it against the opposite side of the throat until it is possible to dislodge it. In the case of a child use a small finger. The risk of pushing the object further down the throat is much greater with a child so use extreme caution.

● If necessary repeat the procedures above:
1. attempt artificial respiration
2. perform four back blows
3. perform four manual thrusts
4. probe the throat

● After removing the object perform more mouth to mouth respiration if necessary and heart massage.

● When the victim recovers he should be seen by a doctor. (Not necessary if the victim recovers fully without any period of unconsciousness).

Prevention

Choking is sixth among the causes of accidental death in the United States; it caused 2,900 deaths in 1976. The causes in adults are often excessive alcohol intake, dentures and large, poorly chewed pieces of food. To prevent choking the American Red Cross recommends the following measures:

● Cut food into small pieces and chew slowly and thoroughly, especially if you wear dentures.

● Do not laugh and talk while chewing and swallowing, and avoid excessive intake of alcohol before and during meals.

● Restrict children from walking, running and playing while they have food or other foreign bodies in their mouths, and keep small objects such as marbles, beads, or thumbtacks out of reach of infants and small children.

Cold Injury

Old people and mountain climbers are most vulnerable to hypothermia – a cooling of the body below normal temperature. If the person is cold to the touch – even their armpits – and appears dopey and confused, then seek expert help. Hospital admission may be necessary. In the meantime, take all possible measures to warm the person up. Remove any wet clothing and dry the sufferer. Cover with blankets and provide warm food and drink (not scalding) but not alcohol. Warm the room. Mild cases will recover by these measures alone.

A baby suffering from cold will be pink, with swollen limbs and a very cold skin. It will be lethargic and unwilling to suck. The body temperature will be below normal.

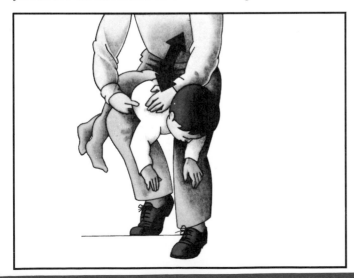

Cold injury can be dangerous and hospital treatment is advisable. Re-warming must be very gradual – increase the room temperature and put more coverings over the baby. Seek help.

Convulsions

Remove the victim from danger. Guide their movements to prevent injury; do not try to stop them. Do not force the mouth open, but if possible put something, such as a knotted handkerchief, between the teeth to prevent the person biting their tongue. On recovering, they will probably not remember what has happened; reassure them and consult a doctor.

Babies and young children may have convulsions or momentary loss of consciousness accompanied by a tremor, as a result of a high fever. Call the doctor and give the baby a tepid sponge with warm water to bring down body temperature. Whether the convulsion is serious or more like a faint, make sure the child has a medical check-up following upon it.

Drowning

Give artificial respiration and heart massage if necessary. Arrange the victim's urgent removal to hospital. There are many recorded cases of people surviving after twenty-five minutes or even longer under water: give artificial respiration even if the person appears completely lifeless, and continue until expert help arrives.

Electric Shock

Switch off the supply, pull out the plug or tear the cable free. If this is impossible, stand on a dry insulating material such as wood or newspaper and push the person away from the supply of current. Be careful not to touch any conducting material with the other hand while doing this. Give artificial respiration and heart massage if necessary. Treat for shock (see below).

Electric shocks may have greater effects than most people expect, since there may be little external signs of damage. Medical advice should always be sought after a serious electric shock. Burns must be treated.

Faints

These are common in illness or when standing in a crowd, and caused by a temporary drop in the blood supply to the brain. There is often some warning: the person may sway, become giddy, his face becomes white and he breaks out in a sweat.

Urge him to breathe deeply and flex his muscles to aid blood circulation. Loosen clothing and lay him down in a current of air with his legs above his head until colour returns. If this is not possible, sit him down with his head between his knees. As he recovers, give him sips of water.

Foreign Bodies

In the ear: An insect in the ear is very distressing; pour in tepid water or olive oil and it should float out. (Do not poke the ears to remove a foreign body: consult a doctor.)

In the nose: Tell the person to breathe through his mouth and consult your doctor or, if possible, rush to the nearest hospital emergency room.

In the eye: Tears may wash the object into the corner of the

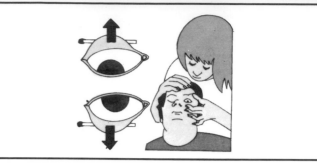

eye so that it can be removed with a clean cloth. Never use a hard object to remove something from the eye. Try lifting the upper lid by the lashes over the lower lid; this draws the lashes of the lower lid over the inside of the upper lid and may brush the object out. Look under the lower lid, and remove any object with a clean cloth or tissue.

If these measures fail, the upper and lower lids may in turn be rolled back over a match, and any grit gently wiped off with a cloth. Never attempt to remove any object from the colored part of the eye (the pupil and iris), but go to major hospital emergency room.

Inhaled: If a foreign body is inhaled it is advisable to consult a doctor without delay.

Gas and Exhaust-Fume Poisoning

Carbon monoxide gas from the domestic gas supply, from a car engine left running in a garage or in fumes coming out of a cracked stove can be lethal. However, natural gas, owing to its lower carbon monoxide content, is much safer than the old coal gas. If the victim is in an enclosed room, take a deep breath before going in and carry them out immediately. The victim may be confused or in a coma. Provide fresh air and give artificial respiration if breathing has stopped. Call a doctor or ambulance; these will provide oxygen if necessary.

Head Injuries

In the case of an injury to the head from a sharp blow causing a wound or any temporary loss of consciousness, consult a doctor. Rest for forty-eight hours after any head injury unless told not to. Report any abnormal drowsiness, persistent vomiting or disturbance of behavior to the doctor. Persistent headache after forty-eight hours which cannot be relieved by aspirin should be reported to a doctor.

Heart Failure (see also Artificial Respiration)

When the heart stops, the victim turns a blue-gray color, has no pulse at wrist or neck and the pupils of the eyes are dilated.

1. Strike the victim's breastbone sharply with the hand once or twice; in the case of babies, tap sharply with two fingers. If the heart does not start, an experienced person can begin external heart massage while continuing artificial respiration. An inexperienced person is not advised to try this as it may cause injury if done incorrectly. Should heart massage prove impossible due to obstruction, or difficult due to inexperience, keep the artificial respiration going as first priority until help arrives, giving any heart massage you are able.

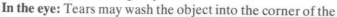

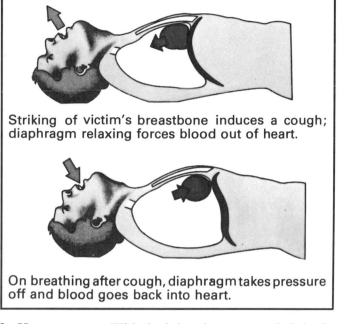

Striking of victim's breastbone induces a cough; diaphragm relaxing forces blood out of heart.

On breathing after cough, diaphragm takes pressure off and blood goes back into heart.

2. Heart massage. With the injured person on their back, place the heel of the hand (use two fingers only for babies) over the breastbone where the ribs meet. Place the other hand over the first hand. Press down on the lower half of the breastbone. Repeat every second for five seconds, then inflate the lungs; repeat this cycle indefinitely until the patient recovers or help arrives.

3. When breathing begins again, lay the person in the coma position and treat for shock.

Heat Stroke

The body can no longer control temperature by sweating. Signs are a high temperature and pulse; hot, dry skin; noisy breathing; unconsciousness. Strip casualty and wrap in wet, cold sheet. Keep wet until his temperature has gone down. Place in recovery position. Fan casualty from above. Send to hospital.

Nose Bleed

Only rarely serious. Ask the sufferer to sit down with their head forward and to breathe through their mouth. Pinch firmly the soft part of the nose for ten minutes. Loosen clothing at neck, chest and waist. Put a bowl or pad under the nose to catch the blood, and place an old towel or sheet around the shoulders to take care of any mess. Seek medical advice if the bleeding is severe or does not stop in an hour. When the person, naturally enough, wants to spit, do not discourage this; but try to discourage sniffing, which will dislodge the blood clots forming over the injured blood vessel.

Poisoning

Ask the person, if conscious, what they have taken. Also, remember that many poisons can be identified by smell.
Non-corrosive poisons such as medicines, weed killers, cigarettes, poisonous plants: do not give the person a drink, and particularly do not give them a salt water drink; this can be dangerous in itself. Seek medical advice.
Corrosive poisons such as disinfectants, cleaning fluid, caustic soda, paraffin, petrol or insect spray: dilute the corrosive by giving water or milk to drink. Do not make the person vomit, as this may lead to more burning. Yellow, gray or

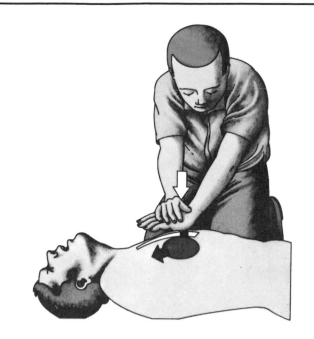

Pressing on indicated part, halfway between middle and end of sternum, expels blood.

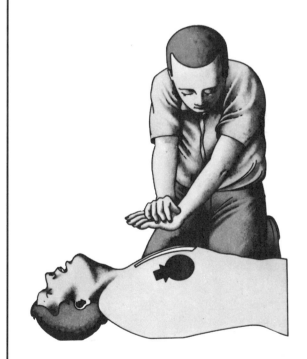

On release, blood goes back into heart.

white burns around the mouth may betray a corrosive poison – do not forget to wipe these away and rinse out mouth. Seek help urgently. Phone your doctor or take the person to the emergency room of the nearest hospital, even if the person appears to have vomited the poison. Some poisons, e.g., aspirin, have serious delayed effects. If the person is unconscious and not breathing, give artificial respiration and, if necessary, heart massage. If unconscious but breathing, lay them on their side in the coma position. Send any particulars of the poison to the hospital with the victim, including any remaining poison, its container or any vomited matter.

Red Urine

Usually due to beetroot, blackcurrant, red wine or candy. Blood in the urine gives it a smoky appearance. This may not be an emergency if the person is otherwise well, but seek medical advice.

Shock

Recognized by rapid, shallow breathing, blurring of vision, deathly pallor, faintness and giddiness, sometimes with a loss of consciousness. This may be caused by bleeding, burns, or injuries, loss of body fluid, a burst appendix, or even by a cut, bad news or fright. Check on bleeding. Send for help. Keep the person warm with blankets and heat the room if cold. Do not give hot water bags and warm drinks, and do not move more than necessary.

Stupor and Coma

If the stupor is not deep, the person may be roused by pressing firmly upwards on the ridge beneath the eyebrows at a point where there is a small dent in the bone. This will cause sufficient pain to rouse the person without hurting them. If the person will not be roused (coma), check that the air-passages are free from any obstruction such as vomit and, if breathing, lay them on their side in the recovery position (see below). If the person is trapped and cannot be moved, keep the air-way clear by tilting the head back. Call the doctor; be ready to give artificial respiration and heart massage. Check that the person is not wearing or carrying any identity discs or cards which may explain the cause of the coma (diabetes, epilepsy, etc.) and give instructions about what to do and whom to contact.

Suffocation

Remove the obstruction, usually a plastic bag, give artificial respiration and heart massage if necessary (see page 195). Seek professional help or take casualty to hospital emergency room.

Strangulation: Lift the person up and cut or loosen cords, ribbons, etc., if hanging. Give artificial respiration and heart massage is necessary. Seek professional help or take casualty to hospital emergency room.

Swallowed Objects

Smooth or round objects such as coins, marbles, buttons or plum stones seldom cause trouble when swallowed. Do not worry unless the person complains of pain, in which case consult the doctor. Pins, needles, safety pins and other sharp objects can be dangerous and you should *call the doctor at once*. But do not panic: many frighteningly sharp objects have been found to pass through the bowel harmlessly. Eat a bulky diet and examine the stools carefully for five days until the object has been passed. X-rays are not generally justified except in an emergency, or if the object cannot be found.

Unconsciousness

If a person is not breathing, give artificial respiration. If breathing, lay them on their side in the recovery position to ensure that vomit is not inhaled. Keep the person quiet and warm, and consult the doctor. If the person recovers, it is quite safe to let them fall asleep provided they remain in the recovery position. Loss of consciousness may be caused by a blow to the head severe enough to shake the brain (concussion).

Recovery Position

This position should be used with unconscious casualties where internal injuries and fractured bones are not suspected. The casualty is kept stable and comfortable, and the position of the head allows any fluid or vomit in the mouth to drain out. Never use a pillow, but the head *can* be placed on a thin cloth or handkerchief.

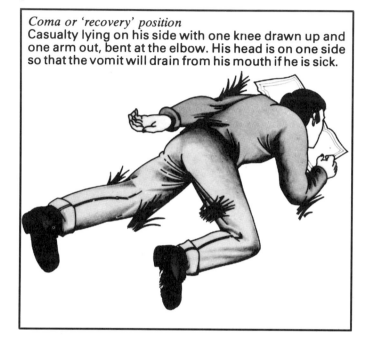

Coma or 'recovery' position
Casualty lying on his side with one knee drawn up and one arm out, bent at the elbow. His head is on one side so that the vomit will drain from his mouth if he is sick.

Appendix 1

How to Get the Best out of your Community Medical Services

How to choose a doctor: A generation ago the majority of doctors were general practitioners dealing as best they could with every problem in medicine. Now only about one in ten doctors are general practitioners. The rest are specialists of one kind or another. Nevertheless, the general practitioner or family doctor is still often the best doctor to go to with a problem unless it is obviously a problem for a pediatrician, obstetrician/gynecologist or psychiatrist – the major specialities other than internal medicine and surgery. The alternative to a general practitioner is the internist (not to be confused with the intern who is a recent medical graduate undergoing hospital training) who has undergone some specialized training in internal medicine but does not necessarily have a diploma. If your problem is a surgical one, then you should usually see a general practitioner or internist first who will assess the problem and refer you to a surgeon.

Most general practitioners have no special qualification other than their MD, and they vary greatly in ability. It is always wise to inquire from friends or people at work about local doctors and their reputation in the community. If you have moved from an area not too far away, your own doctor may be able to recommend someone in your new location. Another good method is to get in touch with the nearest *accredited* hospital (see section on hospitals below) and ask for a list of general practitioners or internists who are on its staff as attending physicians. If you have a medical school in your area, you may also ask them for a similar list. A doctor who is on the list of attending physicians of a medical school or accredited hospital must have good standing among his colleagues, and this guarantees that the doctor will be generally competent.

Another method of finding a doctor is to contact your local county medical society and ask for a list of doctors in your area who are able to take on new patients. But remember the medical society cannot recommend a physician, and the act of giving you a doctor's name does not imply any recommendation. It is up to you to find out more about the doctor. You might begin with one who is located conveniently near your home. Let him know that you want a family doctor and ask him about his hospital affiliations, whether he will do home calls and what arrangements he has for another doctor to cover when he is on holiday or at conferences. You should also be sure to ask about fees – some doctors ask for a deposit in advance of treatment. If the doctor you select does not suit you in the long run, do not hesitate to change but remember that bedside manner is only one aspect of doctoring.

Some general practitioners belong to the American Academy of Family Physicians (AAFP), who have a mandatory program of approved graduate training and continuing study. There are now almost 30,000 members. It would probably be an advantage to get a doctor who belongs to the AAFP if you can.

If you choose an internist you should bear in mind that this term simply means a physician with some graduate training in internal medicine. Some internists have obtained a diploma and are certified by the American Board of Internal Medicine. A larger proportion are "board-eligible" but have not actually obtained a diploma. These physicians are fully experienced, but you may reasonably expect those who have obtained their diplomas to have a wider background knowledge of their subject.

There are now twenty-two divisions of medicine and surgery recognized by the American Board of Medical Specialities. These boards are responsible for establishing proper training in their field and administering examinations. As with internists, other specialists must pass an examination before they can be "board-certified diplomates". Many more do not take the examinations and remain simply board-eligible. In some specialities, doctors may become fellows of a college, an honorary body whose responsibility it is to maintain standards of education in the speciality. Among these organizations are the American College of Obstetrics and Gynecology, the American Academy of Pediatrics, the American College of Physicians, and the American College of Surgeons. Membership of these organizations entitles fellows to use certain initials after their names such as FACOG, FAAP, FACP, and FACS. If you want to check on the status of a doctor, you can refer to the Directory of Medical Specialities (available in some libraries) and see if a particular doctor is a diplomate.

Types of practise: If you live in a rural area you may have no choice of doctor, but in the city you may be able to choose not only the doctor but the type of practise. You can choose a doctor in practise alone or one who is in a group practise. If you choose a doctor in solo practise, then you can be certain that you will have the same person deal with your problem provided the doctor is not on holiday. Group practise has the advantage for the doctor and ultimately the patient that the doctor is in constant close touch with colleagues. The group practise may include a number of different types of specialists who are easily available for you to consult. In such a group practise your notes will be available to whichever doctor you consult, and so the doctor can easily see the history of your problem.

Most doctors charge for each item of service which they supply to the patient. The more the doctor does, the more he charges. Critics of this form of payment say that it encourages the doctor to give the patient too many drugs, too many diagnostic procedures and too much surgery. The alternative is pre-payment, in which a group of doctors offer the patient a plan something like an insurance policy. This means that an individual or family will know in advance what their medical expenses for the year will be. A set fee is paid monthly, regardless of how much the patient uses the doctor. This gives the physician an incentive not to provide any unnecessary facilities and keep the cost of care down, since extra services do not provide him with extra money – yet at the same time such a practise must continue to compete with others for patients.

The overall cost of medical care is decreased by about 20 per cent in pre-paid practises, and studies which have been made to compare the quality of care given by doctors paid in these two ways have failed to find any difference. However, the patient may feel he or she gets less personal attention in a pre-paid practise, and is just another item on the production line. Furthermore, a healthy person using this type of facility is subsidizing people who are ill or people who may be over-using the system. If you want further information about such plans, get in touch with: Group Health Association of America, 1717 Massachusetts Avenue, NW, Washington DC 20036.

Questioning the doctor: The doctor should always give sufficient time to answer your questions, even if the answer is only that he cannot at present discover the cause of your problem. If you have difficulty taking in all the information the doctor gives you, and are afraid that you may forget to ask an important question, take along a close friend or relative. Do not be afraid to question the doctor's advice if it does not appear to make sense to you. It may be that you have forgotten to tell him something important. If the doctor recommends that you take more than three different types of tablet, ask if it is really necessary. Drugs interact with each other, and several drugs taken together can make a person quite ill. Sometimes three or more medications may be necessary, but if at all possible this should be avoided and may mean giving up a sleeping tablet or tranquilizer which is less important than, say, drugs for a heart condition. Be suspicious if the doctor tries to promote to you some remedy which is expensive, and if in doubt about the value of a treatment, particularly surgery, do not hesitate to seek a second opinion. When the Storeworkers' Union of New York City asked for a second opinion before agreeing to pay for elective surgery for its subscribers, it found that there was a 17.5 per cent reduction in operations with a saving of $7.00 per month in premiums apart from the saving in unnecessary pain and disturbance.

Emergency rooms: Often patients go to an emergency room rather than arrange an appointment with a doctor in an office. The emergency staff often do a good job with these non-emergency complaints. However, treatment in an emergency room is likely to be more expensive than in the doctor's office because they are expensively equipped to deal with more severe or pressing health crises. But more important, the emergency doctor thinks in terms of treating the immediate problem. He does not have time to make a complete examination or pursue an underlying complaint to the end. You may end up being told to see a doctor in his office and collect a large bill for emergency treatment not covered by your insurance.

Choosing a hospital: The most important consideration in choosing a hospital is whether the hospital is accredited by the Joint Commission on Accreditation of Hospitals (JCAH). Accreditation by the Commission guarantees a minimum standard of medical care, although it is never possible in any hospital to guarantee completely that there will not be problems which might have been avoided. However, accreditation under this scheme is not required by law.

The JCAH is financially supported and run by four organizations: the American College of Physicians, the American College of Surgeons, the American Hospital Association, and the American Medical Association. To obtain accreditation a hospital must comply with certain published standards and submit to inspection by a team of experts. This team examines the physical plant for safety, checks the hospital by-laws, checks the adequacy of medical records, and examines the hospital's own systems for monitoring its performance. Laboratories, X-ray facilities, pharmacy, dietary services and all the various departments are checked by the JCAH team.

When the examination is complete the hospital will receive either a one- or two-year accreditation or no accreditation. The JCAH may also make recommendations for improvement. Some three-quarters of general hospitals in the US are accredited. The certificate of accreditation is usually displayed in the lobby; alternatively, you can ask the hospital administrator if the hospital is accredited, or write to JCAH, 875 North Michigan Avenue, Chicago, Illinois 60611. If you are dissatisfied with the service or facilities offered by an accredited hospital, then you can complain to the JCAH, who now hold public hearings. You may also complain to the Department of Health, Education and Welfare, which is required to investigate any "substantial allegation" that a hospital in receipt of funds from Medicare is not complying with accepted standards.

Another important guide in choosing a hospital is whether the hospital is associated in any way with a medical school. About 1,000 hospitals in the US are associated with medical schools, and some 400 are members of the Council of Teaching Hospitals of the Association of American Medical Colleges. In order to be a member, the hospitals must have residency programs in at least four or five major fields: internal medicine, obstetrics/gynecology, pediatrics, psychiatry, and surgery. Many more hospitals which do not have formal programs for residents are nevertheless recognized by the American Medical Association Council on Medical Education (535 North Dearborn St, Chicago, Illinois 60610) as suitable for training of residents. Choice of one of these hospitals guarantees an above average standard of competence. Yet other hospitals are approved by the AMA Council for Medical Education for the training of nurses, and again these must have better than average standards to earn that approval.

A final consideration is whether the hospital is voluntary, a privately owned organization aiming at making a profit, or owned by the municipal, county, state or federal government. Ownership in itself tells relatively little about quality of care. Some privately owned hospitals are not run in order to make a profit, and others may specialize in certain relatively straightforward procedures such as appendectomies, abortions, sterilizations which do not require the most expensive backup equipment. They may therefore be able to offer a cheaper and more efficient service. However, proprietary hospitals are likely to be less strict than voluntary or municipal hospitals in selecting staff and in the restrictions they apply in limiting the type of surgery done by general practitioners. It is in this type of hospital that operations may be done by doctors who are not sufficiently experienced or well qualified.

Other health facilities: Long-term care facilities, psychiatric facilities and facilities for the mentally retarded are also accredited by JCAH, and accreditation provides a good guide in choosing one. To find a dentist, consult local or county medical societies, or a nearby dental college if you have one; also ask friends, who will often be the best guide.

Health insurance: Addresses of Blue Cross and Blue Shield are given in Appendix 2, General Section, following. A summary of Medicaid and Medicare is given in Appendix 2, Chapter 10.

HOW TO GET FURTHER INFORMATION ON HEALTH AND HELP WITH HEALTH PROBLEMS

We have listed here some books and organizations which will provide more detailed information on specific health problems. Some organizations are voluntary, some are charities and some are for-profit organizations. Most supply materials which answer individual problems or which may be used in teaching. Sources of general information are listed immediately below, and other more specific sources are arranged chapter by chapter to follow the order of this book.

Books
The Medicine Show. Consumers Union practical guide to some everyday health problems and health products by the editors of Consumer Reports, Consumers Union, Mount Vernon, NY.
Our Bodies, Ourselves. A book by and for women. Boston Women's Health Book Collective. (Simon and Schuster, New York, NY)
Take Care of Yourself. A consumer's guide to medical care. By Donald M. Vickery MD and James F. Fries MD (Addison-Wesley Publishing Co., Reading, MA), provides detailed information on how to deal with illness and when to consult a doctor.

Organizations
American Public Health Association, 1015 18th St., NW, Washington DC 20036. 202-467-5000. Major professional organization of public health workers. Promotes personal and environmental health. Provides a publications service.
American School Health Association, Kent, Ohio 44240. 216-678-1601. Promotes school health programs including teaching of health; publishes booklets.
Association for Advancement of Health Education, 1201 16th St., NW, Washington DC 20036. 202-833-5535. Association for teachers of health education in colleges, schools and communities. Publishes reports, handbooks, guides, educational packages and audiovisual material.
Health Media Association, 1207 De Haro St., San Francisco, CA 94107. 415-282-9318. Provides information and rents films for educational programs on public health.
Medic-Alert Foundation International, 1000 N. Palm, Turlock, CA 95380. 209-632-2371. Provides emblems for members to wear warning of a medical or health problem. Worn by diabetics, epileptics, hemophiliacs, and persons with drug allergies.
National Women's Health Network, 2025 I St., NW, Washington DC 20036. 202-223-6886. Promotes women's health and maintains a national resource file on women's health.

Insurance
Blue Cross Association, 840 N. Lake Shore Drive, Chicago, IL 60611. 312-440-6000.
Blue Shield Association, 211 E. Chicago Ave., Chicago, IL 60611. 312-440-5500.

Appendix 2

Chapter 1. Childhood

PREGNANCY
The National Foundation/March of Dimes produces a comprehensive series of booklets and films about pregnancy and its problems, including some in Spanish language. Especially useful are its booklets entitled: *Be Good to your Baby before it is Born* and *Birth Defects*. Available from: The National Foundation, March of Dimes, 1275 Mamaroneck Ave., White Plains, NY 10605. 914-428-7100.
The American College of Obstetricians and Gynecologists, Suite 2700, One East Wacker Drive, Chicago, IL 60601. 312-222-1600. Also produces a comprehensive series of patient information booklets and leaflets.
International Childbirth Education Association, Supplies Center, PO Box 70258, Seattle, WA 98107. 206-789-4444. Also produces many pamphlets on childbirth preparation, family centered maternity care, breastfeeding, etc.

GENETIC COUNSELING
The National Foundation/March of Dimes (address above) has sponsored genetic counseling and screening programs in many states. If you have had one or more children with an inherited disorder or you have a close relative (parent, brother, sister, cousin) with an inherited condition, you may welcome genetic counseling. It is also possible to detect whether a person is a carrier of certain conditions, such as Tay-Sachs disease, sickle cell anemia and thalassemia (Cooley anemia). If two carriers have children, then the children have a chance, usually one in four, of having the disease. If you have difficulty getting genetic counseling, the National Foundation will be able to tell you of the nearest center able to help. They also have a pamphlet on the subject.
National Genetics Foundation, Nine W. 57th St., New York, NY 10019. Operates a nationwide network of Genetic Counseling and Treatment Centers to give advice on hereditary conditions.

CHILDBIRTH
The following childbirth education associations can provide information, counseling and classes and may be able to put you in touch with local groups:
American Red Cross (National Headquarters address), 17th & D Street, Washington DC 20006
The American Society of Childbirth Educators, Inc., 7113 Lynnwood Drive, PO Box 16159, Tampa, FL 33687. 813-988-2976.
American Society for Psycho-Prophylaxis in Obstetrics, Inc. (Lamaze method), 1411 K Street, NW, Washington DC 20005. 202-783-7050.
Cesarean Birth Association of America, Inc., 125 N. 12th Street, New Hyde Park, NY 11040. 516-997-7394.
Child Welfare League of America, Inc, 67 Irving Place, New York, NY 10003.
Childbirth Without Pain Education Association (Lamaze-Pavlov, psychoprophylactic, method of childbirth), 21034 Snowden, Detroit, MI 48235. 313-345-9850.
C/SEC (Cesareans/Support Education and Concern), 15 Maynard Road, Dedham, MA 02026. 617-326-2534.
International Childbirth Education Association (ICEA), PO Box 20852, Milwaukee, WI 53220. 414-445-7470.
La Leche League, 9616 Minneapolis, Franklin Park, IL 60131. 312-455-7730.
Maternity Center Association, 48 E. 92nd Street, New York, NY 10028. 212-369-7300.
Society for the Protection of the Unborn through Nutrition, 17 N. Wabash, Suite 603, Chicago, IL 60602. 312-332-2334.
If you are interested in alternatives such as home deliveries, you may wish to contact these organizations:
National Association of Parents and Professionals for Safe Alternatives in Childbirth, Dr David Stewart, PO Box 267, Marble Hill, MO 63764.
American Academy of Husband Coached Childbirth, PO Box 5224, Sherman Oaks, CA 91413.
National Women's Health Network (co-ordinates women's groups), PO Box 24192, Washington DC 20024. 202-223-6886.
International Association for Childbirth at Home, PO Box 1219, Cerritoes, CA 90701. 213-802-1020.

CHILD DEVELOPMENT
Pamphlets and further information on child health can be obtained from: American Academy of Pediatrics, 1801 Hinman Ave., Evanston, IL 60204. 312-869-4255.

Books
Taking Care of your Child. A parent's guide to medical care by Robert H. Pantell MD, James F. Fries MD, and Donald M. Vickery MD (Addison-Wesley Publishing Co., Reading, MA).
Ourselves and our Children. A book by and for parents by the Boston Women's Health Book Collective (Random House, New York, NY)
Babyhood: Infant Development from Birth to Two Years by Penelope Leach (Alfred A. Knopf, New York, NY)
Baby and Child Care by Dr Benjamin Spock (Hawthorn Books, New York, NY)
Birth without Violence by Frederick Leboyer (Alfred A. Knopf, New York, NY)

Organizations
Bananas, 6501 Telegraph, Oakland, CA 94609. 415-658-0381 and Child Care Resource Center, 187 Hampshire St., Cambridge, MA 02139. 617-547-9861. Provide free information on welfare policies, practical help in finding child care and referral to other agencies in case of problems.
Coalition for Children and Youth, 815 15th St., NW, Washington DC 20005. 202-347-9380. Provides information and acts as a co-ordinating agency for other organizations interested in problems of children.
Parents Anonymous National Office, 22330 Hawthorne Blvd., Suite 208, Torrance, CA 90505. Toll free 800-421-0353. For parents who abuse their children or fear that they might.
National Organization of Mothers of Twins Club, Inc., 5402 Amberwood Lane, Rockville, MD 20853. 301-460-9108.
Children in Hospitals, 31 Wilshire Park, Needham, MA 02192. 671-482-2915. Helps parents understand the needs of children who are or will be hospitalized.
For parents of handicapped children:
Federation of Children with Special Needs, 120 Boylston St., Room 338, Boston, MA 02116. 617-482-2915.
Handicapped Children's Early Education Program, 400 Maryland Ave., SW Washington DC 20202. 202-245-8710.

CHILDHOOD ACCIDENTS
The National Commission on Product Safety, in Washington DC, produces regular reports on aspects of safety such as playground accidents. *Consumer Reports* is another source of information.

Chapter 2. Nutrition

For more information and recipes on low-fat cookery:
The Prudent Diet by Iva Bennett and Martha Simon (Bantam Books, New York, NY)
How to Eat Well and Stay Well the Mediterranean Way by Ancel and Margaret Keys (Doubleday & Co., New York, NY)
The Benevolent Bean by Margaret and Ancel Keys (Noonday Press, Farrar, Straus & Giroux, Brooklyn, NY)
The American Heart Association Cookbook (David McKay & Co., New York, NY)
Low-fat Cookery by Evelyn S. Stead and Gloria K. Warren (McGraw-Hill, New York, NY)
Middle Eastern Cookery by Claudia Roden (Alfred A. Knopf, New York, NY)

Organizations
Nutrition Today Society, 703 Giddings Ave., Annapolis, MD 21404. 301-267-8616. Provides information about food and nutrition.
National Foundation for Ileitis and Colitis, 295 Madison Ave., New York, NY 10017. 212-685-3440. Provides information on cause and treatment of bowel disease.
American Heart Association, 7320 Greenville Ave., Dallas, TX 75231. 214-750-3500, and also in most states.

DIETING

Here are some useful books which deal with the psychological problems of dieting and explain the best approach:

Permanent Weight Control by Michael and Kathryn Mahoney (W. W. Norton & Co., New York, NY)

Thin from Within By Jack D. Osman PhD (Hart Publishing Co., New York, NY)

Think yourself Thin by Dr Frank J. Bruno (Barnes and Noble, New York, NY)

Organizations

There are many organizations which help dieters to reduce. Not all follow the regime we recommend of reducing fat intake to achieve a healthy as well as a reducing diet. Many reducing programs suggest limiting carbohydrates and eating a relatively high meat diet – we do not recommend this. Diet programs are being modified all the time and so if you want the help of any organization you should ask them what their policy is. Here are some of the larger organizations which you may be interested in contacting:

International Buxom Belles, 27856 Palomino Dr., Warren, MI 48093. 313-754-5731. Assists women to lose weight by group therapy and weight reducing contests.

Lean Line, 151 New World Way, South Plainfield, NJ, 07080. 201-757-7677. Recommends special psychological eating program devised at Rutgers University.

National Council of Obesity, PO Box 35306, Los Angeles, CA 90035. Offers advice, guidance and referral to overweight people. Provides information to individuals, schools and colleges.

TOPS Club (Take Off Pounds Sensibly), 4575 South Fifth Street, Milwaukee, WI 53207. 414-482-4620. Is a noncommercial association using group therapy and competition. Provides information.

Weightwatchers International, 800 Community Drive, Manhasset, LI, NY 11030. Successful commercial organization.

The Diet Workshop Inc., Hearthstone Building, Suite 301, 111 Washington Street, Brookline, MA 02146. Commercial organization, provides classes, information, recipes.

Chapter 3. Fitness

PRE-EXERCISE TESTS

Details of organizations providing EKG stress tests can be obtained from the National Fitness Director, National Council of YMCAs, 291 Broadway, New York, NY 10007, 212-374-2000; National Jogging Association, 1910 K Street, Washington DC 20006, 202-785-8050; and Fitness Finders, 178 E. Harmony, Spring Arbor, MI 49283, 517-750-4131. Your own physician or local public health clinic doctor may also be able to help, and should in any case normally be contacted first. A general return to fitness program is provided by: MR FIT Program, National Heart, Lung and Blood Institute, National Institute of Health, Bethesda, MD 20014. 301-496-4000.

EXERCISE

The President's Council on Physical Fitness and Sports, 400 6th Street, SW, Washington DC 20201. 202-755-7947, is an excellent source of information. Among its many publications are *Jogging/Running* and *The Fitness Challenge in the Later Years*.

An admirable summary of the many exercise and fitness books currently on the US market can be found in *Rating the Exercises* by Charles T. Kunzleman and the editors of *Consumer Guide* (published by William Morrow, New York, NY). Among these specialist books are the works of Dr Kenneth Cooper, published by Bantam Books. His later books – *The New Aerobics, Aerobics for Women* and *The Aerobics Way* – are broadly more satisfactory than his original *Aerobics*, which contains fewer sports and too great an emphasis on the 12-minute fitness test.

Other widely recommended books include:

Jogging by W.J. Bowerman and W.E. Harris (Grosset & Dunlap, New York, NY)

The Complete Book of Running by James F. Fixx (Random House, New York, NY)

Physical Fitness and Dynamic Health by T.K. Cureton (Dial Press, New York, NY)

The Official YMCA Physical Fitness Handbook by C.R. Myers (Popular Library, New York, NY)

Keep Your Heart Running by P.J. Kiell and H.G. Knuttgen (Winchester Press, New York, NY)

The Magic of Walking by Aaron Sussman and Ruth Goode (Simon and Schuster, New York, NY)

Running for Health and Beauty: a Complete Guide for Women by Kathryn Lance (Bobbs-Merrill, New York, NY)

Women's Running by Joan Ullyott (World Publications, Mountain View, CA)

Finally an excellent book, only part of which is devoted to physical fitness, is *The American Way of Life need not be Hazardous to your Health* by John W. Farquar (W. W. Norton & Co., New York, NY). This also contains sections on nutrition, stress, smoking, etc.

(Exercise books or programs devised for senior citizens are detailed in the appendix details for Chapter 10.)

HEALTH CLUBS

Check your telephone directory for location of local YMCAs or write to the National Council of YMCAs, 291 Broadway, New York, NY 10007. Similar organizations such as the YWCA, YMHA, YWHA also organize fitness programs. Private health clubs are listed in Yellow Pages.

Chapter 4. Stress and Relaxation

The Relaxation Response by Herbert Benson (William Morrow, New York, NY)

Learn to Relax: 13 Ways to Reduce Tension by C. Eugene Walker (Prentice-Hall, Englewood Cliffs, NJ)

YOGA

Introduction to Yoga by Richard Hittleman (Bantam Books, New York, NY)

Hathayoga by W. A. Compton (Harper & Row, New York, NY)

The Complete Illustrated Book of Yoga by S. Vishnudavanda (Pocket Books, New York, NY)

Yoga for Beauty and Health: Look Younger and Be Relaxed by E. Rawls and E. Diskin (Warner Books, New York, NY).

Light on Yoga by B.K. Iyengar (Schocken Books, New York, NY).

Lilias Yoga and You by Lilias M. Folan (Bantam Books, New York, NY).

SLEEP

How to Sleep Better: A Drug-Free Program for Overcoming Insomnia by Carl Thoresen and Thomas Coates (Prentice-Hall, Englewood Cliffs, NJ)

SUICIDE AND MENTAL ILLNESS

Mental Health Association, 1800 N. Kent St., Arlington, VA 22209. 703-528-6405. Provides information on mental health and illness and works through hospitals, private agencies and government to aid rehabilitation.

Mental Health Materials Center, 419 Park Ave., South, New York, NY 10016. 212-889-5760. Provides information on mental health to the public.

Save-a-Life League, 815 Second Ave., New York, NY 10017. 212-736-6101. A loose association of organizations known by different names in other areas, such as Stress Centers, Suicide Prevention League, etc.

Chapter 5. Maintaining the Bodywork

BACK

Oh, My Aching Back by Dr Leon Root and Thomas Kiernan (David McKay Co., New York, NY)

Backache, Stress and Tension by Hans Kraus (Simon and Schuster, New York, NY)

FEET

American Pediatry Association, 20 Chevy Chase Circle, NW, Washington DC 20015. 202-537-4900. Provides catalog of audiovisual, informational and educational materials.

SKIN AND HAIR

The AMA Book of Skin and Hair Care edited by Linda Allen Schoen (J.B. Lippincott, Philadelphia, PA). Based on questions answered over the years by the Committee on Cutaneous Health and Cosmetics of the American Medical Association.

Organizations

American Electrolysis Association, PO Box 204, Evanston, IL 60204. 312-623-6100. Maintains referral service for cosmetic removal of hair by qualified personnel.

JOINTS

Arthritis, the Basic Facts. Published by the Arthritis Foundation, New York, NY.

Living with Arthritis by A. B. Corrigan MD (Grosser & Dunlap, New York, NY)

The Arthritis Handbook by Darrell Crane MD (Arco Publishing, New York, NY)

Understanding Arthritis and Rheumatism by Malcolm I. V. Jayson MD and Allan St J. Dixon MD (Pantheon Books, New York, NY)

EYES

Organizations

Better Vision Institute, 230 Park Ave., New York, NY 10017. Professional and manufacturers association. Sponsors pre-school screening program and supplies information.

Auxiliary to American Optometric Association, 7000 Chippewa St., St. Louis, MO 63119. 314-832-5770. Spouses of optometrists. Provide information to the public about vision.

Volunteers for Vision, PO Box 2211, Austin, TX 78767. Encourages screening, supplies information.

DEAFNESS

By law you must now have a medical examination before buying a hearing aid. Ask your family doctor to recommend a specialist, call your county medical society or ask your local crippled children's program. A list of certified audiologists is available from: The American Speech and Hearing Association, 10801 Rockville Pike, Rockville, MD 20852. 202-897-5700.

TEETH

The American Dental Association produces many leaflets, charts and audiovisual kits on dental health. Send for their catalog of materials from: American Dental Association, 211 East Chicago Ave., Chicago, IL 60611. 312-440-2500.

Chapter 6. The Major Hazards

SMOKING

There are a number of useful books which help people who want to give up smoking:

How to Stop Smoking by Herbert Brean (Pocket Books, New York, NY)

How to Stop Smoking in 3 Days by Sidney Petrie (Warner Books, New York, NY)

You Can Quit Smoking in 14 Days by Walter S. Ross (Berkeley Publishing Corp., New York, NY)

Become an Ex-Smoker by Brian G. Danaher and Edward Lichtenstein (Prentice-Hall, Englewood Cliffs, NJ)

And for a summary of the latest facts about smoking, see:

The Smoking Digest published by Office of Cancer Communications, National Cancer Institute, Bldg. 31, Rm 10418, Bethesda, MD 20205. 301-496-4000.

Smoking cessation programs are run by the American Cancer Society, 777 Third Ave., New York, NY 10017. 212-371-2900; American Heart Association, 7320 Greenville Ave., Dallas, TX 75231; American Lung Association, 1740 Broadway, New York, NY 10019. 212-245-8000; American Health Foundation, 320 E. 43rd St., New York, NY 10017. 212-953-1900. Courses vary, but usually involve provision of information about smoking, talking about ways to quit under direction of a leader, group therapy and a buddy system of mutual support.

Profit-making corporations such as SmokEnders of Phillipsburg, NJ, Schick Labs of Los Angeles, and National Association on Smoking and Health of Denver offer courses which claim high success rates, but they do not always take on difficult cases who have failed to stop in other programs. Experts are sceptical of the high success rates sometimes claimed by these organizations, and the Federal Trade Commission has been urged to publish guidelines for evaluation of these programs. The crucial factor in any program is the motivation of participants.

For further information on smoking, apply to: National Clearing House on Smoking and Health, Public Health Service, US Department of Health, Education and Welfare, Center for Disease Control, 1600 Clifton Rd., NE, Atlanta, GA 30333. 404-329-3311.

An integrated fitness program which includes help with smoking cessation is available from: MR FIT Program, National Heart, Lung and Blood Institute, National Institutes of Health, Bethesda, MD 20014. 301-496-4000.

HEART DISEASE

Books

Heart by Dr Sarah R. Riedman. Golden Guide (Golden Press, New York, NY)

The Heart by Donald Longmore, World University Library Service (McGraw-Hill, New York, NY)

I Think I'm Having a Heart Attack by Jerry E. Bishop (Dow Jones Books, Princeton, NJ)

How to Live with your Heart by Arthur Vineberg (Quadrangle, New York, NY)

Living Heart: Two Famous Heart Specialists Tell how your Cardiovascular System Works, Why it Fails and What can be Done about it by Michael DeBakey & Anthony Gotto (David McKay Co., New York, NY)

For further information, contact your local heart association. You can find your nearest branch from: The American Heart Association, 7320 Greenville Ave., Dallas, TX 75231. 214-750-5300.

Other organizations

Heart Disease Research Foundation, 963 Essex Street, Brooklyn, NY 11208. 212-649-9003. Promotes research aimed at early diagnosis, prevention and treatment. Answers questions from public and supplies information. Mended Hearts, 721 Huntington Ave., Boston, MA 02115. 617-732-5609. Association of people who have successfully undergone heart surgery. Provides advice and encouragement to those undergoing heart surgery.

National Heart Education Research Society, 304 San Pablo SE, Suite F, Albuquerque, NM 87108. 505-265-8549. Implements programs of prevention.

CANCER

Books

Preventing Cancer by Dr. Elizabeth Whelan (W.W. Norton & Co., New York, NY). What you can do to cut your risks by up to 50 per cent.

Breast Cancer by Rose Kushner (Harcourt Brace, New York, NY). A personal history and an investigative report.

The Cancer Connection and what we can do about it by Larry Agran (Houghton Mifflin, New York, NY)

The Anti-Cancer Diet by Donald Germann (Wyden Books, New York, NY)

And a Time to Live: Toward Emotional Well-Being during the Crisis of Cancer by R. C. Cantor (Harper & Row, New York, NY)

Getting Well Again: A Step-by-Step, Self-Help Guide to Overcoming Cancer for Patients and their Families by O.C. Simonton, Matthews-S. Simonton, J. Creighton (St. Martin's Press, New York, NY)

The following organizations provide advice and help:

The American Cancer Society, 777 Third Ave., New York, NY 10017. 212-371-2900. Provides special services to cancer patients and supports education.

American Society of Cytology, Health Sciences Center, 130 S. Ninth St., Suite 1006, Philadelphia, PA 19107. 215-922-3880. Promotes cytological method for early cancer detection.

Breast Cancer Advisory Center, PO Box 422, Kensington, MD 20795. 301-949-2530. Disseminates information about breast cancer.

Leukemia Society of America, 211 E. 43rd Street, New York, NY 10017. 212-573-8484. Provides information, aids needy patients, supports research.

National Cancer Cytology Center, 150 Broad Hollow Road, Melville, NY 11746. 516-427-0400. Supports research into early detection of cancer and provides educational programs.

ALCOHOLISM

Treatment

Alcoholism Treatment Facilities Directory: US and Canada. Available from Alcohol and Drug Problems Association of North America, Suite 240, 1101 15th St., NW, Washington DC 20005. 202-452-0990.

Organizations

Alcoholics Anonymous, National Headquarters, 468 Park Avenue South, New York, NY 10016. 212-686-1100.

Books

Living Sober published by Alcoholics Anonymous World Services, New York, NY.

Frontiers of Alcoholism by Morris E. Chafetz, ed., with Howard T. Blane and Marjorie J. Hill (Science House, New York, NY)

The Prevention of Drinking Problems: Alcohol Control and Cultural Influences by Rupert Wilkinson (Oxford University Press, New York, NY)

Chapter 7. Staying Healthy at Work and Play

ALLERGIES

A useful series of booklets on pollen, drug, dust, food, insect, mold, and poison ivy allergies are produced by the National Institute of Allergy and Infectious Diseases, National Institute of Health, 9000 Rockville Pike, Bethesda, MD 20014. 301-496-3454. The Allergy Foundation of America, 801 Second Avenue, New York, NY 10017, 212-867-8875, also produces a series of useful booklets including a list giving the ragweed pollen index for hundreds of locations in N. America. However, if you are thinking of moving first obtain detailed advice from your allergist, who can advise about your type of allergy. Also seek local advice about the place you are thinking of moving to, because pollen conditions can sometimes vary greatly within an area. The local medical society or local chamber of commerce may be able to help you. The National Climatic Center, Federal Building, Asheville, NC 28801, 704-258-2850, can advise where particular climates can be found in the USA if you know which climate is most suitable to your condition.

Your allergist may recommend that you install air conditioning or an air filter at home. However, sometimes such devices can make matters worse, especially if they are not kept scrupulously clean. The US Food and Drug Administration recommends that before purchasing such a device, one should be rented first and tried out to see if it brings relief. A unit capable of producing an air change in the room five to six times per hour is desirable. However, most air conditioners on the market are not capable of removing dust or pollen.

Books
Allergies: Questions and Answers about Allergies & your Child by Doris J. Rapp MD (Drake Publishers Inc., New York, NY) provides useful further information.

Organizations
Allergy Foundation of America, 801 Second Ave., New York, NY 10017. 212-867-8876. A national voluntary health agency aimed at solving allergy problems.

International Allergy Association, 133 E. 58th Street, New York, NY 10022. 212-355-1005. Society of allergists and laymen interested in treatment and control of allergy.

National Foundation for Asthma, PO Box 50304, Tucson, AZ 85703. 602-624-7481. Provides medical and social rehabilitation for chronic asthmatics.

Medic-Alert Foundation International, 1000 N. Palm, Turlock, CA 95380. 209-632-2371. Provides warning bracelet or neck chain to alert medical personnel in case of emergency.

COLDS AND FLU

For further information on home treatment, consult *The Medicine Show*, Chapter 2 (The Common Cold), Chapter 3 (Coughs and Cold Remedies), Chapter 4 (Sore Throats), published by editors of Consumer Reports, Consumer's Union of US, Inc., Mount Vernon, NY.

HEADACHES
Books
Control of Migraine by John B. Brainard MD (W.W. Norton & Co., New York, NY) Organizations:

National Migraine Foundation, 5214 N. Western Ave., Chicago, IL 60625. 312-878-7715. Provides information about migraine and headache to the public.

HAZARDS AT WORK

Most American workers are protected by The Occupational Safety and Health Act of 1970. Both employers and employees have obligations under this Act.

Employers: "Each employer shall furnish to each of his employees employment and a place of employment free from recognized hazards that are causing or are likely to cause death or serious harm to his employees, and shall comply with occupational safety and health standards issued under the Act."

Employees: "Each employee shall comply with all occupational safety and health standards, rules, regulations and orders issued under the Act that apply to his own actions and conduct on the job."

The only workers or workplaces *not* covered by the Act are self-employed persons; family owned and operated farms; and workplaces already protected by other Federal agencies under other Federal statutes.

The 1970 Act created three new governmental agencies. The Occupational Safety and Health Administration (OSHA), within the Department of Labor, sets and enforces safety and health safety standards; the National Institute for Occupational Safety and Health (NIOSH), within the Department of Health, Education and Welfare, conducts scientific research into occupational safety and health (notably in the area of toxic substances) and recommends standards for OSHA's adoption; and the Occupational Safety and Health Review Commission (OSHRC) settles disputes arising from enforcement of the Act.

Employers are obliged to inform their employees about any OSHA standard that applies to their work. Workers can also obtain copies of the relevant standards from their nearest OSHA office (see telephone directory for address). OSHA officers conduct job site inspections to ensure compliance with its regulations and also to investigate alleged safety or health hazards.

If you detect or suspect hazardous conditions, you have the right to request an OSHA inspection (again via the area office listed in your local telephone directory). You should always report the potential hazard to your supervisor or employer first, but if you believe that the hazard remains, you can then approach OSHA directly. OSHA will withhold your name from your employer at your request.

If you believe the hazard is so great as to cause "imminent danger" of death or serious injury, then you can walk off the job. The leaflets listed below detail the circumstances in which this becomes a legal right, but broadly the Act protects you against discrimination for walking off the job so long as you can demonstrate that you had no alternative and had acted "reasonably". The Act also protects you from discrimination for reporting suspected hazards.

If the hazard you suspect concerns a toxic substance, contact NIOSH – again via the area offices listed in the telephone directory and again after approaching your employer or supervisor if at all possible. Except in situations of extreme danger, OSHA and NIOSH prefer to allow employers an opportunity to act first.

OSHA and NIOSH each publish a mass of leaflets detailing aspects of the 1970 Act. Some are specialist (like the OSHA Safe Work Practises Series covering such topics as *Machine Guarding* and *Handling Hazardous Materials*), others are more general and these include:
Workers' Rights under OSHA (OSHA 2253)
A Worker's Guide to NIOSH (DHEW–NIOSH Publication No. 78-171)
All about OSHA (OSHA 2098)
OSHA Inspections (OSHA 2098)
A good general book is *Crisis in the Workplace: Occupational Disease and Injury* by Nicholas A. Ashford (The MIT Press, Cambridge, MA)

Chapter 8. Sex and Health

SEX DIFFICULTIES
Organizations
American Association of Sex Educators, Counselors and Therapists, Suite 304, 5010 Wisconsin Avenue, NW, Washington DC 20016. 202-686-2523. Is able to advise you of a reputable sex therapist in your locality.

Books
Becoming Orgasmic, A Sexual Growth Program for Women by Julia Heiman, Leslie LoPiccolo and Joseph LoPiccolo (Prentice-Hall, Englewood Cliffs, NJ)
Learning to Love by Paul Brown and Carolyn Faulder (Universe Books, New York, NY)
Dr William Masters and Virginia Johnson have produced two books, *Human Sexual Response* (Little-Brown, Boston, MA), which details the exact physiology of sexual response, and *Human Sexual Inadequacy* (also Little-Brown), which details their techniques in dealing with sex difficulties. An authorized popularization of their work has been published called *Understanding Human Sexual Inadequacy* by Fred Belliveau and Lin Richter (Bantam Books, New York, NY)
The Joy of Sex, A Gourmet Guide to Lovemaking edited by Alex Comfort (Crown Publishers Inc., New York, NY)
The Hite Report, by Shere Hite (Dell/paperback, Macmillan/hardcover, both New York, NY)

HOMOSEXUALITY

The following organizations provide help for homosexuals and their families:
Parents and Friends of Gays, PO Box 24528, Los Angeles, CA 90024. 213-472-8952.
The National Gay Task Force, Suite 1601, 80 Fifth Avenue, New York, NY 10011. The information line is on 212-741-5815.
Gay National Educational Switchboard, Pacific Center, Berkeley, CA. 415-444-5555.

CONTRACEPTION

Planned Parenthood Federation of America Inc., 810 Seventh Avenue, New York, NY 10010. 212-541-7800. Has 188 affiliated groups nationwide and some 900 clinics. Look in the white pages of local telephone directory under Planned Parenthood. Many local groups run hotlines. Booklets and brochures are available from local groups or from national headquarters above.

For Catholics wanting non-contraceptive methods of family planning: The Human Life and National Family Planning Foundation, 1511 K Street, NW, Washington DC 20005. 202-393-1380. Provides advice on family planning, originally set up by grant from Catholic bishops.

VENEREAL DISEASES

For practical advice and where to find your nearest free clinic, telephone this hotline toll free: 800-523-1885. The hotline is run by Operation Venus, 1218 Clover Street, Philadelphia, PA 19107, which also provides written material. Alternatively contact your local municipal health department, which will be listed in the white pages of the telephone directory under the name of your town or city.
American Social Health Association, 260 Sheridan Ave., Suite 307, Palo Alto, CA 94306. 415-321-5134. Provides information, education about veneral disease, dedicated to prevention.
Gay Men's VD Clinic, 1556 Wisconsin Ave., NW, Washington DC 20007. 202-338-3363. Provides VD testing and referral, and compiles statistics.

Chapter 9. Holiday Health

For information on vaccination requirements, quarantine measures, US Public Health Service recommendations on vaccination, health hints for the traveler, reentry or importation of pets, importation or exportation of human remains, see *Health Information for International Travel* published by US Department of Health, Education and Welfare, Center for Disease Control, Bureau for Epidemiology, Quarantine Division, Atlanta, GA 30333.

Organizations

International Association for Medical Assistance to Travelers, 350 Fifth Avenue, New York, NY 10001. 212-279-6465. Publishes directory of English-speaking doctors abroad.

Chapter 10. A Healthy Old Age

Many of the problems which afflict senior citizens are not confined to people over the age of sixty. Therefore, further information on topics such as heart disease or arthritis, for instance, will be found elsewhere in this appendix, just as the topics themselves were covered separately in the book itself.
The growing numbers of Americans in retirement has also encouraged the development of many specialist organizations devoted to their varying needs. It is always usually sensible to contact such organizations locally: many community family and social welfare agencies, which offer counseling and information services, are listed in the telephone directory. However, we give below details of some larger organizations specializing in the care of the elderly, and other useful sources of information.

EDUCATION

Adult Education Association of USA, 810 18th Street, NW, Washington DC 20006. 202-347-9574.
National Home Study Council, 1601 18th Street, NW, Washington DC 20009. 202-234-5100.

EXERCISE

Senior Sports International, 5670 Wilshire Boulevard, Suite 360, Los Angeles, CA 90036. 213-938-5548. Runs Senior Olympics program through local clubs.
The Fitness Challenge . . . in the Later Years devised and published by the President's Council on Physical Fitness and Sports. (For address, see appendix details for Chapter 3 above)
Vigor Regained by H.A. de Vries (Prentice-Hall, Englewood Cliffs, NJ)

HEALTH (General)

American Public Health Association, 1015 18th Street, NW, Washington DC 20036. 202-467-5000.
National Health Council, 1740 Broadway, New York, NY 10019. 202-582-6040.

National Association for Mental Health, 1800 N. Kent Street, Rosslyn, VA 22209. 703-528-6405.
(Local public health organizations are likely to offer more immediate help, however, than these national bodies. Many senior citizen clubs or veterans' associations can also provide advice.)
Health in the Later Years by Robert Rothenberg (Signet Books, New York, NY) is a paperback encyclopedia-style book of advice on health problems as they affect the elderly. It also contains a useful summary of medicare, social security benefits and details of 200 agencies specializing in the problems of senior citizens.
A Good Age by Dr Alex Comfort (Crown Publishers Inc., New York, NY)

HOMES FOR THE AGED

American Association of Homes for the Aged, 1050 17th Street, NW, Suite 770, Washington DC 20036. 202-296-5960.
National Council on the Ageing, 60 E. 42nd Street, New York, NY 10017. 212-687-6815.
National Geriatrics Society, 212 W. Wisconsin Ave., 3rd Floor, Milwaukee, WI 53203. 414-272-4130. Provides long-term care of the chronically-ill aged and promotes proper standards of care.

MEDICARE AND SOCIAL SECURITY

The principle behind Medicare and Social Security is simple enough. People pay Social Security contributions during their working lives in order to receive benefits when they retire; the system also ensures benefits for the family if the breadwinner dies or is disabled. Part of the contributions made by workers goes into a separate hospital insurance trust fund, so that people have help in meeting their medical bills when they are over 65 (for men) or 62 (for women).

But there the simplicity ends, since the benefits received by any individual or family depends on their own individual circumstances – how long he or she has been working, how much was earned, for instance. Employers and labor unions can often help disentangle the complications of the system, but obviously the best source is your local Social Security office. The Social Security Administration has more than 850 offices located throughout the country, and each of these offices has people who visit neighboring communities to help explain the system. For the address of your local office, look in the telephone directory or ask at the post office.

The Medicare program is a part of the overall Social Security program. It falls into two parts. The first section, or Part A, helps pay for your care in hospital; Part B helps pay your doctor's bills or costs of certain other medical services you may need. In both cases there are some medical services which are *not* covered by Medicare, so it is important to know when you can or cannot expect financial help. Again, local Social Security offices will advise.

RETIREMENT

American Association of Retired Persons, 1909 K Street, NW, Washington DC 20049. 202-872-4700.
(Also Golden Age Clubs, listed in telephone directories).

RECREATION AND SOCIAL WELFARE

Again, use community sources such as public health clinics or simply identify potential organizations through the white pages. There are a mass of special organizations now reflecting the interests and needs of senior citizens. Most religious groups, for instance, have a section caring for the elderly. The branch of the federal government most responsible for care of the elderly is the Department of Health, Education and Welfare, 200 Independence Ave., SW, Washington DC 20201. 202-245-6296.
Council of the Golden Ring Clubs, 201 W. 52nd Street, New York, NY 10019. 212-265-7000.
The National Council of Senior Citizens, 1511 K Street, NW, Washington DC. 202-783-6850.
American Legion, 1608 K Street, NW, Washington DC 20006. 202-393-4811.
American Veterans Committee, Suite 930, 1346 Connecticut Ave., NW, Washington DC 20036. 202-293-4890.
Veterans of Foreign Wars of the United States (Ladies Auxiliary), 406 W. 34th Street, Kansas City, MO 64111. 816-561-8655.

Chapter 11. Emergency!

The American National Red Cross organizes first aid classes: call your local chapter for details. It also produces a useful manual, *Standard First Aid and Personal Safety*, published by Doubleday and Co., New York, NY. Also useful for reference: *Emergency Medical Guide* by John Henderson MD (McGraw-Hill Paperbacks, New York, NY).

Organizations

The American National Red Cross (National Headquarters), 17th and D Streets, NW, Washington DC 20006. 202-737-8300.
ACT Foundation, PO Box 911, Basking Ridge, NJ 07920. 201-766-2273. Provides guidance to local communities in establishing and improving emergency medical systems and in teaching resuscitation and emergency aid. International Rescue and First Aid Association, 3200 Valleyview Drive, Columbus, OH 43204. Fosters teaching of first aid and rescue to volunteers and paid workers.

This book has been written by journalists, not doctors, but we are indebted to the many medical experts who have helped us in its compilation. Sometimes they provided much of the original material, sometimes they read our draft manuscripts to check that our layman's language was not achieved at the expense of accuracy. But if any errors have survived the processes of checking and double-checking, the blame does not rest with the individuals and organizations whose help we acknowledge. Not even this distinguished panel of consultants could ensure that every reader will agree with every word in the book. Medical knowledge is rarely a question of absolute truth; much is inevitably a matter of opinion or interpretation. And responsibility for any opinions expressed within a book naturally rests with its editors rather than its advisers.

We cannot pretend that we will please everyone. The more devoted adherents of individual medical theories will be disappointed that we do not embrace their beliefs. We have strived constantly not to sensationalize, but some readers will doubtless accuse us of being alarmist. Some facts, though, *are* alarming: the needless suffering and death caused by smoking, the manifest dangers of unfitness, and so on. We are sorry if any doctors disapprove of our attempts at explaining current medical thinking in simple terms. We believe that most people will welcome a simple and dispassionate presentation of the facts. It is then up to you to decide what, if anything, you propose to do.

Health knows no national boundaries and so this book draws upon the latest international research. The links between medical specialists in the United States and those in Britain have always been especially strong, and they are reflected in this book. It began life in Britain, taking its inspiration from a series in the color magazine section of the London *Sunday Times*. It swiftly became a best-seller. This edition has been totally revised for the United States although some British research remains, just as American thinking can be found in the UK book. At all stages the book has been a team effort, but this edition owes a particular debt to several individuals.

Dr John Knowles, the late President of the Rockefeller Foundation to whom this book is dedicated, was a source of great encouragement and advice before his death earlier this year. Edward Miller, in the New York Office of Times Newspapers, co-ordinated all our researches with quiet yet spectacular efficiency. Starling Laurence, at W. W. Norton in New York, and Alan Samson, at Michael Joseph in London, were perceptive editors at our two publishing houses and coped painstakingly with the marriage of the two languages, American and English.

Other individuals and organizations to whom we are indebted are Dr Dan Horne, of the National Clearing House for Smoking and Health; Dr Morris Chafetz, of the Gail Dickersin Health Education Foundation; Dr Christopher Tietze, of The Population Council; Dr Ernest L. Wynder, of the American Health Foundation; the Occupational Safety and Health Administration; the US Department of Agriculture; the President's Council on Physical Fitness and Sports; the Federal Trade Commission; the US Department of Labor; the American and Michigan Heart Associations; and, of course, the US Department of Health, Education and Welfare.

In addition there are the thirty-two individuals whose help in compiling the original version of this book was acknowledged in the British edition. We are also grateful to several publishers for allowing us to reproduce material from their books. The weight tables for babies on page 23 are taken from *Babyhood: Infant Development from Birth to Two Years* by Penelope Leach and reprinted by permission of Alfred A. Knopf, New York; the noise table on page 150 is taken from *Noise*, by Rupert Taylor, pages 55–6, copyright Rupert Taylor 1970, and reprinted by Penguin Books of Great Britain. Crown Publishers Inc., the Consumers' Association, the Government Printing Office and Churchill Livingstone also gave us permission to reproduce material in this book.

The book has been co-edited by Oliver Gillie and Derrik Mercer. Gillie, who has a PhD from Edinburgh University, is medical correspondent of the London *Sunday Times* and a frequent visitor to the United States to investigate medical research. He is the author of several books, including *Living Cell* and *Who Do You Think You Are, Man or Superman?: The Genetic Controversy*, and is married with two daughters. Mercer is managing editor (news) of *The Sunday Times* and was formerly deputy editor of its color magazine section. He is currently working on a new *Sunday Times* book on the British countryside to be published in America in 1980. He is married with twin sons and, like Gillie, is an enthusiastic if unspeedy jogger.

The three other main authors are Caroline Conran, cookery correspondent of *The Sunday Times Magazine*; Celia Haddon, a former Magazine staff writer now concentrating on books; and Tony Osman, the Magazine's science editor. Clive Crook, art editor of *The Sunday Times Magazine*, was art editor and designer of this book. Other contributors to the text include Dr Margaret Ashwell, a member of the scientific staff at the Clinical Research Centre of the British Medical Research Council; Professor Jeremy Morris, of the Department of Community Health, and Dr Mervyn Davies, of the Department of Environmental Physiology, both at the London School of Hygiene and Tropical Medicine at the University of London; and Rosemary Atkins, Michael Bateman, Mimi Errington, Alex Finer, Paul Flattery and Norman Harris, who are all either present or past writers for *The Sunday Times Magazine*. Photographers and artists whose work appears in this book are listed below.

We all owe an enormous debt to colleagues here in New York and London, not only Edward Miller whose contribution to this edition has already been acknowledged but also Harold Evans, the editor of *The Sunday Times*, for allowing us the time to complete the book, and Robert Ducas, the President of Times Newspapers of Great Britain in America, for the efficiency and élan which he always brings to these marriages between journalism and book publishing.

New York, March 1979

Index

Page numbers in *italics* refer to the illustrations

Acknowledgments

The illustrations in this book are reproduced by kind permission of the following (numbers refer to page numbers):

Candy Amsden: 106, 110–11, 155; Barnaby's Picture Library: 77; Ian Beck: 153; Paul Bevitt: 35, 58–9; Carol Binch: 26–7; Liz Butler: 32; David Case: 185; Leslie Chapman: 67; Colorific: 75; Richard Draper: 101, 189, 190–1, 192, 193, 194, 195, 196; Duffy: 82–3; Dan Fern: 171; Alain le Garsmeur: 177; Lyn Gray: 29, 33; Dr D. A. Griffiths/Vivienne Cowper, Crown Copyright: 146; Susan Griggs: 13; Brian Grimwood: 65, 147; Hargrave Hands: 73, 115, 117 (*above*); John Kobal: 121 (*centre*);

Ken Lewis: 102, 103, 112, 113, 173; Alan Manham: 166–7; Mansell Collection: 184; Sarah Midda: 127; Duncan Mill: 123; David Montgomery: 181, 186; Parents Magazine: 20; Popperfoto: 121 (*right*); QED: 15, 17, 23, 61, 90–1, 117 (*below*); Ray Rathborne: 39; David Reed: 62–3; Arthur Robins: 87, 88, 89; *The Sunday Times*: 84, 85, 121 (*top right*), 133, 149; Joan Thompson/Garden Studio: 14, 78, 79, 80, 81, 92, 93, 105, 134, 182; Diane Tippell: 45, 46, 48, 49, 51, 54; Topix: 98; David Watson: 31; James Wedge: 107; Ann Winterbotham: 143, 162, 163, 164; Ian Wright: 178.